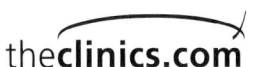

SURGICAL CLINICS OF NORTH AMERICA

Hereditary Cancer Syndromes

GUEST EDITOR
Ismail Jatoi, MD, PhD

CONSULTING EDITOR
Ronald F. Martin, MD

August 2008 • Volume 88 • Number 4

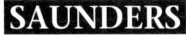

An Imprint of Elsevier, Inc.
PHILADELPHIA   LONDON   TORONTO   MONTREAL   SYDNEY   TOKYO

W.B. SAUNDERS COMPANY
A Division of Elsevier Inc.

1600 John F. Kennedy Blvd., Suite 1800, Philadelphia, PA 19103-2899

http://www.theclinics.com

SURGICAL CLINICS OF NORTH AMERICA
August 2008
Editor: Catherine Bewick

© 2008 Elsevier ■ All rights reserved.

Volume 88, Number 4
ISSN 0039–6109
ISBN-10: 1-4160-6356-0
ISBN-13: 978-1-4160-6356-8

This journal and the individual contributions contained in it are protected under copyright by Elsevier, and the following terms and conditions apply to their use:

Photocopying

Single photocopies of single articles may be made for personal use as allowed by national copyright laws. Permission of the Publisher and payment of a fee is required for all other photocopying, including multiple or systematic copying, copying for advertising or promotional purposes, resale, and all forms of document delivery. Special rates are available for educational institutions that wish to make photocopies for non-profit educational classroom use. For information on how to seek permission visit www.elsevier.com/permissions or call: (+44) 1865 843830 (UK)/(+1) 215 239 3804 (USA).

Derivative Works

Subscribers may reproduce tables of contents or prepare lists of articles including abstracts for internal circulation within their institutions. Permission of the Publisher is required for resale or distribution outside the institution. Permission of the Publisher is required for all other derivative works, including compilations and translations (please consult www.elsevier.com/permissions).

Electronic Storage or Usage

Permission of the Publisher is required to store or use electronically any material contained in this journal, including any article or part of an article (please consult www.elsevier.com/permissions). Except as outlined above, no part of this publication may be reproduced, stored in a retrieval system or transmitted in any form or by any means, electronic, mechanical, photocopying, recording or otherwise, without prior written permission of the Publisher.

Notice

No responsibility is assumed by the Publisher for any injury and/or damage to persons or property as a matter of products liability, negligence or otherwise, or from any use or operation of any methods, products, instructions or ideas contained in the material herein. Because of rapid advances in the medical sciences, in particular, independent verification of diagnoses and drug dosages should be made.

Although all advertising material is expected to conform to ethical (medical) standards, inclusion in this publication does not constitute a guarantee or endorsement of the quality or value of such product or of the claims made of it by its manufacturer.

Surgical Clinics of North America (ISSN 0039–6109) is published bimonthly by Elsevier Inc., 360 Park Avenue South, New York, NY 10010-1710. Months of publication are February, April, June, August, October, and December. Business and Editorial Offices: 1600 John F. Kennedy Blvd., Suite 1800, Philadelphia, PA 19103-2899. Customer Service Office: 6277 Sea Harbor Drive, Orlando, FL 32887-4800. Periodicals postage paid at New York, NY and additional mailing offices. Subscription prices are $238.00 per year for US individuals, $382.00 per year for US institutions, $119.00 per year for US students and residents, $292.00 per year for Canadian individuals, $466.00 per year for Canadian institutions, $309.00 for international individuals, $466.00 per year for international institutions and $154.00 per year for Canadian and foreign students/residents. To receive student/resident rate, orders must be accompanied by name of affiliated institution, date of term, and the *signature* of program/residency coordinator on institution letterhead. Orders will be billed at individual rate until proof of status is received. Foreign air speed delivery is included in all *Clinics* subscription prices. All prices are subject to change without notice. POSTMASTER: Send address changes to *Surgical Clinics*, Elsevier Journals Customer Service, 6277 Sea Harbor Drive, Orlando, FL 32887-4800. **Customer Service: 1-800-654-2452 (US). From outside of the United States, call 1-407-563-6020. Fax: 1-407-363-9661. E-mail: JournalsCustomerService-usa@elsevier.com.**

Reprints. For copies of 100 or more of articles in this publication, please contact the commercial Reprints Department, Elsevier Inc., 360 Park Avenue South, New York, New York 10010-1710; Tel. (212) 633-3812, Fax: (212) 462-1935, E-mail: reprints@elsevier.com.

The *Surgical Clinics of North America* is also published in Spanish by McGraw-Hill Interamericana Editores S.A., P.O. Box 5-237 06500 Mexico D.F. Mexico; and in Portuguese by Interlivros Edicoes Ltda., Rua Comandante Coelho 1085, CEP 21250, Rio de Janeiro, Brazil; and in Greek by Paschalidis Medical Publications, Athens Greece.

The *Surgical Clinics of North America* is covered in *MEDLINE/PubMed (Index Medicus)*, *EMBASE/Excerpta Medica*, *Current Contents/Clinical Medicine*, *Current Contents/Life Sciences*, *Science Citation Index*, and *ISI/BIOMED*.

Printed in the United States of America.

HEREDITARY CANCER SYNDROMES

CONSULTING EDITOR

RONALD F. MARTIN, MD, Staff Surgeon, Marshfield Clinic, Marshfield; and Clinical, Associate Professor, University of Wisconsin School of Medicine and Public Health, Madison, Wisconsin; Lieutenant Colonel, Medical Corps, United States Army Reserve

GUEST EDITOR

ISMAIL JATOI, MD, PhD, FACS, Department Head, Breast Care Center, National Naval Medical Center, Uniformed Services University, Bethesda, Maryland

CONTRIBUTORS

WIGDAN AL-SUKHNI, MD, Resident, Division of General Surgery, Department of Surgery, University of Toronto; and MSc candidate, Samuel Lunenfeld Research Institute, Toronto, Ontario, Canada

WILLIAM F. ANDERSON, MD, MPH, Senior Investigator, Biostatistics Branch, Division of Cancer Epidemiology and Genetics, National Cancer Institute, National Institutes of Health, Department of Health and Human Services, Bethesda, Maryland

MELYSSA ARONSON, MSc, (C) CGC, Senior Genetic Counsellor, Dr. Zane Cohen Digestive Disease Clinical Research Centre, Toronto, Ontario, Canada

JOHN R. BENSON, MA, DM (oxon), FRCS (Eng), FRCS (Ed), Consultant Breast Surgeon, Cambridge Breast Unit, Addenbrooke's Hospital; and Fellow of Selwyn College, Cambridge, United Kingdom

GLENDA G. CALLENDER, MD, Fellow, Department of Surgical Oncology, The University of Texas M. D. Anderson Cancer Center, Houston, Texas

DANIEL CALVA, MD, Resident in Surgery, Roy J. and Lucille A. Carver University of Iowa College of Medicine, Iowa City, Iowa

KATHLEEN A. CALZONE, MSN, RN, APNG, FAAN, Senior Nurse Specialist, Research, National Institutes of Health, National Cancer Institute, Center for Cancer Research, Genetics Branch, Bethesda, Maryland

STEVEN GALLINGER, MD, MSc, Professor, Division of General Surgery, Department of Surgery, University of Toronto; and Senior Investigator, Samuel Lunenfeld Research Institute, Toronto, Ontario, Canada

JOHAN HANSSON, MD, PhD, Associate Professor of Oncology, Department of Oncology-Pathology, Cancer Center Karolinska, Karolinska Institute, Karolinska University Hospital Solna, Stockholm, Sweden

PAMELA HEBBARD, MD, General Surgery, Memorial University of Newfoundland, St. John's, Newfoundland, Canada

JAMES R. HOWE, MD, Professor of Surgery, Chief, Division of Surgical Oncology and Endocrine Surgery, Roy J. and Lucille A. Carver University of Iowa College of Medicine, Iowa City, Iowa

DAVID G. HUNTSMAN, MD, Associate Professor of Pathology, University of British Columbia; and Genetic Pathologist, Department of Pathology, British Columbia Cancer Agency, Vancouver, British Columbia, Canada

ISMAIL JATOI, MD, PhD, FACS, Department Head, Breast Care Center, National Naval Medical Center, Uniformed Services University, Bethesda, Maryland

SIONG-SENG LIAU, MBChB (Ed), MRCS (Ed), Surgical Registrar, Cambridge Breast Unit, Addenbrooke's Hospital, Cambridge, United Kingdom; Formerly Kenneth Warren Fellow, Harvard Medical School, Boston, Massachusetts

JANE LYNCH, BSN, Instructor, Department of Preventive Medicine and Public Health, Creighton University School of Medicine, Omaha, Nebraska

HENRY T. LYNCH, MD, Chairman and Professor of Preventive Medicine, Medicine, and Public Health, Department of Preventive Medicine and Public Health, Creighton University School of Medicine, Omaha, Nebraska

TAWAKALITU OSENI, MD, Department of Surgical Oncology, Fox Chase Cancer Center, Philadelphia, Pennsylvania

NANCY D. PERRIER, MD, Associate Professor, Department of Surgical Oncology, The University of Texas M. D. Anderson Cancer Center, Houston, Texas

THEREASA A. RICH, MS, CGC, Certified Genetic Counselor, Department of Surgical Oncology, The University of Texas M. D. Anderson Cancer Center, Houston, Texas

EDIBALDO SILVA, MD, PhD, Associate Professor of Surgery, Cancer Center, Creighton University Medical Center, Omaha, Nebraska

LOUISE M. SLAUGHTER, MSPH, United States Representative from New York's 28th District, U.S. House of Representatives, Washington, District of Columbia

PETER W. SOBALLE, MD, FACS, William R. Drucker Professor of Surgery, Uniformed Services University, Bethesda, Maryland

DEBRAH WIRTZFELD, MD, Associate Professor of Surgery and Clinical Genetics, Memorial University of Newfoundland, St. John's, Newfoundland, Canada

HEREDITARY CANCER SYNDROMES

CONTENTS

Foreword xi
Ronald F. Martin

Preface xiii
Ismail Jatoi

Cancer Genetics: A Primer for Surgeons 681
John R. Benson and Siong-Seng Liau

> Contemporary ideas of carcinogenesis envisage a series of stochastic genetic changes that confer a selective growth advantage over healthy cells. These changes collectively lead to the disruption of coordinated networks of intercellular communication and cause a fundamental change in cellular behavior, which affects processes, such as proliferation, differentiation, and apoptosis. This progressive dysregulation of cellular function implies that cancer is not a morphologic entity, but a process in which the malignant phenotype is gradually acquired.

Genetic Testing for Cancer Susceptibility 705
Kathleen A. Calzone and Peter W. Soballe

> Genetic testing for mutations in genes associated with an inherited predisposition to cancer is rapidly moving outside specialty genetic services and into mainstream health care. Surgeons, as front-line providers of cancer care, are uniquely positioned to identify those who may benefit from genetic testing and institute changes to their health care management based on those results. This article provides an overview of the critical elements of the process of genetic testing for cancer susceptibility.

The Genetic Information Nondiscrimination Act: Why Your Personal Genetics are Still Vulnerable to Discrimination 723
Louise M. Slaughter

> Genetic research offers great potential for early treatment and the prevention of numerous diseases. As technology continues to advance, ethical, legal, and social challenges continue to present themselves. The Genetic Information Nondiscrimination Act (GINA) looks to protect an individual's genetic information from employer and insurance discrimination while encouraging Americans to take advantage of genetic testing to prevent and prepare for potential diseases. GINA will do more than stamp out a new form of discrimination: it will help the United States be a leader in a field of scientific research that holds as much promise as any other in history.

An Overview of the Role of Prophylactic Surgery in the Management of Individuals with a Hereditary Cancer Predisposition 739
Tawakalitu Oseni and Ismail Jatoi

> Genetic testing for cancer susceptibility has been implemented widely in recent years, with the hope that it eventually will lead to a reduction in cancer-related mortality. Asymptomatic individuals who have a genetic predisposition for cancer can be identified, and many may benefit from early intervention. Not all of these individuals will develop cancer, however, and the penetrance varies among individuals with different mutations. Surveillance, chemoprevention, and prophylactic surgery are accepted options for managing individuals who have a genetic predisposition for cancer. Yet, there are no randomized prospective trials that have assessed the impact of these interventions specifically in mutation carriers. The decision to undergo prophylactic surgery therefore should be made after all other management options are considered, and the patient is informed of the potential risks and benefits of surgery. This article provides an overview of the role of prophylactic surgery for managing patients who have a genetic predisposition for cancer. It specifically discusses the potential role of surgery in preventing breast, colon, thyroid, and gastric cancers. Additionally, it discusses the types of prophylactic surgical procedures that are performed commonly, and their expanding role in cancer prevention.

Hereditary Diffuse Gastric Cancer: Prophylactic Surgical Oncology Implications 759
Henry T. Lynch, Edibaldo Silva, Debrah Wirtzfeld, Pamela Hebbard, Jane Lynch, and David G. Huntsman

> Hereditary diffuse gastric cancer (HDGC) is an autosomal dominantly inherited syndrome attributed to mutations of the E-cadherin gene, *CDH1*. There is no proven effective screening for

early HDGC, and symptomatic disease is almost universally fatal. The only available effective option for *CDH1* carriers is prophylactic total gastrectomy, but the variable age of onset of HDGC and the reduced penetrance (about 70%) of the *CDHI* gene further complicate patients' decision making.

Hamartomatous Polyposis Syndromes 779
Daniel Calva and James R. Howe

Since the histologic description of the hamartomatous polyp in 1957 by Horrilleno and colleagues, descriptions have appeared of several different syndromes with the propensity to develop these polyps in the upper and lower gastrointestinal tracts. These syndromes include juvenile polyposis, Peutz-Jeghers syndrome, hereditary mixed polyposis syndrome, and the phosphatase and tensin homolog gene (PTEN) hamartoma tumor syndromes (Cowden and Bannayan-Riley-Ruvalcaba syndromes), which are autosomal-dominantly inherited, and Cronkhite-Canada syndrome, which is acquired. This article reviews the clinical aspects, the molecular pathogenesis, the affected organ systems, the risks of cancer, and the management of these hamartomatous polyposis syndromes. Although the incidence of these syndromes is low, it is important for clinicians to recognize these disorders to prevent morbidity and mortality in these patients, and to perform presymptomatic testing in patients at risk.

Hereditary Colorectal Cancer Syndromes: Familial Adenomatous Polyposis and Lynch Syndrome 819
Wigdan Al-Sukhni, Melyssa Aronson, and Steven Gallinger

Familial colorectal cancer (CRC) accounts for 10% to 20% of all cases of CRC. Two major autosomal dominant forms of heritable CRC are familial adenomatous polyposis (FAP) and Lynch syndrome (also known as hereditary nonpolyposis colorectal cancer). Along with the risk for CRC, both syndromes are associated with elevated risk for other tumors. Improved understanding of the genetic basis of these diseases has not only facilitated the identification and screening of at-risk individuals and the development of prophylactic or early-stage intervention strategies but also provided better insight into sporadic CRC. This article reviews the clinical and genetic characteristics of FAP and Lynch syndrome, recommended screening and surveillance practices, and appropriate surgical and nonsurgical interventions.

Management of Women Who Have a Genetic Predisposition for Breast Cancer 845
Ismail Jatoi and William F. Anderson

The management of women who have a genetic predisposition for breast cancer requires careful planning. Women who have *BRCA 1* and *BRCA 2* mutations are at increased risk for breast cancer and for other cancers as well, particularly ovarian cancer. Screening, prophlyactic surgery, and chemoprevention are commonly utilized strategies in the management of these patients, and women may choose more than one of these strategies. No randomized prospective trials have assessed the impact of these strategies specifically in mutaiton carriers. All patients should be informed that screening, prophylactic surgery, and chemoprevention have the potential for harm as well as benefit.

Multiple Endocrine Neoplasia Syndromes 863
Glenda G. Callender, Thereasa A. Rich, and Nancy D. Perrier

The multiple endocrine neoplasia (MEN) syndromes are rare autosomal-dominant conditions that predispose affected individuals to benign and malignant tumors of the pituitary, thyroid, parathyroids, adrenals, endocrine pancreas, paraganglia, or non-endocrine organs. The classic MEN syndromes include MEN type 1 and MEN type 2. However, several other hereditary conditions should also be considered in the category of MEN: von Hippel-Lindau syndrome, the familial paraganglioma syndromes, Cowden syndrome, Carney complex, and hyperparathyroidism jaw-tumor syndrome. In addition, researchers are becoming aware of other familial endocrine neoplasia syndromes with an unknown genetic basis that might also fall into the category of MEN. This article reviews the clinical features, diagnosis, and surgical management of the various MEN syndromes and genetic risk assessment for patients presenting with one or more endocrine neoplasms.

Familial Melanoma 897
Johan Hansson

Approximately 5% to 10% of cases of cutaneous melanoma occur in families that have a hereditary predisposition for this disease. In 20% to 40% of such melanoma families, germline mutations in the *CDKN2A* gene have been identified. Apart from a high risk of melanoma, a proportion of kindreds that have familial melanoma also have an increased risk of pancreatic carcinoma. Guidelines for management of familial melanoma and the issue of genetic testing for *CDKN2A* germline mutations are discussed.

Index 917

FORTHCOMING ISSUES

October 2008
Advances and Controversies in Minimally Invasive Surgery
Jon Gould, MD, and Scott Melvin, MD, *Guest Editors*

December 2008
Biliary Surgery
John L. Munson, MD, *Guest Editor*

RECENT ISSUES

June 2008
Soft Tissue Sarcomas
Matthew T. Hueman, MD, and Nita Ahuja, MD, *Guest Editors*

April 2008
OB/GYN for the General Surgeon
Charles Dietrich, III, MD, *Guest Editor*

February 2008
Advances in Abdominal Wall Hernia Repair
Kamal FMF Itani, MD, and Mary Hawn, MD, *Guest Editors*

The Clinics are now available online!

www.theclinics.com

Foreword

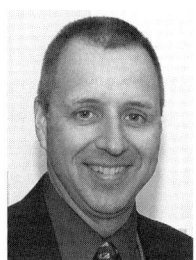

Ronald F. Martin, MD
Consulting Editor

This issue of the *Surgical Clinics of North America* might represent a departure to some from our usual discourse, but I would submit that this is absolutely in line with where we ought to be focusing our attention. Surgeons have been treating cancer since before we could spell DNA, let alone understand what it was. Our understanding of cancer and its causes has until recently been profoundly primitive and it still might be. Yet, we as surgeons have been called to do our bit and historically have been the leaders in the management of patients with cancer. That position of leadership has certainly changed over the past few decades, but surgery as a significant component of cancer management is in no immediate peril of extinction. I would, however, suggest that the reason for surgical intervention and the nature of surgical intervention is likely to become barely recognizable to its previous form.

To be sure, it is easy to write a foreword suggesting "the future aint what it used to be" (with apologies to Mr. Berra) regarding cancer—we all know that things are changing. At this time though, I think we have enough writing on the wall to make our claims about how things are changing and why.

Among Halsted's great contributions to surgery was his suggestion of wide resection of cancer to include nodal drainage and other organs or structures deemed expendable to improve survival. In his time this made a huge difference, but it also set the stage for a fairly dogmatic approach to a disease that we knew almost nothing about. The best we could think was that tumor cells must go to lymph nodes and so on to other organs. Of course, that progression was found to represent a subset of patterns of cancer spread and the concept of cancer being a systemic disease took greater hold. Yet all the while we basically clung to the idea of TNM staging as a proxy for classifying the level of de-differentiation of cancers. Now in the era of polymerase chain reaction, micro-array technology, the human genome project, and the ability to share and compare information at extremely rapid rates, the capacity to develop a more sophisticated understanding of the genetic derangement of cancers is likely to exceed what we can glean from an anatomic proxy that is horrifically prone to sampling error and failed analysis. The collection of articles in this issue represents a marker along the path towards a fundamentally different approach to the patient with cancer. These articles, focused on known inherited cancer syndromes, provide an insight into the larger topic of collected inherited and acquired genetic alterations. The articles all contain themes in common: what are the known recurrent genetic changes are there for a given syndrome, how do we use that knowledge to guide patients and families, how do we screen patients for the genetic abnormality or the end state condition, and for whom do we consider a preemptive or prophylactic option? Assuming we gather enough information about enough cancers, we could likely extrapolate these principles to patients at risk for sporadic cancers as well.

One of our roles as surgeon has been to provide locoregional control with intent to "cure" when thought feasible, or palliate, both of which are noble goals no doubt. But armed with better information, our role may shift into targeted prevention, which at present is best seen in these patients or kindreds with identifiable high-risk genetic abnormalities.

I would encourage the reader to consider these articles as very useful information in the practical sense of patient care (additionally, professors and test writers dearly love to quiz people over factoids about inherited disorders of all sorts), but also with an eye to what to expect as we move forward to a more sophisticated approach in general to the patient with a genetic problem. We are deeply indebted to Dr. Jatoi and his colleagues for the excellent work they have submitted for your consideration.

Ronald F. Martin, MD
Department of Surgery
Marshfield Clinic
1000 North Oak Avenue
Marshfield, WI 54449, USA
E-mail address: martin.ronald@marshfieldclinic.org

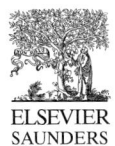

Preface

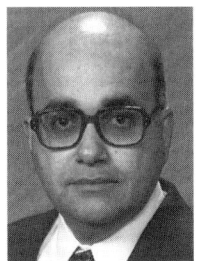

Ismail Jatoi, MD, PhD, FACS
Guest Editor

Genetic testing for cancer susceptibility is now widely utilized. Clinicians can identify individuals with a genetic predisposition for cancer and provide options to reduce cancer risk. Increasingly, surgeons are playing a key role in the management of these patients. Thus, surgeons should be fully aware of the various strategies that are available for the management of individuals with a genetic predisposition for cancer, including screening, chemoprevention, and prophylactic surgery. However, collaboration with physicians of other disciplines remains essential.

This issue of *Surgical Clinics of North America* contains 10 articles, written by experts from North America and Europe. These articles review various topics relevant to the surgical management of patients with hereditary cancer syndromes. In these articles, the authors also provide their personal perspectives on controversial issues. I am deeply grateful to all the authors for their excellent contributions. I would also like to thank Catherine Bewick, Dr. Ronald Martin, and the editorial staff at Elsevier for their valuable assistance in assembling this issue of *Clinics*. I hope that this issue serves as a valuable guide for the management of patients with hereditary cancer syndromes.

Ismail Jatoi, MD, PhD, FACS
Department of Surgery
National Naval Medical Center
Uniformed Services University
4301 Jones Bridge Road
Bethesda, MD 20814, USA

E-mail address: ismail.jatoi@us.army.mil

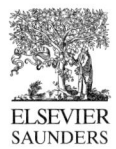

Cancer Genetics: A Primer for Surgeons

John R. Benson, MA, DM (oxon),
FRCS (Eng), FRCS (Ed)[a,b,*],
Siong-Seng Liau, MBChB (Ed), MRCS (Ed)[a,c]

[a]Cambridge Breast Unit, Addenbrooke's Hospital, Hills Road,
Cambridge CB2 0QQ, UK
[b]Selwyn College, Grange Road, Cambridge, CB3 9DQ, UK
[c]Harvard Medical School, 25 Shattuck Street, Boston, MA 02115, USA

Contemporary ideas of carcinogenesis envisage a series of stochastic genetic changes that confer a selective growth advantage over healthy cells. These changes collectively lead to the disruption of coordinated networks of intercellular communication and cause a fundamental change in cellular behavior, which affects processes, such as proliferation, differentiation, and apoptosis. This progressive dysregulation of cellular function implies that cancer is not a morphologic entity, but a process in which the malignant phenotype is gradually acquired. Rates of proliferation and differentiation are stringently regulated within normal tissues of a multicellular organism such that organs do not exceed a specific size and tissue renewal is proportionate and confined to replacement of damaged or effete cells only. An important mechanism for growth control in multicellular organisms is density-dependent growth inhibition, which ensures that no single cell has unrestrained growth and competition for space and nutrients is "fair." This mechanism may be mediated by an increase in cellular requirements for macromolecular growth factors. As confluency is reached with crowding of cells, their innate sensitivity to these growth factors decreases, perhaps as a result of a reduction in the density of cell surface receptors [1]. Polypeptide growth factors are a group of regulatory molecules that have been well characterized from serum and cell tissue extracts. There seems to be a close relationship between growth factor production and growth of many types of tumor. They are functionally divided into positive and negative growth

---

* Corresponding author. Cambridge Breast Unit, Addenbrooke's Hospital, Hills Road, Cambridge CB2 0QQ, United Kingdom.
  E-mail address: john.benson@addenbrookes.nhs.uk (J.R. Benson).

factors depending on whether epithelial proliferation is stimulated (mitogenic) or inhibited, respectively. Control of the cell cycle and hence rate of tumor growth is determined by the balance of growth factors acting on a cell. Although cells have an inherent program that influences rates of proliferation, differentiation, and cell death, this sea of soluble growth factors represents a principle mechanism for modulation and regulation of cellular activity by exogenous stimuli. Aberrant function of autocrine and paracrine growth factor loops leads to excessive proliferation and promotes neoplastic development [2].

Cancer genes

The existence of multiple mitogenic growth factors may guarantee a rapid growth phase during the early stages of embryogenesis thereby maximizing the chances of sustained viability. A consequence of this collective mitogenic potential of cells may be a lower threshold for development of hyperproliferative states that presage cancer. The sequence of events leading to formation of a tumor is ultimately attributable to genetic mutations and changes in gene expression, although the latter can be modified by host factors. Concepts of carcinogenesis over the past 2 decades have been dominated by the paradigm of oncogenes and more recently tumor suppressor genes [3]. The malignant phenotype is considered to arise from an accumulation, either randomly or sequentially, of alterations within these two operational classes of genes at the somatic cell level. Oncogenes are derived from normal cellular counterparts termed proto-oncogenes, which have some sequence homology with tumor-producing viruses. Activated oncogenes represent a positive or "gain-of-function" change resulting in a growth advantage over normal cells in possession of the inactivated proto-oncogene. The latter code for various proteins, including polypeptide growth factors and their receptors, together with several key components of the signal transduction process and nuclear regulators of the cell cycle. The normal proto-oncogene product may simply be produced in excessive amounts rather than activation being associated with an abnormal gene product. In both scenarios, there are increased rates of cell proliferation and persistence of genetically aberrant cells. By contrast, tumor suppressor genes are characterized by mutations that lead to loss of function. Tumor suppressor genes are natural elements of a cell's genetic code and products of these genes exert a negative (suppressive) influence on cellular proliferation but promote pathways leading to programmed cell death. In addition to acting as a kind of brake on the cell cycle, they have a crucial role in maintenance of genomic integrity and fidelity of DNA replication. Mutations within these tumor suppressor genes essentially produce tumors by default, whereas oncogenic events within a cell tend to have an executive influence on malignant change.

Inherited and sporadic forms of cancers

The genetic alterations within a cell that form the basis for malignant transformation can be either inherited or acquired [4]. Germline mutations are present within all cells, whereas somatic mutations affect individual cells within a particular tissue. Although most cancers arise from changes in gene expression consequent to acquired mutations within somatic cells, a minority (5%) of tumors develop within the setting of an inherited genetic predisposition. The cells of such individuals possess a pre-existing germline mutation and require fewer subsequent events for induction of carcinogenesis. Occasionally a genetic susceptibility may be manifest as a systemic effect whereby spontaneous mutations within all tissues become more frequent or carcinogens are metabolized less efficiently. Table 1 shows examples of specific tumors resulting from an inherited genetic predisposition that are associated with various familial cancer syndromes.

Epidemiologic studies of inherited and sporadic forms of certain cancers have provided much insight into the genetic initiation process. Knudson [5,6] proposed a "two-hit" hypothesis in which mutations in both alleles of a gene pair were a prerequisite for cancer development (Fig. 1). Individuals who have an inherited predisposition already possessed a mutation in one allele (present in all cells) and thus required only one further somatic mutation for tumor formation. Sporadic forms of the cancer depended on two somatic mutations, the chances of which were correspondingly smaller for any equivalent mutation rate. Knudson's hypothesis is especially applicable to those tumors arising from loss of function in tumor suppressor genes; usually inactivation of both alleles is essential before levels of the gene product decrease sufficiently to induce malignant change. By contrast, oncogenes behave in a dominant manner and mutation within a single allele may be sufficient for tumor development. Sometimes heterozygosity at an oncogene locus (eg, 5q21) results in a premalignant phenotype, such as colonic polyps, with malignant transformation once mutation occurs in the second allele. Fearon and Vogelstein [7] proposed a model for colorectal carcinogenesis based on sequential genetic changes and progression from normal to dysplastic epithelium, polyp formation, and eventual colon cancer (see discussion of cytoplasmic tumor suppressor genes).

Carcinogenesis

Carcinogenesis is a multistage process with the sequential acquisition of mutations within the genome [8]. It remains unclear whether invasive malignancy develops once a critical number and type of mutations are present within a cell, or whether serial accumulation is mandatory, whereby mutations are acquired in a particular order. Many genetic changes are already present in premalignant and in situ forms of cancer. The incidence of

Table 1
Genes involved in familial cancer syndromes

Syndrome	Gene	Tumors
Ataxia telangiectasia	ATM	Lymphoma
		Breast cancer in heterozygotes
Bloom syndrome	BLM	Solid tumors
Cowden syndrome	PTEN1	Breast cancer
		Hamartoma
Familial adenomatous polyposis	APC	Colorectal cancer
		Desmoids
		Osteomas
		Duodenal cancer
Familial breast ovarian cancer	BRCA1, BRCA2	Breast cancer
		Ovarian cancer
		Male breast cancer (BRCA2)
Familial retinoblastoma	RB1	Retinoblastoma
		Osteosarcoma
Fanconi anemia	FACC, FACA	AML
Gorlin syndrome (basal cell nevus syndrome)	PATCHED	Basal cell cancer
		Medulloblastoma
		Ovarian fibroma
Hereditary nonpolyposis colon cancer (HNPCC or Lynch syndrome)	hMLH1, hMSH2, hPMS2, hMSH6	Colorectal cancer
		Endometrial cancer
		Gastric cancer
		Ovarian cancer
		Uroepithelial cancer
Hereditary papillary renal cancer	MET	Papillary renal cancer
		Other cancers
Juvenile polyposis	SMAD4	Hamartomatous polyps
		Colorectal cancer
Li Fraumeni syndrome	p53, hCHK2	Soft tissue sarcoma
		Breast cancer
		Brain tumors
		Leukemia
Multiple endocrine neoplasia 1 (MEN1)	MEN1	Parathyroid hyperplasia
		Endocrine pancreatic tumors
		Pituitary tumors
Multiple endocrine neoplasia 2 (MEN2)	RET	Medullary thyroid cancer
		Pheochromocytoma
Neurofibromatosis	NF1, NF2	Neurofibroma
		Acoustic neuroma
		Meningioma
		Schwannoma
Peutz-Jeghers syndrome	LKB1	Hamartomatous polyps
		Breast cancer
		Other tumors
Tuberous sclerosis	TSC1, TSC2	Renal angiomyolipomas
		Rhabdomyoma
von Hippel–Lindau syndrome	VHL	Renal cell cancer
		Hemangioblastoma
		Retinal angioma
		Pheochromocytoma
Wilms tumor	WT1	Wilms tumor
Xeroderma pigmentosum	XPB, XPD, XPA	Skin cancer

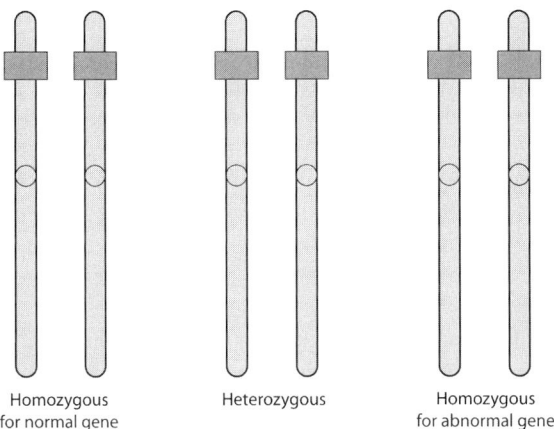

Fig. 1. Knudson proposed that the genetic changes within a somatic cell that underlie development of cancer are related to germline mutations, which are inherited in a Mendelian pattern. Individuals who have a familial predisposition already possess a mutation in one of a pair of alleles and require only one further mutation for malignancy to develop. By contrast, those individuals who do not have a genetic predisposition must acquire a mutation in each allele of a pair. Identification of the genes involved in hereditary susceptibility would provide insight into somatic cell mutations within sporadic tumors.

many common cancers (such as those of the breast, prostate, colon, or skin) increases with age with kinetics dependent on the fourth or fifth power of elapsed time. This observation suggests that a minimum of four or five events must occur before tumor development [9]. Moreover, the association of cancer with increasing age suggests that continuous exposure to low levels of environmental or endogenous carcinogens may have a cumulative effect and perhaps act on tissues more susceptible to neoplastic change.

Among those cancers that are attributable to inheritable forms of the disease, the development of malignancy is almost inevitable. In such cases, either the homozygous (tumor suppressor genes) or heterozygous state (oncogenes) confers a high level of genetic susceptibility and no further genetic mutation may be necessary for tumor initiation (eg, retinoblastoma). In other circumstances, the chance of developing cancer depends on a balance of genetic predisposition and acquired mutations. For most human cancers there is no inherited risk and these are termed sporadic tumors. They depend exclusively on somatic mutations. These latter genetic alterations result from one of two interrelated processes.

> There is an intrinsic error rate for DNA synthesis and repair within normal tissues, which results in acquired mutations that are passed on to the cell progeny during replication. This phenomenon leads to a background rate of spontaneous mutation that has been estimated to be a 1 in 1 million chance for any particular gene each time a cell divides. This figure represents a very low baseline somatic mutation rate and the

chance of a key cancer gene being mutated spontaneously must be extremely low. A powerful positive selection pressure operates from the outset for cancer-promoting mutations, however, and this effectively magnifies the impact of low-frequency events. Once a mutation has occurred in a stem cell, a malignant clone of cells arises that replicates the initial mutation thousands of times. As the clone size approaches about 100 cells, the chance of a second mutation within this primary clone increases significantly, which in turn enhances any selective growth advantage and this new clone outgrows the first one. This process is continued and leads to acquisition of a collection of cellular features typical of the malignant phenotype.

This baseline rate of spontaneous somatic mutation is augmented by environmental factors interacting with cellular DNA either directly or indirectly. These include not only exposure to agents, such as radiation and chemical carcinogens, but also the genotoxic effects of endogenous agents, such as free radicals, which induce oxidative stress. Various chemicals are known to be carcinogenic and some of the mechanisms for induction of tumors have been elucidated. Although many of the well-documented industrial cancer risks have been minimized in recent years, several potential sources of carcinogens exist within the environment of contemporary western society. Most of these involve low levels of exposure, including low-density ionizing radiation and ultraviolet irradiation. These contribute to the background rate of somatic mutation and in some cases can greatly increase rates of malignancy.

The origin of cancer cells

One of the most challenging aspects in the research and treatment of cancer is tumor heterogeneity. Not only is there variation between individuals with respect to a designated tumor type, but cells composing a single tumor are far from homogeneous. Any theory for the origin of cancer cells must provide an explanation for cellular heterogeneity and address the questions of whether cancer is monoclonal or polyclonal in origin and whether cancers originate from stem cells or differentiated somatic cells.

Stem cells

Growth and development of normal tissues proceeds to a point at which the rate of cell proliferation is balanced by cell loss. Some tissues undergo hypertrophy or hyperplasia in response to normal physiologic processes (eg, breast and uterine tissues), but regress spontaneously on withdrawal of an external stimulus. Furthermore, during the process of normal development and tissue renewal, the progeny of stem cells differentiate into mature cells that have characteristic biochemical and functional properties. Stem cells themselves originate from multipotential precursor cells that give rise to stem cells with a degree of genetic restriction and reduced potential. All stem cells have the capacity for self-renewal and can proliferate indefinitely. They undergo asymmetric cell divisions to produce a pool of identical progenitor cells or transit amplifying cells that differentiate into the cellular type appropriate for a particular location (Fig. 2). Stem cells for one particular lineage cannot differentiate into cells of another lineage and are "determined" once formed. The phenotype of these stem cells is influenced by environmental factors that control replacement of senescent cells from undifferentiated stem cells [10].

Monoclonal theory

Much evidence has accrued supporting a monoclonal origin for most human cancers. This theory implies that a single cell undergoes malignant transformation and forms a primary clone from which further subclones are derived. This process of clonal evolution has been described earlier and is predicated on a selective growth advantage for mutated cells that permits them to bridge bottlenecks imposed by restrictions of space, nutrients, and oxygen [11]. A polyclonal origin for cancer might be feasible for some

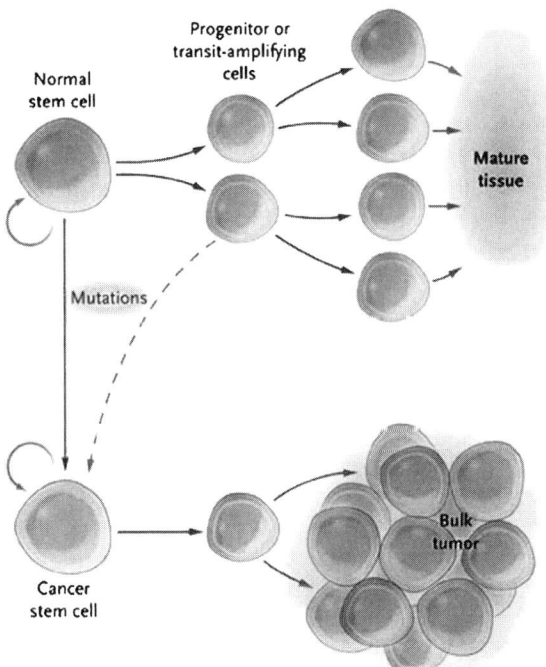

Fig. 2. All stem cells undergo asymmetric cell divisions to produce a pool of identical progenitor cells or transit amplifying cells that differentiate into the cellular type appropriate for a particular location.

inherited forms of cancer in which there are germline mutations in both alleles and genetic susceptibility operates as a field effect. For most sporadic cancers and inherited forms that depend on a further somatic mutation, however, polyclonality is highly improbable; multiple cells in close proximity would have to be transformed concurrently or within a relatively short time frame to form a single tumor.

The sequential acquisition of mutations during clonal evolution not only provides a positive selection pressure but also generates a degree of instability within the genome. This genetic instability favors further mutational change among individual cells of a clone. These additional and random mutations result in phenotypic differences between cells that are manifest as variations in rates of proliferation, cell motility, and metastatic potential, and sensitivity/resistance to therapeutic interventions. The mature tumor thus contains cells of monoclonal origin but phenotypic and genetic diversity. This process generates subclones of cells with different functional properties, some of which have the capacity to metastasize [12].

Cancer stem cell hypothesis

Many tumors are grossly similar to their tissue of origin, which is most evident for well-differentiated lesions. It was previously believed that cancers arose from dedifferentiation of the mature phenotype with reversion to a more primitive state to a greater (poorly differentiated) or lesser (well differentiated) degree. It is unlikely that a mature somatic cell would exist within tissues for a sufficiently long period to accumulate a mandatory number of mutations for malignant transformation. By contrast, stem cells have greater longevity and have the capacity for self-renewal. The cancer stem cell hypothesis proposes that the stem cell is the target for carcinogenesis and not mature somatic cells [13]. A tumor would arise from differentiation of rapidly proliferating, undifferentiated stem cells and contain varying proportions of these two stem cell types. Furthermore, the proportion of malignant stem cells that have undergone differentiation (and apoptosis) relative to those that continue to proliferate determines histologic grade. A cell may thus possess the typical features of a malignant phenotype yet still have gone through a sequential process of differentiation to a comparable point as the normal cell lineage. Cancer stem cells have now been identified in tumors of the breast and nervous system and are the focus for novel and more targeted forms of treatment. Cancer stem cells thus form a functional group of cells that initiate tumor formation and can differentiate into heterogeneous progeny that sustain tumor growth. A relatively small population of quiescent or slowly dividing cancer stem cells is responsible for the continued expansion of a tumor by spawning more differentiated cells. These latter cells constitute the bulk of the tumor (epithelial component) and have short-term proliferative capacity. The development of cancer therefore parallels normal tissue development with origin from a hierarchical lineage of cells [10].

Genetic alterations

The process of mitosis with division of a cell to produce progeny with identical genetic content is extremely complex. Although cell division is well orchestrated with a high degree of fidelity, there is an innate fallibility that leads to errors in DNA replication. The cell possesses multiple mechanisms for ongoing repair of inappropriate alterations in base-pair sequences, and can activate programmed cell death when there is overwhelming DNA damage or gross chromosomal changes. Some of the enzymes involved in these repair processes can be susceptible to mutational events and indirectly cause malignant transformation of cells by allowing persistence and propagation of gene alterations. Individuals who have Bloom syndrome's have a deficiency of DNA ligase I and are highly susceptible to developing cancer (see Table 1).

Types of mutation

In recent years there has been major progress in understanding and unraveling the genetic alterations that lead to disruption and dislocation of molecular and biochemical pathways. Although no single genetic change has been identified that causes cancer, it is now appreciated that cancer cells display a finite number of aberrant pathways and the defective portion of the DNA is relatively small in proportion to overall genome size. Exogenous agents, such as chemicals and irradiation, induce direct DNA damage, but a background mutation rate occurs from the hydrolytic interaction of water itself with DNA. This interaction results in the cleavage of glycosidic bonds which can depurinate or depyrimidate nucleotide bases or cause strand breaks. Genetic alterations associated with malignant change can be broadly divided into the following five categories:

- Changes in nucleotide sequence resulting from base pair substitutions, deletions, or insertions. Deletions and insertions can lead to major problems with gene transcription and are sometimes referred to as mis sense mutations. These often result in a truncated protein because the altered DNA sequence cannot be read. Up to 90% of pancreatic adenocarcinomas contain missense mutations. Tautomeric changes within individual nucleotides may have minimal impact and cause minor changes in protein structure and function. Indeed, a codon with a single base alteration could be "silent" and not effect any change in amino acid sequence.
- Changes in the normal diploid number of chromosomes are common in cancer. Aneuploid cells usually have a reduced complement of chromosomal material (up to 50%) and result from inappropriate segregation of chromosomes during mitosis.
- Chromosomal translocations are the most common structural rearrangement in cancer cells and involve fusion of different chromosomes or

segments of a single chromosome that are noncontiguous. This interchange of chromosomal material can result in an oncogene being positioned next to transcription regulatory sequences leading to overexpression. Alternatively, a fusion gene may be formed from combination of coding sequences on either side of the breakpoint. A classic example of the latter is formation of the Philadelphia chromosome in chronic myelogenous leukemia (Fig. 3) [14]. This chromosome results from fusion of the carboxy terminus of the c-abl gene on chromosome 9 and the amino terminus of the bcr gene on chromosome 22 (bcr-abl gene product).

Gene amplifications result from multiple copies of an amplicon containing 0.5 to 10 megabases of DNA. This phenomenon occurs relatively late in the pathogenesis of cancer and probably reflects acquired genetic instability. When an amplicon encodes an oncoprotein, this is overexpressed and promotes tumorigenesis. Many oncogenes derive enhanced expression from this mechanism and are associated with particularly aggressive phenotypes. For example, the n-myc gene is frequently amplified in neuroblastomas, which are highly lethal tumors [15].

Epigenetic changes represent a nonmutational pathway for modulation of gene expression. Instead of changes in nucleotide sequence, DNA methylation and histone modification are used to maintain a gene in a closed confirmation such that it cannot be accessed by DNA polymerase. Hypermethylation is a method for gene silencing and can prevent expression of tumor suppressor genes (eg, BRCA-1) even when the gene sequence is intact [16].

Genetic instability

The process of clonal selection amplifies the rate of spontaneous mutation in somatic cells to permit emergence of tumors. The frequency of mutational events is further enhanced by the existence of genetic instability which occurs pari-passu with clonal evolution. As cells progressively acquire cancer-related mutations, the genome becomes more unstable and prone to

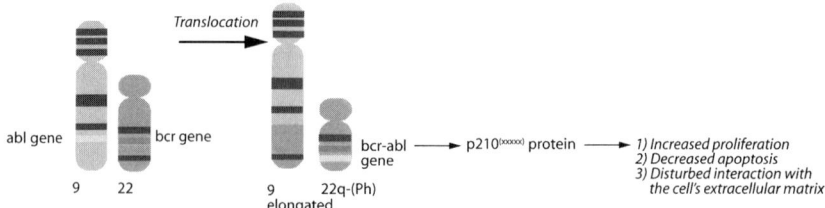

Fig. 3. Formation of the Philadelphia chromosome in chronic myelogenous leukemia resulting from fusion of the carboxy-terminus of the c-abl gene on chromosome 9 and the amino-terminus of the bcr gene on chromosome 22 (bcr-abl gene product).

genetic alteration, which is a general property of the cellular DNA and not attributable to specific mutations. Genetic instability seems to be inherent in a large proportion of cancers and greatly increases the probability of further spontaneous mutations that contribute to neoplastic development. Although cells are vulnerable to genetic damage, there are specific mechanisms that serve to maintain the integrity of the genome [17].

Caretaker genes: These genes are involved in recognition and repair of nucleotide base pair abnormalities or DNA strand breaks. Base excision and nucleotide excision repair are two general mechanisms that may be involved and have been implicated in BRCA-1 and BRCA-2 defects and their interaction with the repair protein Rad51 [18].

Gatekeeper genes: These genes control entry of cells into the replicative cycle and activate cell cycle arrest in the presence of damaged DNA. This set of gatekeeper genes works in collaboration with caretaker genes so that sufficient time and opportunity exist for repair of damaged DNA before onset of cell division. If this gatekeeper function fails, there is a risk that damaged portions of DNA will be passed on to daughter cells as potential cancer-promoting mutations. Gatekeepers operate around the cell cycle control or checkpoints (G1/S and G2/M) and interact with signal transduction pathways that are rapidly integrating stimulatory and inhibitory signals from within and outside the cell during the gap periods of the cell cycle (G1 and G2). The cell assesses the final polarity of the net signaling and together with an analysis of DNA integrity directs gatekeeper activities. Activation of gatekeeper pathways influences one or another of these checkpoints and prevents either the onset of DNA synthesis or entry into mitosis. Specific defects in caretaker and gatekeeper genes can lead to dramatic rates of genetic instability and rapid progression to a lethal phenotype.

Genetic instability can be manifest at one of two levels. Most instability is observed at the level of the chromosome, with large-scale deletions, duplication, or interchange of whole or large segments of chromosomes. Less commonly, nucleotide instability results from substitution, deletion, or insertion of nucleotides. Interestingly, there is an inverse relationship between instability at the chromosomal and nucleotide levels suggesting that these pathways may be mutually exclusive.

Chromosomal instability

Karyotypic analyses indicate that most cancers of epithelial origin display aneuploidy [19]. This finding suggests that several genes, when mutated, lead to this form of instability, which is at least 10-fold higher in aneuploid compared with diploid tumors. The molecular basis for this chromosomal instability is heterogeneous, but defects in specific checkpoints discussed earlier promote this form of genetic instability [20]. "Spindle checkpoint" genes ensure that segregation of chromosomes on the mitotic spindle proceeds without error, but mutations in these genes are commonly detected in human cancer [21].

Defects in a second checkpoint, referred to as a "DNA damage checkpoint," are probably a more frequent cause of chromosomal instability. This checkpoint prevents cells with damaged DNA from entering mitosis; replication of damaged DNA results in abnormalities of chromosomal segregation and mitotic recombination. Gross structural alterations in chromosomes occur if DNA replication goes ahead in the presence of either a single or double strand break. Some inherited forms of cancer predisposition are linked to these DNA strand break pathways and genes such as ATM (ataxia telangiectasia mutated), ATR (ATM and Rad-3 related), BRCA-1, BRCA-2, and p53 are DNA damage checkpoint genes that have been implicated in human malignancy [22]. Within normal cells, functional p53 prompts cell cycle arrest in G1 in the presence of inappropriate chromosomal segregation. By contrast, a defective p53 protein allows cells to progress through the G1/S transition and eventually aneuploidy occurs in daughter cells. A further mechanism for chromosomal instability is abnormal number and function of centrosomes. Centrosomes act to nucleate the ends of the mitotic microtubule spindle along which sister chromosomes separate during mitosis [23]. A final mechanism for chromosomal instability is by way of dysfunctional telomeres [24]. The latter are ribonuclear protein complexes located at the ends of all functional eukaryotic chromosomes. Telomeric dysfunction promotes end-to-end fusions and fusion-bridge-breakage cycles that result in gross structural chromosomal abnormalities [25]. Several mechanisms exist, therefore, whereby cells may become aneuploid with chromosomal instability. Collectively, these are responsible for the relatively frequent occurrence of these complex lesions.

Nucleotide instability

Instability at the nucleotide level is relatively uncommon in cancers and probably reflects the impact of environmental carcinogens or the background rate of somatic mutation. Defects in two main cellular DNA repair systems can lead to significant levels of genetic instability, however.

Nucleotide excision repair: This process is responsible for detection and repair of bulky DNA lesions induced by exogenous mutagens [26] and was first recognized in individuals who had xeroderma pigmentosum. The latter possess an inherited defect in this DNA repair system characterized by severe UV photosensitivity and susceptibility to skin cancers [27]. The disease is autosomally recessive and heterozygotes are not at increased risk for malignancy. The disease thus poses a significant clinical risk only in the context of an inherited predisposition.

DNA mismatch repair: This system is responsible for correction of DNA replication errors, including base–base mismatches and abnormal nucleotide loops resulting from insertions/deletions of DNA and incorporated during the replicative process. Base–base mismatches typically affect nonrepetitive DNA sequences, whereas insertional/deletion loops occur at sites of repetitive DNA sequences. These lesions lead to gains or losses of short mono- or dinucleotide repeat units (eg, poly(A) or poly(CA) repeats) within sections of the genome called microsatellite regions. The microsatellite sequences are characterized by identical nucleotide repeats and are frequently observed in the coding regions of genes. This type of nucleotide replication error is known as microsatellite instability and has been identified in most tumors developing in patients who have hereditary nonpolyposis coli (HNPCC), otherwise known as Lynch syndrome [28,29]. This disease is caused directly by mutations in genes required for DNA mismatch repair that were initially investigated in yeast; human homologs were later identified [30]. Mismatch repair defects accelerate the mutation rate for hereditary and sporadic forms of colon cancer, however. Furthermore, mismatch repair defects can be detected in more than 10% of all colorectal, stomach, and endometrial cancers. It is now recognized that at least 95% of HNPCC cases are attributable to mutations in the human homologs of two mismatch repair genes (MSH2 and MLH1) [31]. A correspondingly lower proportion (15%) of sporadic colorectal cancers exhibit microsatellite instability and this often results from a nonmutational event (epigenetic inactivation of the MLH1 gene) [29].

Chromosomal translocations

Two principle forms of chromosomal translocations occur in human cancers:

- Complex translocations: These are the more common type of translocation and probably represent a stochastic event with no predictable pattern of repetition within tumors of the same histopathologic subtype.
- Simple translocations: These seem to be non-stochastic events and are characterized by distinctive patterns of breakpoints and chromosomal rearrangements in specific cancers. These simple types of translocation are most likely not due to any underlying genetic instability but instead may reflect low-frequency aberrations in normal physiologic recombination events. Translocations provide the opportunity for an oncogene to come under the influence of a strong promoter, either from repositioning next to regenerating sequences or fusion of two disparate coding regions.

Gene amplification

Gene amplification occurs toward the later stages of the neoplastic continuum and is a further manifestation of genetic instability. Gene amplification results in exaggerated expression of otherwise normal genes, although the term oncogene encompasses overexpression of a normal gene and an intrinsic gene abnormality that leads to enhanced functional activity of the gene. Defects in the apoptotic pathway may permit cells with amplified chromosomal segments to survive (eg, p53 abnormalities).

Cell cycle checkpoints and cancer

The progression of cells through the normal cell cycle is closely regulated as part of the complex process of cell division. The aforementioned checkpoints exert a restraining influence on cell cycle progression and help ensure fidelity of DNA replication and that DNA repair processes are not compromised by time limitation. These control mechanisms minimize propagation of heritable mutations and reduce the risk for cancer development. Genes encoding proteins that promote cell cycling are frequently subject to activation in human cancers through gain-of-function mutation or gene amplification.

Oncogenes

It is now acknowledged that human cancer is a multifactorial process with several key steps being prerequisite for development of cancer. The original term "oncogene" implied that cancer might be caused by change in a single gene, but this is an oversimplified and outdated concept. A revolution in understanding carcinogenesis at the molecular level originated from work on RNA tumor viruses, which can rapidly induce tumors after inoculation into animal cells [32,33]. These viruses contain reverse transcriptase and can synthesize DNA with a complementary base pair sequence to viral RNA. This DNA can then be incorporated into host DNA and cause malignant transformation. Both normal and malignant cells contain DNA sequences that are homologous or identical to the oncogenic segments of these so-called "retroviruses." These are termed cellular proto-oncogenes and correspond to viral (v-onc) oncogenes. These have probably arisen during evolution from incorporation of the cellular counterparts into viral structures. There is a remarkable level of conservation of these ancestral oncogenes.

The cellular homolog of viral oncogenes, the proto-oncogenes, are clearly not functioning in a tumorigenic capacity in most cells within animal tissues. These genetic sequences have oncogenic potential and this is expressed when the sequence is part of the viral genome—v-onc as opposed to c-onc. It may be surmised that cellular proto-oncogenes become activated either by overexpression of the normal gene product (quantitative change) or by alteration of the proto-oncogene to yield an abnormal product with oncogenic activity (qualitative change).

Not all cellular oncogenes have a viral homolog and other methods have been used to identify these other oncogenes. These include gene transfer, insertional mutagenesis, and analysis of chromosomal translocation and sites of amplification. In the former process, viruses activate cellular oncogenes (for which there is no viral counterpart, v-onc) by insertion of viral replicative sequences adjacent to the cellular DNA. These function as a promoter or enhancer and promote malignant transformation [34]. Most oncogenes code for protein products that form components of mitogenic growth signaling pathways. Stimulation of these pathways leads to increased rates of proliferation and promotes tumor formation. One of the earliest oncogene products to be characterized was from the src gene [35]. The protein product of the cellular homolog (c-src) is located mainly on the cytoplasmic side of the plasma membrane and is capable of autophosphorylation and phosphorylation of other proteins [36]. Phosphorylation occurs on tyrosine residues and these so-called "tyrosine protein kinases" can be divided into two main classes: those forms that are membrane associated but without any obvious transmembrane or extracellular domains, and those with a prominent extracellular domain that constitute a potential site for ligand binding. These are members of the growth factor receptor family and play an important role in mediation of external growth stimulatory signals (eg, erbB1, erbB2, PDGFR, IGFR1). These two types of tyrosine kinases constitute distinct ways in which mutant forms of the protein can function as an oncogene. A third category of oncogene is represented by nuclear proteins that are more proximate effectors in cell cycle control.

Receptor protein tyrosine kinases as oncogenes

Amplification of the genes controlling receptor protein tyrosine kinase is common in human cancers, resulting in overexpression and enhanced responsiveness to positive growth factor signals. This overexpression of receptors tends to promote ligand-independent dimerization with constitutive activation of the receptor, which can lead to stimulation of downstream mitogenic pathways in the absence of any external stimulus [37]. Epidermal growth factor receptor (EGFR) and HER2/neu are otherwise known as erbB1 and erbB2, respectively, and belong to a family of receptor protein tyrosine kinases (erbB 1–4), so-called because of their homology to the erythroblastoma viral gene product v-erbB [38]. Genes for both of these growth factor receptors are frequently amplified in breast, pancreas, and lung cancers. Furthermore, EGFR/erbB1 is overexpressed in up to 80% of head and neck cancers with levels of expression correlating inversely with survival [39]. Ligand binding to receptor protein tyrosine kinase usually leads to downstream activation of Ras and the mitogen-activated protein kinase cascades. The binding of EGF and similar ligands (TGFα) to the EGFR is a classic example of this [40]. Interestingly, HER2/neu (erbB2) has no natural ligand and functions as an amplifier by forming heterodimers with other members of the erbB family. Overexpression results in formation of homodimers of erbB2, which have constitutively active tyrosine kinase activity. In contrast to EGFR, this activated HER2/neu has a much broader range of potential downstream substrates that can transduce mitogenic, growth stimulatory signals [41]. Mutations in the c-ret and c-met receptor protein tyrosine kinase oncogenes are found in some familial cancer syndromes, such as multiple endocrine neoplasia (MEN) 2A and 2B and familial forms of medullary thyroid cancer (c-ret) [42].

Cytoplasmic protein tyrosine kinases as oncogenes

The cytoplasmic portion of receptor protein tyrosine kinases converge on a common second messenger system called ras proteins. The primary role of these proteins is to act as shuttling molecules that couple receptor activation to downstream effector pathways involved in regulation of cellular proliferation, differentiation, and survival. Ras proteins are small GTPases that oscillate between inactive guanosine diphosphate (GDP)–bound and active guanosine triphosphate (GTP)–bound forms. This activated form of GTP-bound ras can interact with multiple downstream effectors to influence a spectrum of cellular processes varying from DNA synthesis to cell morphology and adhesion. The system is switched off by GTPase-activating proteins (GAPs) that hydrolyze GTP-bound ras to its GDP-bound form. Activating mutations of ras are found in approximately 30% of human cancers and permit cells to partially bypass receptor protein tyrosine kinase–signaling pathways [43]. Oncogenic sequences usually result from a missense point mutation and the ras protein is maintained in the activated GTP-bound state. A single amino acid substitution can render the GTP-bound form resistant to hydrolysis by GAPs. Generation of a continuous mitogenic signal provides a powerful driver for tumorigenesis. K-ras mutations are common in solid tumors: pancreatic (>90%), colorectal, endometrial, biliary tract, lung, and cervical. They occur together with H-ras mutations in about one third of leukemias and other myeloid malignancies, whereas H-ras mutations alone are found in bladder tumors. Downstream targets include Raf, which is a serine/threonine kinase that coordinates with ras to phosphorylate the kinase MEK, which in turn phosphorylates MAP kinase [44].

Nuclear proteins as oncogenes

Oncogene products residing within the nucleus itself might be expected to have a more direct influence on gene expression through binding to segments of DNA that contain gene regulatory elements. The myc oncogene is well characterized as a nuclear oncogene with growth stimulatory properties. Distinct forms of the gene exist in neuroblastoma/retinoblastoma (N-myc) and small cell lung carcinomas (L-myc) and all three forms of the gene have been implicated in human malignancy [45]. The myc gene is universally expressed in cells and participates in a highly conserved pathway that is shared by most cells. Levels of the myc product are generally increased in actively dividing cells and the myc gene encodes transcriptional factors controlling proliferation, differentiation, and apoptosis. Abnormal expression within tumor cells may result from breakdown of a negative feedback loop whereby the myc product fails to appropriately regulate activity of the gene. Oncogenic forms of myc may result from various changes, including point mutation, amplification, and translocation.

Tumor suppressor genes

Although ultimately oncogenic growth stimulatory activities may become dominant within malignant cells, defects in tumor suppressor genes may lead to excessive proliferation and neoplastic progression by default. These genes are thus sometimes referred to as anti-oncogenes; this term implies that mutations within these genes can be the primary driving force for malignant transformation, rather representing a suppressor response to an established tumorigenic phenotype.

Tumor suppressor gene products are integral components of cell cycle regulatory pathways and have both gatekeeper and caretaker functions. Some tumor suppressor genes possess functional duality and inactivation leads to major disruption of cell cycle regulation. It is thus absence of a normal gene function rather than the presence of an abnormal gene per se that characterizes tumor suppressor gene disorders. A significant advance in understanding the concept of tumor suppressor genes came from studies into the genetic basis of retinoblastomas [46]. Familial cases who had bilateral tumors were noted to have loss of part of chromosome 13 (13q14). Sporadic cases who had unilateral tumors also showed a similar chromosomal loss and Knudson [5,6,47] proposed his famous two-hit hypothesis; in familial cases of the disease, one hit is inherited as a germline mutation, whereas the second hit is acquired early in life (perhaps in utero). It is now known that these two hits each correspond to allelic loss of a tumor suppressor gene—the retinoblastoma gene Rb-1. This gene was mapped to the chromosomal region 13q14 and its normal product is present in all cells except those of retinoblastoma tissue. Tumor formation is thus related to absence of the retinoblastoma gene product.

The breast cancer susceptibility genes BRCA-1 and BRCA-2 are tumor suppressor genes that display an autosomal dominant pattern of inheritance with variable penetrance. Mutations within these two genes account for approximately three quarters of hereditary breast cancer cases and confer a lifetime risk of between 80% and 85% by age 70 years [48] (ie, a 10-fold increase). At the cellular level, the effects of BRCA-1 and BRCA-2 are recessive and both copies of an allele must be lost or mutated for cancer progression. Individuals who have a germline mutation in these genes have a dominantly inherited susceptibility and the second hit occurs in the somatic copy. Tumors from genetically predisposed patients show loss of heterozygosity in the wild-type BRCA-1 allele [49] but interestingly mutations of BRCA-1 and BRCA-2 are uncommon in sporadic breast cancers. The latter do not seem to result from acquired somatic mutations in both alleles and in this respect breast cancer genes differ from p53 and RB, which behave as classic tumor suppressor genes (mutations in both inherited and sporadic forms of cancer).

Transcriptional factors as tumor suppressor genes

The Rb gene product is a universally expressed nuclear protein that has a fundamental role in controlling progression of cells through the G1 checkpoint at the transition from G1 to S-phase entry [50]. Levels of the Rb protein are critical determinants of overall functional status and when the amount of protein decreases below a threshold value, suppressor activity is lost and the cell acquires an oncogenic phenotype. Transfection of the Rb gene into tumor cells lacking Rb expression reasserts normal features and cell behavior.

Like the Rb protein, the p53 gene product is present in a wide variety of normal cells and levels of expression are increased in up to half of all cancers. Moreover, the protein product seems to be more stable with a longer half-life in transformed cells. The p53 protein is often referred to as the guardian of the genome and has an important cell cycle checkpoint function that helps protect cells from genotoxic damage. It causes cells to arrest in the G1 phase of the cell cycle and can act as a homotetrameric transcriptional factor that is activated in response to cellular insults, such as irradiation, hypoxia, and drug-induced DNA damage. Although levels of p53 are increased in some tumors, the protein product is abnormal and p53 mutations are usually inactivating and associated with loss of gene function. Moreover, the p53 gene can act in a dominant negative manner whereby the presence of any abnormal protein product can impair function of normally expressed protein. Defective p53 introduced into the germline of transgenic mice leads to augmented tumorigenesis in the offspring of these p53-deficient mice [51]. p53 therefore functions as a tumor suppressor gene at the transcriptional level rather like the Rb gene. Indeed, the two proteins form part of a signaling network that regulates progression through the cell cycle and exerts a restraint on inappropriate growth-promoting signals. Mutations of the p53 gene occur in the Li-Fraumeni syndrome, which is associated with breast cancer, sarcomas, and adrenocortical tumors [52]. Two further key components of this network include p16 ink4a and p14ARF. The former binds and inhibits the cyclin D–dependent kinases CDK4 and CDK6 and thereby induces Rb-dependent G1 arrest [53,54]. Mutations of this gene are commonly found in familial and sporadic forms of melanoma, pancreatic, lung, and bladder cancers. p14ARF is also a potent tumor suppressor capable of activating p53 by binding directly to the p53 inhibitor MDM2. Mutations within this gene frequently occur in T-cell leukemias.

Cytoplasmic tumor suppressor genes

The development of colorectal cancers may be attributable to absence of a normal gene product. One form of colorectal cancer is associated with the hereditary condition familial adenomatous polyposis coli (FAP), which results in formation of hundreds of polyps within the colon and rectum. A proportion of these will become dysplastic and thereafter progress to carcinoma [7]. An abnormality on chromosome 5 was originally identified in one of these patients and the defective segment localized to 5q21. Furthermore, mutations at this site (the APC gene) can be found in more than three quarters of cases of sporadic colorectal cancer. By analogy with retinoblastoma, a two-hit mechanism may apply; individuals who have FAP inherit a germline mutation of APC and require one further hit for development of cancer (heterozygosity predisposes to polyp formation alone). Sporadic forms of colorectal cancer require two somatic hits for tumor formation. Loss of function of tumor suppressor genes thus seems to be an important mechanism for carcinogenesis. The APC gene and protein product has been characterized and the latter interacts with β-catenin, which is a component of the Wnt/Wingless signaling pathway [55]. Wild-type APC protein associates with β-catenin and targets it for proteasomal degradation. When APC is mutated, however, it is no longer able to negatively regulate β-catenin. Accumulated β-catenin translocates to the nucleus where it promotes cell cycle progression by interaction with transcriptional factors LEP/TCP (lymphoid enhancer factor/T-cell factor). Mutations in β-catenin have been identified in colorectal cancer and could be linked to abnormalities on chromosomes 17 and 18, which are frequently found in familial (nonpolyposis) and sporadic forms of the disease. Chromosome 17 mutations might lead directly to p53 dysfunction and impact on the (Rb/p53/p16/p14) signaling network [53].

Receptor tumor suppressor genes

TGFβ represents a family of multifunctional regulatory peptides involved in a range of processes, including development, wound healing, and carcinogenesis. The peptides are a component of the complex language of intercellular communication and potentially act as a switch that permits a biphasic functional profile. TGFβ is a preeminent inhibitory growth factor and in the premalignant and early stages of cancer this tumor suppressor activity is sustained. As cells pass along the neoplastic continuum, however, functional disruption occurs and malignant epithelial cells show a reduced or absent response to the growth inhibitory effects of TGFβ. Despite a dominance of growth inhibition in the early stages of carcinogenesis, during growth of a tumor there is a shift in the balance between tumor suppressor and potential pro-oncogenic activity. In the more advanced stages of malignant disease, TGFβ might promote tumor growth indirectly through the collective effects of stromal formation, angiogenesis, and immune suppression [56]. The tumor suppressor activity of TGFβ has generated much interest in the potential role of this growth factor in the process of carcinogenesis and the mediation of response to some therapies. The exact function of TGFβ depends on tumor stage and cellular context with relative amounts of ligand and receptor being a crucial determinant of response. TGFβ receptors jointly coordinate a cellular response and mutations in the type II receptor gene lead to loss of a growth inhibitory response in colon cancer cell lines, which can be restored by transfection of the type II receptor subunit. The type II receptor is mutated in HNPCC through a mismatch repair error. Mutations within the TGFβ1 gene have been found in familial breast cancer and represent one of several low-risk genes (relative risk <1.5) that together with BRCA-1 and BRCA-2 (and other higher-risk genes, such as PTEN and p53) contribute to approximately 25% of familial predisposition.

Mutations in genes regulating apoptosis and cell death pathways

Programmed cell death or apoptosis is an essential feature of normal development and is an ongoing process throughout the life of a complex multicellular organism. For example, selective removal of cells during the phase of tissue remodeling in organogenesis is achieved by coordinated activation of cell death programs. This process leads to generation of digits and body cavities, for example. Apoptosis is also activated when cells are subjected to an insult, such as DNA damage [57]. Cancer cells possess the ability to evade mechanisms of programmed cell death. Overexpression of the anti-apoptotic protein bcl-2 has been found in 85% of more aggressive lymphomas [58]. The bcl-2 gene is up-regulated by a chromosomal translocation (14:18) and elevated levels of bcl-2 protein bind to various proapoptotic factors (bad, bax, bid). Bcl-2 is a potent cell survival factor and prevents cytochrome c release, which in turn inhibits cell death. Inactivating mutations of p53 lead to impaired apoptotic pathways, with downstream effectors interacting with proapoptotic members of the bcl-2 family. Functioning p53 protein increases transcription of the bax gene, which promotes release of cytochrome c from mitochondria and promotes apoptosis.

Epigenetics

Most cancers display epigenetic changes that are reversible and heritable changes in gene expression without DNA sequence alterations. They act as translators between the environment and the genome and represent an interface between genotype and phenotype. Cancer cells have an imbalance of DNA methylation; although there is widespread loss of genomic DNA methylation with neoplastic progression, there is aberrant hypermethylation of cytosine residues in CpG islands in the promoter region of genes [59]. These CpG islands are highly conserved segments of DNA with a GC content in excess of 50%. They are found in the promoter regions of almost half of mammalian genes. These CpG islands are normally protected from methylation, but aberrant methylation is widespread in human cancers and leads to selective gene silencing. Each tumor has its own pathways of methylation and hypermethylation profile. Epigenetic silencing tends to promote genetic instability with 5-methylcytosine being highly mutagenic and predisposing to C:G → A:T transitions. For example, in sporadic colon cancers there is evidence of hypermethylation and silencing of the DNA mismatch repair gene MLH1 leading to microsatellite instability [60]. Epigenetic silencing represents an important mechanism for inactivation of tumor suppressor genes. The BRCA-1 and APC genes can be inactivated by hypermethylation and in the case of the former this can act as a second hit in hereditary forms of breast cancer [61]. In sporadic cancers, there can be hypermethylation of one allele and genomic loss of the other allele. Various novel genes that can be epigenetically silenced are likely to be discovered in the future. Furthermore, it may be possible to restore normal gene expression by pharmacologic manipulation of epigenetic changes without the need for genetic engineering.

Summary

There have been great advances in our understanding of the molecular basis of carcinogenesis over the past 2 decades. Increasing understanding of the pathobiology and genetics of cancer has led to advances in treatment and risk prediction. Cancers are caricatures of normal tissues; their component cells are not foreign and genetically disparate like endogenous pathogens, but rogue cells with a finite number of genetic changes [62]. Newer forms of biologic therapies focus on blocking, bypassing, or re-regulating aberrant pathways and aim to control rather than kill cancer cells with improvement of disease-free survival and quality of life [63]. Targeting of specific growth factor pathways that drive tumor growth has become a clinical reality and this approach is consonant with the paradigm of control rather than cure.

The cellular heterogeneity of individual tumors presents a continued therapeutic challenge. There is increasing recognition that phenotypic heterogeneity for some cancers may reflect an accumulation of mutations in a large number of less highly penetrant genes rather than being attributable to simple changes in one or two dominant genes. The sophisticated methods of genetic profiling with DNA microarrays and their integration with proteomics may ultimately allow individual tailoring of treatments and more accurate risk estimation for patients who have a hereditary predisposition. If tumors arise from transformation of stem cells (or a closely related progenitor) into malignant stem cells, then the latter must be targeted therapeutically; these cells are either quiescent or cycle relatively slowly and are resistant to conventional chemotherapy. The ability of stem cells to self-renew provides the opportunity for regeneration and clinical recurrence of cancer. Cancer stem cells retain programs for invasion and metastases together with protective mechanisms that favor survival despite exposure to potentially noxious therapies. Future research will focus on identification of biochemical pathways that are unique to cancer stem cells and thereby permit selective targeting of this important subpopulation of tumor cells.

References

[1] Frank LM, Teich NM. Introduction to the cellular and molecular biology of cancer. New York: Oxford University Press; 1995.
[2] Benson JR, Baum M, Colletta AA. Role of TGF beta in the anti-estrogen response/resistance of human breast cancer. J Mammary Gland Biol Neoplasia 1996;1(4):381–9.
[3] Bishop JM, Weinberg RA. Molecular oncology. New York: Scientific American Inc.,; 1996.
[4] Bodmer WF. Inherited susceptibility to cancer. In: Frank LM, Teich NM, editors. Introduction to the cellular and molecular biology of cancer. 2nd edition. New York: Oxford University Press; 1995. p. 98–124.
[5] Knudson AG Jr. Genetics of human cancer. Annu Rev Genet 1986;20:231–51.
[6] Knudson AG Jr. Hereditary cancer, oncogenes, and antioncogenes. Cancer Res 1985;45(4): 1437–43.
[7] Fearon ER, Vogelstein B. A genetic model for colorectal tumorigenesis. Cell 1990;61(5): 759–67.
[8] Hanahan D, Weinberg RA. The hallmarks of cancer. Cell 2000;100(1):57–70.
[9] Stewart SA, Weinberg RA. Telomeres: cancer to human aging. Annu Rev Cell Dev Biol 2006;22:531–57.
[10] Jordan CT, Guzman ML, Noble M. Cancer stem cells. N Engl J Med 2006;355(12):1253–61.
[11] Greaves M. Cancer causation: the Darwinian downside of past success? Lancet Oncol 2002; 3(4):244–51.
[12] Dalerba P, Cho RW, Clarke MF. Cancer stem cells: models and concepts. Annu Rev Med 2007;58:267–84.
[13] Reya T, Morrison SJ, Clarke MF, et al. Stem cells, cancer, and cancer stem cells. Nature 2001;414(6859):105–11.
[14] Rowley JD. Letter: a new consistent chromosomal abnormality in chronic myelogenous leukaemia identified by quinacrine fluorescence and Giemsa staining. Nature 1973;243(5405): 290–3.
[15] Brodeur GM. Molecular pathology of human neuroblastomas. Semin Diagn Pathol 1994; 11(2):118–25.
[16] Catteau A, Morris JR. BRCA1 methylation: a significant role in tumour development? Semin Cancer Biol 2002;12(5):359–71.
[17] Kinzler KW, Vogelstein B. Cancer-susceptibility genes. Gatekeepers and caretakers. Nature 1997;386(6627):761–3.
[18] Sharan SK, Morimatsu M, Albrecht U, et al. Embryonic lethality and radiation hypersensitivity mediated by Rad51 in mice lacking Brca2. Nature 1997;386(6627):804–10.

[19] Weaver BA, Cleveland DW. Aneuploidy: instigator and inhibitor of tumorigenesis. Cancer Res 2007;67(21):10103–5.
[20] Kastan MB, Bartek J. Cell-cycle checkpoints and cancer. Nature 2004;432(7015):316–23.
[21] Kops GJ, Weaver BA, Cleveland DW. On the road to cancer: aneuploidy and the mitotic checkpoint. Nat Rev Cancer 2005;5(10):773–85.
[22] Lobrich M, Jeggo PA. The impact of a negligent G2/M checkpoint on genomic instability and cancer induction. Nat Rev Cancer 2007;7(11):861–9.
[23] Mountzios G, Terpos E, Dimopoulos MA. Aurora kinases as targets for cancer therapy. Cancer Treat Rev 2008;34:175–82.
[24] Hahn WC. Role of telomeres and telomerase in the pathogenesis of human cancer. J Clin Oncol 2003;21(10):2034–43.
[25] Artandi SE, Attardi LD. Pathways connecting telomeres and p53 in senescence, apoptosis, and cancer. Biochem Biophys Res Commun 2005;331(3):881–90.
[26] Saldivar JS, Wu X, Follen M, et al. Nucleotide excision repair pathway review I: implications in ovarian cancer and platinum sensitivity. Gynecol Oncol 2007;107(1 Suppl 1):S56–71.
[27] Leibeling D, Laspe P, Emmert S. Nucleotide excision repair and cancer. J Mol Histol 2006;37(5–7):225–38.
[28] Soreide K, Janssen EA, Soiland H, et al. Microsatellite instability in colorectal cancer. Br J Surg 2006;93(4):395–406.
[29] Vasen HF. Review article: the Lynch syndrome (hereditary nonpolyposis colorectal cancer). Aliment Pharmacol Ther 2007;26(Suppl 2):113–26.
[30] Li GM. Mechanisms and functions of DNA mismatch repair. Cell Res 2008;18(1):85–98.
[31] Fishel R, Lescoe MK, Rao MR, et al. The human mutator gene homolog MSH2 and its association with hereditary nonpolyposis colon cancer. Cell 1993;75(5):1027–38.
[32] Butel JS. Viral carcinogenesis: revelation of molecular mechanisms and etiology of human disease. Carcinogenesis 2000;21(3):405–26.
[33] Rous P. Viruses and tumour causation. An appraisal of present knowledge. Nature 1965;207(996):457–63.
[34] Toren A, Ben-Bassat I, Rechavi G. Infectious agents and environmental factors in lymphoid malignancies. Blood Rev 1996;10(2):89–94.
[35] De Larco JE, Todaro GJ. Growth factors from murine sarcoma virus-transformed cells. Proc Natl Acad Sci U S A 1978;75(8):4001–5.
[36] Turner CE, Burridge K. Transmembrane molecular assemblies in cell-extracellular matrix interactions. Curr Opin Cell Biol 1991;3(5):849–53.
[37] Zwick E, Bange J, Ullrich A. Receptor tyrosine kinase signalling as a target for cancer intervention strategies. Endocr Relat Cancer 2001;8(3):161–73.
[38] Perona R. Cell signalling: growth factors and tyrosine kinase receptors. Clin Transl Oncol 2006;8(2):77–82.
[39] Cruz JJ, Ocana A, Del Barco E, et al. Targeting receptor tyrosine kinases and their signal transduction routes in head and neck cancer. Ann Oncol 2007;18(3):421–30.
[40] Lo HW, Hsu SC, Hung MC. EGFR signaling pathway in breast cancers: from traditional signal transduction to direct nuclear translocation. Breast Cancer Res Treat 2006;95(3):211–8.
[41] Baselga J, Albanell J. Mechanism of action of anti-HER2 monoclonal antibodies. Ann Oncol 2001;12(Suppl 1):S35–41.
[42] Marx SJ. Molecular genetics of multiple endocrine neoplasia types 1 and 2. Nat Rev Cancer 2005;5(5):367–75.
[43] Malumbres M, Barbacid M. RAS oncogenes: the first 30 years. Nat Rev Cancer 2003;3(6):459–65.
[44] Mirza AM, Gysin S, Malek N, et al. Cooperative regulation of the cell division cycle by the protein kinases RAF and AKT. Mol Cell Biol 2004;24(24):10868–81.
[45] Nesbit CE, Tersak JM, Prochownik EV. MYC oncogenes and human neoplastic disease. Oncogene 1999;18(19):3004–16.

[46] Vogel F. Genetics of retinoblastoma. Hum Genet 1979;52(1):1–54.
[47] Knudson AG. Cancer genetics. Am J Med Genet 2002;111(1):96–102.
[48] Ford D, Easton DF. The genetics of breast and ovarian cancer. Br J Cancer 1995;72(4): 805–12.
[49] Merajver SD, Pham TM, Caduff RF, et al. Somatic mutations in the BRCA1 gene in sporadic ovarian tumours. Nat Genet 1995;9(4):439–43.
[50] Harbour JW, Dean DC. Rb function in cell-cycle regulation and apoptosis. Nat Cell Biol 2000;2(4):E65–7.
[51] Blackburn AC, Jerry DJ. Knockout and transgenic mice of Trp53: what have we learned about p53 in breast cancer? Breast Cancer Res 2002;4(3):101–11.
[52] Malkin D, Li FP, Strong LC, et al. Germ line p53 mutations in a familial syndrome of breast cancer, sarcomas, and other neoplasms. Science 1990;250(4985):1233–8.
[53] Sherr CJ, McCormick F. The RB and p53 pathways in cancer. Cancer Cell 2002;2(2):103–12.
[54] Sherr CJ. The INK4a/ARF network in tumour suppression. Nat Rev Mol Cell Biol 2001; 2(10):731–7.
[55] Clevers H. Wnt breakers in colon cancer. Cancer Cell 2004;5(1):5–6.
[56] Benson JR. Role of transforming growth factor beta in breast carcinogenesis. Lancet Oncol 2004;5(4):229–39.
[57] Viktorsson K, Lewensohn R, Zhivotovsky B. Apoptotic pathways and therapy resistance in human malignancies. Adv Cancer Res 2005;94:143–96.
[58] Sanchez-Beato M, Sanchez-Aguilera A, Piris MA. Cell cycle deregulation in B-cell lymphomas. Blood 2003;101(4):1220–35.
[59] Miremadi A, Oestergaard MZ, Pharoah PD, et al. Cancer genetics of epigenetic genes. Hum Mol Genet 2007;16 Spec No 1:R28–49.
[60] Esteller M. Epigenetic lesions causing genetic lesions in human cancer: promoter hypermethylation of DNA repair genes. Eur J Cancer 2000;36(18):2294–300.
[61] Esteller M. Epigenetic gene silencing in cancer: the DNA hypermethylome. Hum Mol Genet 2007;16 Spec No 1:R50–9.
[62] Pierce GB, Speers WC. Tumors as caricatures of the process of tissue renewal: prospects for therapy by directing differentiation. Cancer Res 1988;48(8):1996–2004.
[63] Schipper H, Goh CR, Wang TL. Shifting the cancer paradigm: must we kill to cure? J Clin Oncol 1995;13(4):801–7.

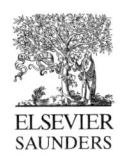

Genetic Testing for Cancer Susceptibility

Kathleen A. Calzone, MSN, RN, APNG, FAAN[a],*,
Peter W. Soballe, MD, FACS[b]

[a]*National Institutes of Health, National Cancer Institute, Center for Cancer Research, Genetics Branch, 8901 Wisconsin Avenue, Building 8, RM 5101, Bethesda, MD 20889-5105, USA*
[b]*Department of Surgery, Uniformed Services University, 4301 Jones Bridge Road, Bethesda, MD 20814-4799, USA*

Over the past 15 years, advances in molecular genetics have resulted in the development of many commercially available genetic tests for cancer susceptibility. The ongoing rapid translation of this technology to the clinical setting provides an extraordinary opportunity to improve health outcomes by enabling providers to identify those individuals at the greatest level of risk who may benefit from aggressive surveillance and risk-reducing interventions. Direct-to-consumer marketing is becoming a challenge for the medical community [1–3]. With increased insurance coverage, some legislative protection against genetic discrimination, and marketing directly to primary-care and oncology providers, genetic tests for cancer susceptibility are moving beyond specialty genetic services and into the health care mainstream. As a consequence, providers need to understand the clinical validity of these tests as well as the critical elements of the genetic assessment, education, counseling, and testing process [2,4,5].

Establishing a differential diagnosis

Performing an assessment and establishing a list of differential diagnoses are the first steps in evaluating an individual with a personal or family history of cancer. Without this core evaluation, the tendency may be to test only for mutations in the most common genes linked to a given cancer. For example, in breast cancer, one would certainly consider *BRCA1* and *BRCA2*, but should also consider less frequent genetic mutations, such as Cowden (*PTEN*) or Li-Fraumeni (*TP53*) syndromes, depending on the

---

* Corresponding author.
E-mail address: calzonek@mail.nih.gov (K.A. Calzone).

constellation of cancers in the individual and family [6]. The personal and family cancer history is the first step in establishing a list of differential diagnoses, which is then used to select candidate gene or genes and determine what type of test, if any, is indicated. Even when evaluating individuals in which a deleterious mutation has already been identified in the family, the family history is essential because more than one gene mutation can be segregating in any given family, especially in those of common ancestral origin, such as Ashkenazi Jewish, where the prevalence of three founder *BRCA* mutations is increased.

The optimal family history is illustrated in the form of a pedigree, uses standard nomenclature (Fig. 1), and includes a minimum of three generations [7,8]. The graphic illustration of the family history facilitates analysis for patterns of disease and permits assessment for the various patterns of transmission. Pedigree information is ascertained on all individuals from both maternal and paternal lineages. Information collected includes race and ethnicity, current health status, current age or age at and cause of death, type of each primary cancer, age at diagnosis for each primary, bilaterality for paired organs, and carcinogen exposure, such as smoking or asbestos. Adoption, consanguinity, and any assisted reproductive technology, such as donor egg or sperm, are also documented. Lastly, information on surgeries that could modify cancer risk, such as prophylactic mastectomy or bilateral salphingo oophorectomy, is recorded.

It may be a challenge for healthcare providers to find sufficient time to collect such a detailed family history so the US Surgeon General launched Web site "My Family Health Portrait" (http://www.hhs.gov/familyhistory) in 2004 to assist providers, individuals, and families in collecting pedigree information on common hereditary diseases, including cancers of the colon, breast, and ovary. Available in both English and Spanish versions, the tool is designed to be completed by lay individuals. The tool produces a report and limited pedigree but not a full three-generation pedigree and not in the detail described above [9]. Even though the pedigree may require expansion, this tool may decrease the time needed to collect a detailed family history.

Interpretation of a family history can be complicated by such factors as missing or unavailable family information, small family size, and inaccurately reported histories [10–12]. Certain malignancies, such as breast cancer, are usually accurately reported [13]. However, rarer cancers and all gynecologic malignancies are often inaccurately identified [14]. Increased geographic or relationship distance from the reporting individual also increases the chance for errors [15]. There are even reports of fabricated family histories [16]. Therefore, when critical decisions are being made based on a family's history alone, some confirmation with pathology reports or death certificates may be necessary.

Once a list of differential diagnoses of genetic syndromes is established, it can be used to determine whether there is a gene for which mutation testing would be of value. If testing is being considered, attempts to estimate the

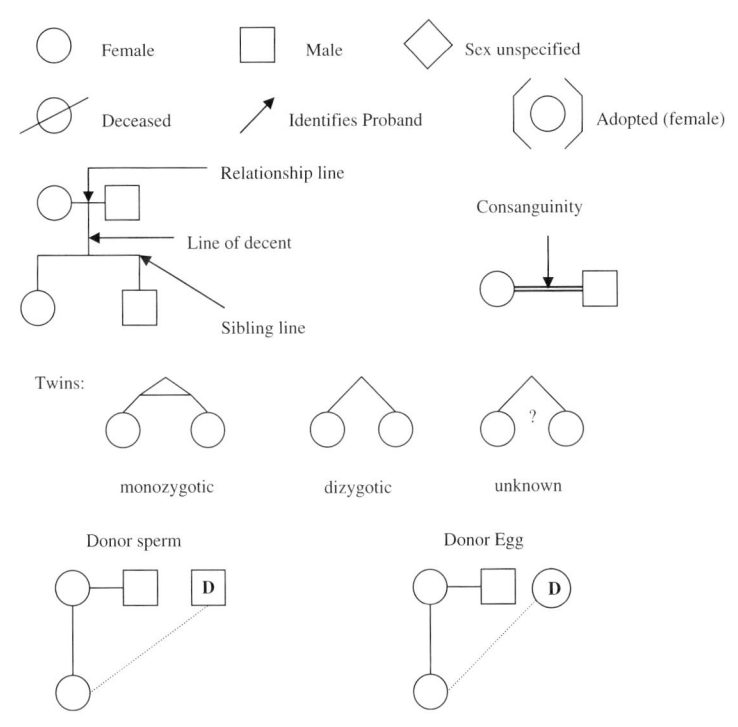

Fig. 1. Standard pedigree nomenclature. (*Data from* Bennett RL, Steinhaus KA, Uhrich SB, et al. Recommendations for standardized human pedigree nomenclature. Pedigree Standardization Task Force of the National Society of Genetic Counselors. Am J Hum Genet 1995; 56(3):745–52.)

individual's or family's likelihood of harboring a specific gene mutation (prior probability) should be undertaken [17]. Different strategies are used to calculate a prior probability, including statistical models, prevalence data from specific populations, penetrance data for specific mutations, Mendelian inheritance, and Bayesian analysis. These strategies all have different levels of performance, ease of use, optimal applications, and limitations [17–19].

Most statistical models are specific to a given gene or genes and not every gene has a model available for use. When calculating prior probabilities using models, the user must first determine whether the model is calculating a family or an individual probability. This is especially important when the individual for whom testing is being considered has not been affected with cancer. Prior probability models are limited by the assumption inherent in the mathematical construct as well as by specific family constructs. Small family sizes, high proportions of individuals of the opposite gender in cancers that are gender specific (eg, prostate, breast, or ovary), adoptions, and early deaths from unrelated causes all influence the reliability of prior probability estimates [12].

The pedigree in Fig. 2 illustrates a family in which a paternal cousin and paternal great aunt are affected with breast or ovarian cancer. Other

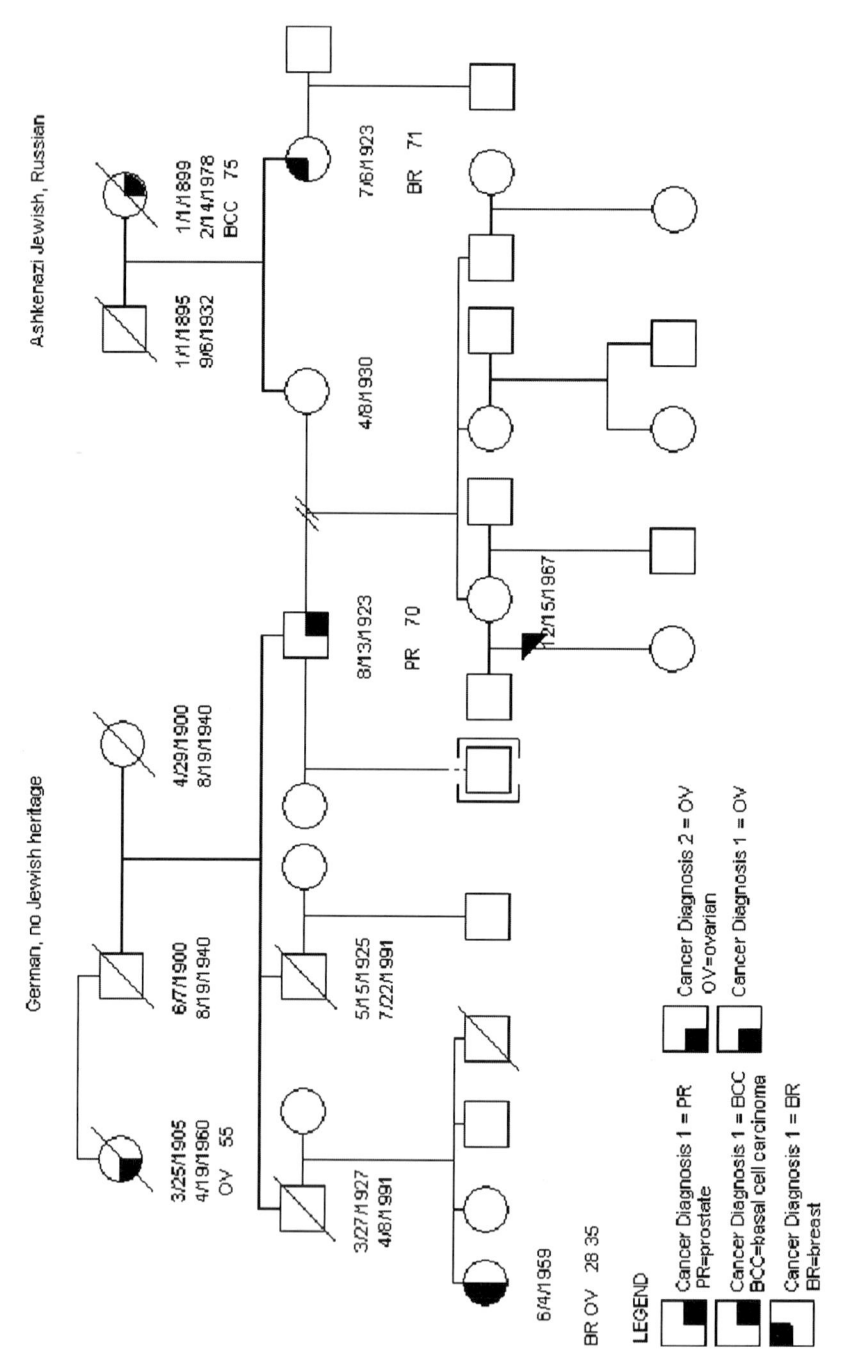

Fig. 2. Case example.

instances of breast or ovarian cancer are obscured due to male dominance in the paternal lineage. A prior probability model, such as BRCAPro [20,21], would underestimate the proband's risk of harboring a *BRCA* mutation because third-degree relatives are not incorporated into the calculations. Subsequently, the paternal cousin was found to have a deleterious *BRCA1* mutation. The proband then tested positive for the same mutation, revealing that her father is an obligate carrier.

In circumstances in which a specific mutation has been identified in a family, prior probabilities can be determined using the appropriate Mendelian pattern of inheritance associated with that gene (eg, autosomal dominant for *BRCA1/2*). However this approach does not account for age of the individual being considered for testing. Living without cancer beyond the expected age that cancer would occur if a person were a mutation carrier decreases the probability that an individual actually harbors the family's known mutation.

Bayes theorem is a mathematical calculation that combines Mendelian inheritance laws with other conditional information, such as age. For example, Bayesian analysis is useful to calculate prior probabilities in older, unaffected individuals being considered for testing. In these instances, Mendelian inheritance alone will overestimate the actual probability of an individual's being a carrier [22,23].

For some specific syndromes, tumor-specific characteristics are emerging as an adjunct to family history as indications for genetic testing. Colon cancer associated with the Lynch syndrome (hereditary nonpolyposis colon cancer [HNPCC]) is characterized by microsatellite instability (MSI) in the tumor. MSI is a finding on polymerase chain reaction of multiple repeats of small snippets of DNA segments, an indication of cells with a DNA-mismatch-repair defect. MSI is frequently complemented by immunohisotchemical staining for the protein products of these DNA-repair genes. The Bethesda guidelines (Box 1), which are used for identifying families or individuals who are candidates for genetic testing for the Lynch syndrome, have been revised to include criteria for MSI testing [24]. When colorectal [25] and endometrial [26] cancers of patients who would not have been candidates for genetic testing based on family history alone are screened for MSI and immunohistochemical evidence of defective DNA-repair proteins at the time of diagnosis, many individuals are identified as candidates for genetic testing. Subsequent genetic testing has confirmed germline mutations in many of these cases.

Breast cancers from individuals with a deleterious mutation in *BRCA1* have a greater likelihood of being estrogen and progesterone receptor negative and HER-2 negative ("triple negative") [27]. Preliminary data from testing women selected based on the diagnosis of triple-negative breast cancer has demonstrated frequent deleterious mutations in *BRCA1* [28].

Decision support tools for health care providers, such as the Genetic Risk Assessment on the Internet with Decision Support, are under development, but careful assessment of family and personal histories and sound clinical

> **Box 1. Revised Bethesda Guidelines (2004) for testing for the Lynch syndrome**
>
> Colorectal cancer diagnosed in a patient less than 50 years of age
>
> Presence of synchronous, metachronous colorectal, or other tumors associated with Lynch syndrome (HNPCC) regardless of age[a]
>
> Colorectal cancer with the MSI-high histology diagnosed in a patient less than 60 years of age (MSI-high refers to peaks in more than one of the recommended microsatellites [BAT25, BAT26, D2S123, D5S346, and D17S250])
>
> Colorectal cancer diagnosed in one or more first-degree relatives with an HNPCC-related tumor and with one of the cancers being diagnosed at less than 50 years of age.
>
> Colorectal cancer diagnosed in two or more first- or second-degree relatives with HNPCC-related tumors, regardless of age
>
> ---
>
> [a] Lynch syndrome–related tumors include cancers of the colon, rectum, endometrium, stomach, ovaries, pancreas, ureter, renal pelvis, biliary tract, small bowel, and brain, usually glioblastomas (Turcot syndrome), sebaceous gland adenomas, or keratoacanthomas (Muir–Torre syndrome).
>
> *Data from* Umar A, Boland CR, Terdiman JP, et al. Revised Bethesda Guidelines for hereditary nonpolyposis colorectal cancer (Lynch syndrome) and microsatellite instability. J Natl Cancer Inst 2004;96(4):261–8.

judgment remain critical to the evaluation of any individual and to the use of these tools to calculate prior probabilities [17,29].

When should genetic testing be considered?

The decision to offer genetic testing extends beyond evidence of a possible inherited susceptibility to cancer to include the interpretation and potential uses of the test results. The American Society of Clinical Oncologists (ASCO) recommends all of the following before considering any genetic testing [4]:

- Evidence from an individual or that person's family of a cancer susceptibility syndrome
- Ability to interpret the results of the contemplated test
- Certainty that testing will facilitate a diagnosis or influence medical management

Pre- and post-test genetic education and counseling are an integral part of this process and include explanation of essential information on the suspected syndrome and gene; exploration of issues of psychosocial vulnerability associated with testing; review of the risks, benefits, and limitations of testing; consideration of possible test outcomes and the implications of each outcome for future medical management; and discussion of the dissemination of results and their implications to other family members.

Determining the optimal person to test

For any family suspected of an inherited predisposition to cancer, the genetic basis for that cancer must first be established. The best way to do that, whenever possible, is to first test a family member who already has a cancer associated with the identified syndrome. Testing an unaffected family member without knowing the specific mutation in a family decreases the information yielded and may make the interpretation of test results misleading when no mutation is detected. Failure to find a mutation could be because the individual has not inherited the family's mutation, but it also could be because there is a mutation that is not detectable by the method used for testing, in which case the individual is still at an increased risk for cancer. Not finding a mutation may also be because some genes associated with an inherited susceptibility to cancer have yet to be identified, so the cancer in the family could be due to a different susceptibility syndrome and therefore a different gene. None of the techniques for genetic testing, in the absence of a specific known mutation, have 100% accuracy; the patient may be a false negative. Also, we are only beginning to understand that gene modifiers can confound genetic testing results. For example, in a small study in the Kathleen Cuningham Foundation Consortium for Research into Familial Breast Cancer (kConFab) familial cancer repository of mutation-negative individuals with breast cancers resembling those found in *BRCA1* carriers, methylation of the *BRCA1* promoter was identified and was associated with the characteristic breast cancer phenotype [30]. In the absence of a known genetic mutation in a family, negative test results in an unaffected relative are considered "uninformative," which means the presence of a cancer susceptibility gene mutation and an increased risk of cancer have not been ruled out.

If there is no available living family member affected with a relevant cancer, an alternative is to consider testing a stored biologic specimen, such as a tissue block from a deceased relative. This kind of analysis may be difficult or even impossible and not all laboratories will perform tests on stored specimens. But, testing for a limited number of mutations, such as the three Ashkenazi Jewish founder mutations, may be more technically feasible.

Once all efforts to find and test an affected individual have been unsuccessful, an unaffected individual can be tested. However, this necessitates careful genetic education and counseling about the limitations of this testing and the uninformative nature of a "negative" test.

Genetic education and counseling

Genetic testing for single-gene disorders, such as a cancer predisposition, is done in the context of genetic education, counseling, and autonomous informed decision-making. Genetic counseling involves assessment of the individual and family, education and communication about the specific genetic condition, and the personal and familial implications of that condition [31]. The assessment extends beyond the medical and family history to an evaluation of the individual's perceived risk, understanding of genetic testing, motivation for testing, and intended use of the information [32]. The primary aim of genetic counseling is to assist people in understanding and adapting to the medical, psychologic, and familial implications of genetic information and genetic disease [33]. Genetic counseling is performed by various providers, including genetic and oncologic physicians, genetic counselors, and nurses. Genetic counseling should facilitate individual informed autonomous decision-making regarding the genetic test. Box 2 provides a summary of the critical elements of pretest genetic counseling.

Box 2. Elements of pretest genetic education and counseling

Provide information on the suspected cancer syndrome, gene or genes, cancer risks and other health risks
Explain the genetics of the syndrome, the risk of harboring a mutation, and the patterns of transmission
Discuss alternatives to genetic testing
Discuss the risks, benefits, and limitations of genetic testing, including psychologic and discriminatory risks
Explain the possible test outcomes, including likelihood of uninformative results and the identification of variants of uncertain significance
Present information about the accuracy of the genetic test
Identify of health care management options based on possible test results
Discuss implications for children and other family members based on pattern of transmission and importance of disseminating risk and genetic information to family members
Provide an estimate of costs associated with testing, counseling, and medical management, and identify options for insurance coverage
Discuss how genetic information and genetic test results will be recorded and stored in the medical record
Discuss specimen storage and reuse if applicable

Data from Geller G, Botkin J, Green M, et al. Genetic testing for susceptibility to adult-onset cancer: the process and content of informed consent. JAMA 1997;277:1467–74; and Offit K, Thom P. Ethical and legal aspects of cancer genetic testing. Semin Oncol 2007;34:435–43.

The underlying principles of genetic counseling are education, autonomous decision-making, and assessment of and attention to psychosocial issues that may have an impact on making adjustments to test outcomes. Facilitating autonomous decision-making is especially important when there is no evidence that any one approach is clearly efficacious. For example, it is often unclear what benefits may be gained by testing for mutations in *TP53*, which is associated with the severe and complex Li-Fraumeni phenotype, for which there are limited screening options and limited risk-reduction measures available [4].

The process of genetic education and counseling may involve multiple visits to address all the pre- and post-test issues, including medical implications. Many services are multidisciplinary and include genetic counselors, nurses, physicians, and behavioral health professionals [34,35]. Delivery of genetic education and counseling can take several forms. Face-to-face encounters have been the traditional method. Recently, other approaches, including supplementation with computer-assisted education or group-education sessions, have been shown to be effective adjuncts to the encounter [36–38]. Such strategies as telephone counseling or telemedicine may be useful to increase access to genetic services, especially for those who reside in remote areas [39–42].

Informed consent

ASCO and genetic experts agree that informed consent is an essential component of genetic testing for cancer susceptibility. While a genetic test is not drastically different from other medical tests, the potential for discrimination, implications for both the individual and the family, and the predictive nature of the information has resulted in a well-defined approach to consenting for these tests [32]. The consent for genetic testing may be written and provided by the commercial laboratory or developed by an individual institution's program, or it may be a verbal assent documented in the medical record following pretesting counseling. Regardless of the method, ASCO has summarized the basic elements of informed consent (Box 3) and these are complementary to the critical elements of pretest genetic counseling in Box 2 [4]. Before disclosure of test results, some programs obtain a second consent, in writing or verbally, confirming that the individual still wants to know the results.

Genetic education, counseling, and testing in children

Some inherited cancer syndromes include the risk for pediatric malignancies. Most experts agree that, unless there are cancer risks for children or evidence supporting changes in medical management that should be implemented while the individual is a child, cancer susceptibility testing should be deferred until at least legal adulthood [4,43]. Putting off testing until the child matures minimizes concerns about autonomous informed decision-making, risks of discrimination, negative impact on family relationships,

> **Box 3. Basic elements of informed consent**
>
> Information on the specific test being performed
> Implications of a positive and negative result
> Possibility that the test will not be informative
> Options for risk estimation without genetic testing
> Risk of passing a mutation to children
> Technical accuracy of the test
> Fees involved in testing and counseling
> Psychologic implications of tests results (benefits and risks)
> Risks of insurance of employer discrimination
> Confidentiality issues
> Options and limitations of medical surveillance and strategies for prevention following testing
> Importance of sharing genetic test results with at-risk relatives so that they may benefit from this information
>
> ---
>
> *Data from* Oncology ASOC. American Society of Clinical Oncology policy statement update: genetic testing for cancer susceptibility. J Clin Oncol 2003;21(12):2397–406.

and psychologic issues [43]. Unfortunately, the time of maturity differs for each child, which means the application of these guidelines must be tailored to the specific family or child [44]. For cancer syndromes that include pediatric cancers, such as familial adenomatous polyposis, neurofibromatosis, and multiple endocrine neoplasia, testing of children is less controversial and is routinely offered because of the established medical benefits. Genetic testing in children is most controversial in the setting of cancer syndromes that confer risks for pediatric cancers, such as with Li-Fraumeni syndrome (*TP53*), where evidence is lacking regarding options for risk management or risk reduction. Decisions in this circumstance are based on minimizing harm while balancing the parents' wishes [44].

Genetic education and counseling for children requires special considerations. First, the parent, parents, or legal guardian are present for the counseling sessions and are responsible for consenting to genetic testing [45]. In cases involving very young children, the counseling session addresses how test results will be shared with the child when the child is older [4]. After about age 10, children may be more involved in the decision to pursue testing and older children often feel they should make their own choice about testing [46].

Selecting the testing laboratory

Currently, regulatory oversight of clinical genetic testing laboratories is limited. As a consequence, the quality assurance for these tests is highly variable. The Clinical Laboratory Improvement Act (CLIA) regulates any clinical laboratory testing that generates diagnostic or other health information by specifying personnel qualifications, quality assurance standards, documentations, and validation of tests and procedures [47]. CLIA mandates that laboratories undergo periodic proficiency testing at defined intervals to verify their capacity to perform and interpret highly complex tests [48,49]. However, because a specialty area for molecular and biologic genetic tests has not been established, there is no mandated proficiency testing for genetic testing [49]. In addition, the majority of genetic tests are developed and assembled within individual laboratories. The Food and Drug Administration (FDA) only regulates test kits manufactured for use by multiple laboratories. As a consequence, most tests are subject to no FDA oversight [48].

In this minimally regulated environment, careful laboratory selection has emerged as an important component of the genetic testing process and forces the health care provider to judge the analytic and clinical validity of the genetic tests they order. There is no mandatory registration for genetic testing laboratories. However, one related resource for health care providers, GeneTests (http://www.geneclinics.org/), includes an international laboratory directory. Online information about each laboratory includes a list of testing services, method or methods used for analysis, senior laboratory staff credentials, and contact information, including Web site links. This resource also provides information about available research studies and up-to-date reviews on many inherited cancer syndromes.

Interpretation of test results

Interpretation of germline testing for gene mutations depends on whether there is a known deleterious mutation in the family. Fig. 3 [50] provides an algorithm outlining test interpretation.

Testing performed in a family in which a deleterious mutation is known is most informative and produces one of two possible results:

1. The laboratory detects the mutation that is known to be in the family. In this instance, individual cancer risks are based on the penetrance associated with specific mutations in that gene. In addition, a targeted discussion and encouragement about disclosure of test results and the option for genetic testing to family members is needed [51].
2. The laboratory does not detect the family mutation. These individuals have not inherited the family's cancer risks. In most instances, their risks are no higher than those of the general population. However, the individual may have other personal cancer risk factors or may have inherited a mutation in another cancer susceptibility gene not tested, perhaps from another branch of the family. Also there has been some recent evidence in *BRCA* families that women testing negative for a familial *BRCA* mutation may still harbor an increased risk above that of the general population [52]. This finding remains controversial because

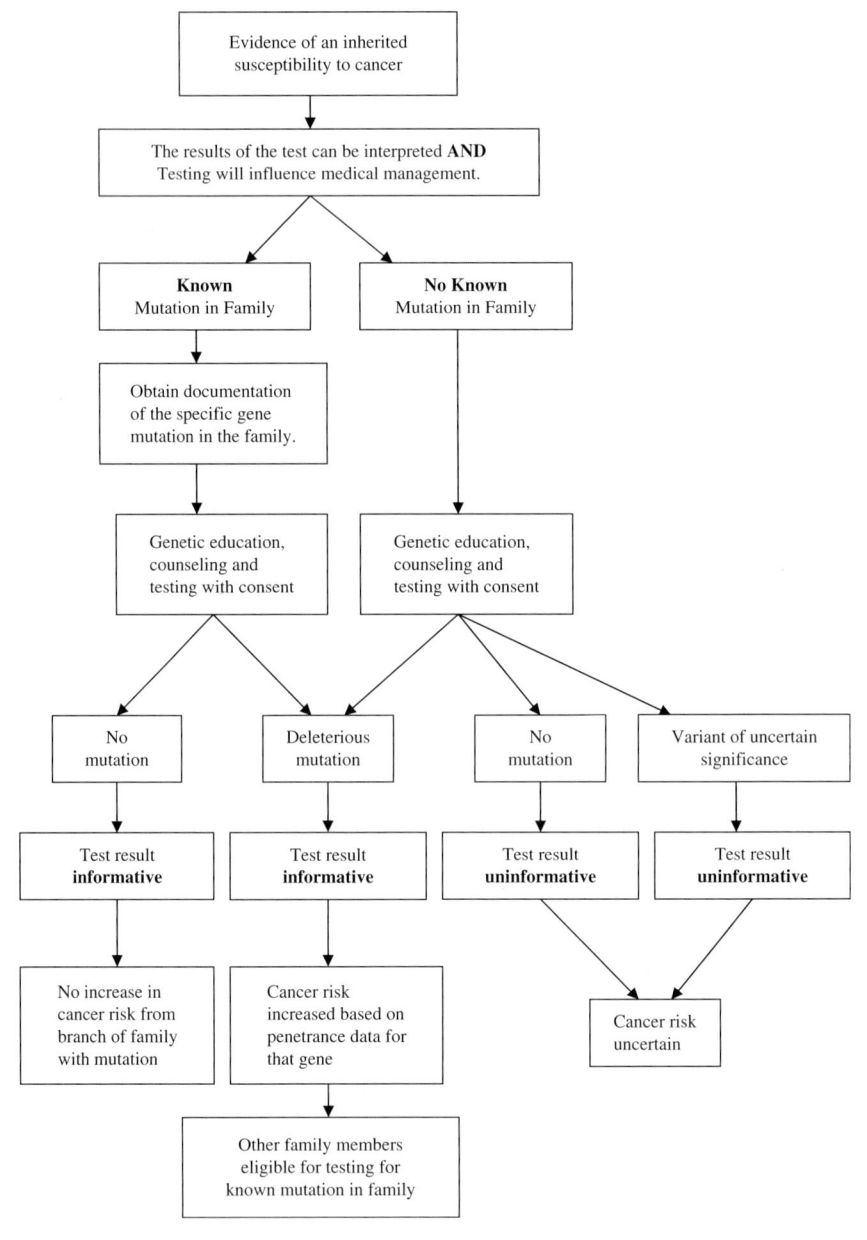

Fig. 3. Genetic testing algorithm for cancer susceptibility. (*Data from* NCI PDQ Cancer Genetics Editorial Board. Elements of cancer genetics risk assessment and counseling 2008. Available at: http://www.cancer.gov/cancertopics/pdq/genetics/risk-assessment-and-counseling/healthprofessional. Accessed March 6, 2008.)

of concerns about ascertainment bias. Analyses in other cohorts, however, suggest a polygenic model modulating breast cancer risk even in mutation-positive families [53]. Further research is needed to clarify risk in women testing negative for a familial *BRCA* mutation.

Interpretation of genetic test results is more complex when no familial mutation has been identified. In this case there are three possible results for each individual:

1. A mutation is identified and there is evidence that the mutation results in an increased risk for cancer. Discovery of a deleterious mutation confers cancer risks based on the penetrance associated with specific mutations in specific genes. In addition, a targeted discussion and encouragement about disclosure of test results and the option for genetic testing to family members is needed [51].
2. No mutation is identified ("uninformative"). Not finding a mutation in the absence of a known mutation in the family is uninformative because a genetic basis for the cancer in the family has not been established and, therefore, a genetic predisposition to cancer in this individual cannot be ruled out. Reasons that the test was negative include (1) the tested individual has not inherited a mutation, (2) the test itself is inadequately sensitive (false negatives), (3) a different gene, not the one tested for, is responsible for the cancer in the family, (4) DNA sequencing is normal even though epigenetic factors have made an impact on a gene's expression, and finally (5) the cancers apparently tracking in this family may be due to shared environmental conditions and not with a germline mutation at all. Individuals affected with the disease that runs in the family mutation may sometimes not be carriers of the familial mutation. This is termed a "phenocopy," an individual with the same phenotype (the disease) but a normal genotype. This is especially common in familial syndromes that include otherwise common cancers. Examples could include a woman diagnosed with breast cancer who tests negative for the known *BRCA* mutation in her family or the individual with MSI-negative colon cancer in a Lynch syndrome family.
3. A variant of uncertain significance (VUS) is identified. Variants are mutations for which the impact on the gene and subsequent health risks are uncertain. Many such variants are missense mutations that result in a single amino acid change in the resulting protein. As our knowledge increases, these variants may be reclassified as either a benign polymorphism or a deleterious mutation, but this may take years. During the interval of uncertainty, health care providers must cope both with how to track these variants and individuals and how to clinically minimize the patient's risks. One strategy employed to clarify the meaning of a VUS is to test for it in other family members to see if it correlates with the incidence of cancer in the pedigree. This approach is often informative if the cancers are clearly arising from only one branch of the family

(maternal or paternal). If analysis reveals that the VUS has been passed down from the opposite branch, the likelihood that it is deleterious is markedly reduced. Unfortunately, if the VUS is being passed down from the cancer side of the family, this is insufficient evidence either for or against its impact on anyone's cancer risk. In addition, a variant's tracking with cancer does not establish whether it is the responsible mutation. It must also be shown to alter the function of the relevant protein enough to have an impact and thereby increase the individual's cancer risk [54].

Future challenges

In addition to direct-to-consumer marketing, the health care community will be increasingly challenged by the availability of genetic tests for cancer susceptibility for lower penetrant genes. These discoveries are often made and translated to commercially available tests so rapidly that they are being marketed before there is sufficient or even any evidence for clinical utility. Recently, three companies (deCODE genetics, 23andMe, and Navigenics) launched direct-to-consumer genetic testing for different genome-wide scans for multiple single nucleotide polymorphisms and other genetic variants for such things as ancestry information and common individual traits, but also common health conditions, including cancer [55–57]. The public interest and uptake in these tests is still uncertain. However, the burden of interpretation and management of any findings from these genetic tests will certainly fall on health care providers.

Summary

Considering the significant amount of healthcare provider time associated with the delivery of cancer genetic testing services, the rapidly changing information about these genes, and the need for careful laboratory selection, many providers refer patients who may be candidates for testing to those who specialize in cancer genetics. A wide range of health professionals are trained in cancer genetics, including physicians, nurses, and genetic counselors. The National Cancer Institute maintains an online directory for health professionals who specialize in cancer genetics and who are willing to accept referrals. The online directory (http://www.cancer.gov/search/geneticsservices/) can be searched by provider name or by city, state, country, cancer type, and cancer syndrome. Listing in this directory is voluntary and is not a reflection of government endorsement. However, to be listed in the directory, each professional must be licensed, certified, or eligible for profession-specific certification and have completed cancer genetics training.

The surgical community is a pivotal and front-line provider of health care services for cancer patients and is uniquely positioned to help narrow the gap between genetic research discoveries and their use to improve the efficacy of cancer care and risk reduction. The translational research continuum requires planning to integrate genetic considerations into clinical practice [58]. Genetic testing for cancer susceptibility challenges the provider by both the complexity and urgency of the assessment, genetic education, counseling, test interpretation, and results disclosure. Simple modifications to practice, such as expanding to a more detailed family history or use of the Surgeon General's Family History Tool can facilitate the identification of individuals who are optimum candidates for multidisciplinary genetic evaluation and counseling.

References

[1] Gray S, Olopade OI. Direct-to-consumer marketing of genetic tests for cancer: Buyer beware. J Clin Oncol 2003;21(17):3191–3.
[2] Hudson K, Javitt G, Burke W, et al, American Society of Human Genetics Social Issues Committee. ASHG Statement on direct-to-consumer genetic testing in the United States. Obstet Gynecol 2007;110(6):1392–5.
[3] Wolfberg A. Genes on the Web—Direct-to-Consumer Marketing of Genetic Testing. N Engl J Med 2007;355(6):543–5.
[4] American Society of Clinical Oncology. American Society of Clinical Oncology Policy Statement Update: genetic testing for cancer susceptibility. J Clin Oncol 2003;21(12):2397–406.
[5] Freedman AN, Wideroff L, Olson L, et al. US physicians' attitudes toward genetic testing for cancer susceptibility. Am J Med Genet 2003;120(1):63–71.
[6] Robson M. Seizing the opportunity: recognition and management of hereditary cancer predisposition. Semin Oncol 2007;34(5):367–8.
[7] Bennett RL, Steinhaus KA, Uhrich SB, et al. Recommendations for standardized human pedigree nomenclature. Pedigree Standardization Task Force of the National Society of Genetic Counselors. Am J Hum Genet 1995;56(3):745–52.
[8] Wattendorf D, Hadley D. Family history: the three-generation pedigree. Am Fam Physician 2005;72(3):441–8.
[9] Yoon PW, Scheuner MT, Gwinn M, et al. Awareness of family health history as a risk factor for disease—United States, 2004. MMWR Morb Mortal Wkly Rep 2004;53(44):1044–7.
[10] Mitchell RJ, Brewster D, Campbell H, et al. Accuracy of reporting of family history of colorectal cancer. Gut 2004;53(2):291–5.
[11] Chang ET, Smedby KE, Hjalgrim H, et al. Reliability of self-reported family history of cancer in a large case-control study of lymphoma. J Natl Cancer Inst 2006;98(1):61–8.
[12] Weitzel JN, Lagos VI, Cullinane CA, et al. Limited family structure and BRCA gene mutation status in single cases of breast cancer. JAMA 2007;297(23):2587–95.
[13] Schneider KA, DiGianni LM, Patenaude AF, et al. Accuracy of cancer family histories: comparison of two breast cancer syndromes. Genet Test 2004;8(3):222–8.
[14] Murff HJ, Spigel DR, Syngal S. Does this patient have a family history of cancer? An evidence-based analysis of the accuracy of family cancer history. JAMA 2004;292(12):1480–9.
[15] Ziogas A, Anton-Culver H. Validation of family history data in cancer family registries. Am J Prev Med 2003;24(2):190–8.
[16] Evans DG, Kerr B, Cade D, et al. Fictitious breast cancer family history. Lancet 1996; 348(9033):1034.
[17] Lindor NM, Lindor RA, Apicella C, et al. Predicting BRCA1 and BRCA2 gene mutation carriers: comparison of LAMBDA, BRCAPRO, Myriad II, and modified Couch models. Fam Cancer 2007;6(4):473–82.
[18] Domchek SM, Eisen A, Calzone K, et al. Application of breast cancer risk prediction models in clinical practice. J Clin Oncol 2003;21(4):593–601.

[19] Barcenas CH, Hosain GM, Arun B, et al. Assessing BRCA carrier probabilities in extended families. J Clin Oncol 2006;24(3):354–60.
[20] Berry DA, Parmigiani G, Sanchez J, et al. Probability of carrying a mutation of breast-ovarian cancer gene BRCA1 based on family history [see comments]. J Natl Cancer Inst 1997; 89(3):227–38.
[21] Parmigiani G, Berry D, Aguilar O. Determining carrier probabilities for breast cancer–susceptibility genes BRCA1 and BRCA2. Am J Hum Genet 1998;62(1):145–58.
[22] Offit K, Brown K. Quantitating familial cancer risk: a resource for clinical oncologists. J Clin Oncol 1994;12(8):1724–36.
[23] Trepanier A, Ahrens M, McKinnon W, et al, National Society of Genetic Counselors. Genetic cancer risk assessment and counseling: recommendations of the National Society of Genetic Counselors. J Genet Couns 2004;13(2):83–114.
[24] Umar A, Boland CR, Terdiman JP, et al. Revised Bethesda Guidelines for hereditary nonpolyposis colorectal cancer (Lynch syndrome) and microsatellite instability. J Natl Cancer Inst 2004;96(4):261–8.
[25] Hampel H, Frankel WL, Martin E, et al. Screening for the Lynch syndrome (hereditary nonpolyposis colorectal cancer). N Engl J Med 2005;352(18):1851–60.
[26] Hampel H, Frankel W, Panescu J, et al. Screening for Lynch syndrome (hereditary nonpolyposis colorectal cancer) among endometrial cancer patients. Cancer Res 2006;66(15): 7810–7.
[27] Lakhani SR, Van De Vijver MJ, Jacquemier J, et al. The pathology of familial breast cancer: predictive value of immunohistochemical markers estrogen receptor, progesterone receptor, HER-2, and p53 in patients with mutations in BRCA1 and BRCA2. J Clin Oncol 2002;20(9): 2310–8.
[28] Kandel MJ, Stadler Z, Masciari S, et al. Prevalence of BRCA1 mutations in triple negative breast cancer (BC). ASCO Annual Meeting Proceedings Part I. Atlanta, GA; June 2–6, 2008. J Clin Oncol 2006;24(18S):508.
[29] Emery J, Morris H, Goodchild R, et al. The GRAIDS Trial: a cluster randomised controlled trial of computer decision support for the management of familial cancer risk in primary care. Br J Cancer 2007;97(4):486–93.
[30] Snell C, Krypuy M, Wong EM, et al. BRCA1 promoter methylation in peripheral blood DNA of mutation negative familial breast cancer patients with a BRCA1 tumour phenotype. Breast Cancer Res 2008;10:R12.
[31] Biesecker BB. Goals of genetic counseling. Clin Genet 2001;60(5):323–30.
[32] Geller G, Botkin J, Green M, et al. Genetic testing for susceptibility to adult-onset cancer: the process and content of informed consent. JAMA 1997;277:1467–74.
[33] National Society of Genetic Counselors' Definition Task Force, Resta R, Biesecker BB, Bennett RL, et al. A new definition of genetic counseling: National Society of Genetic Counselors' Task Force report. J Genet Couns 2006;15(2):77–83.
[34] Calzone KA, Stopfer J, Blackwood A, et al. Establishing a cancer risk evaluation program. Cancer Pract 1997;5(4):228–33.
[35] Daly MB, Stearman B, Masny A, et al. How to establish a high-risk cancer genetics clinic: limitations and successes. Curr Oncol Rep 2005;7(6):469–74.
[36] Green MJ, Biesecker BB, McInerney AM, et al. An interactive computer program can effectively educate patients about genetic testing for breast cancer susceptibility. Am J Med Genet 2001;103(1):16–23.
[37] Green MJ, Peterson SK, Baker MW, et al. Use of an educational computer program before genetic counseling for breast cancer susceptibility: effects on duration and content of counseling sessions. Genet Med 2005;7(4):221–9.
[38] Calzone KA, Prindiville SA, Jourkiv O, et al. A randomized comparison of group versus individual genetic education and counseling for familial breast and/or ovarian cancer. J Clin Oncol 2005;23:3455–64.

[39] Lea DH, Johnson JL, Ellingwood S, et al. Telegenetics in Maine: successful clinical and educational service delivery model developed from a 3-year pilot project. Genet Med 2005;7(1):21–7.
[40] Jenkins J, Calzone KA, Dimond E, et al. Randomized comparison of phone versus in-person BRCA1/2 predisposition genetic test result disclosure. Genet Med 2007;9:487–95.
[41] Coelho JJ, Arnold A, Nayler J, et al. An assessment of the efficacy of cancer genetic counseling using real-time videoconferencing technology (telemedicine) compared to face-to-face consultations. Eur J Cancer 2005;41:2257–61.
[42] Sangha KK, Dircks A, Langlois S. Assessment of the effectiveness of genetic counseling by telephone compared to a clinic visit. J Genet Couns 2003;12(2):171–84.
[43] Wertz DC, Fanos JH, Reilly PR. Genetic testing for children and adolescents. Who decides? JAMA 1994;272(11):875–81.
[44] Offit K, Thom P. Ethical and legal aspects of cancer genetic testing. Semin Oncol 2007;34: 435–43.
[45] Tischkowitz M, Rosser E. Inherited cancer in children: practical/ethical problems and challenges. Eur J Cancer 2004;40:2459–70.
[46] Bernhardt BA, Tambor ES, Fraser G, et al. Parents' and children's attitudes toward the enrollment of minors in genetic susceptibility research: implications for informed consent. Am J Med Genet 2003;116:315–23.
[47] Schwartz MK. Genetic testing and the clinical laboratory improvement amendments of 1988: present and future. Clin Chem 1999;45:739–45.
[48] Javitt GJ, Hudson K. Federal neglect: regulation of genetic testing. Issues Sci Technol 2006; 22:58–66.
[49] Hudson KL, Murphy JA, Kaufman DJ, et al. Oversight of US genetic testing laboratories. Nat Biotechnol 2006;24:1083–90.
[50] NCI PDQ Cancer Genetics Editorial Board. Elements of cancer genetics risk assessment and counseling. Available at: http://www.cancer.gov/cancertopics/pdq/genetics/risk-assessment-and-counseling/healthprofessional. Accessed March 6, 2008.
[51] Offit K, Groeger E, Turner S, et al. The "duty to warn" a patient's family members about hereditary disease risks. JAMA 2004;292:1469–73.
[52] Smith A, Moran A, Boyd MC, et al. Phenocopies in BRCA1 and BRCA2 families: evidence for modifier genes and implications for screening. J Med Genet 2007;44:10–5.
[53] Katki HA, Mitchell H, Gail MH, et al. Breast-cancer risk in BRCA-mutation-negative women from BRCA-mutation-positive families. Lancet Oncol 2007;8(12):1042–3.
[54] Easton DF, Deffenbaugh AM, Pruss D, et al. A systematic genetic assessment of 1,433 sequence variants of unknown clinical significance in the BRCA1 and BRCA2 breast cancer–predisposition genes. Am J Hum Genet 2007;81(5):873–83.
[55] deCODE genetics. Available at: http://www.decodeme.com/index. Accessed March 6, 2008.
[56] 23 and me. Available at: https://www.23andme.com/. Accessed March 6, 2008.
[57] Navigenics. Available at: http://www.navigenics.com/corp/Main/. Accessed March 6, 2008.
[58] Khoury MJ, Gwinn M, Yoon PW, et al. The continuum of translation research in genomic medicine: How can we accelerate the appropriate integration of human genome discoveries into health care and disease prevention? Genet Med 2007;9(10):665–74.

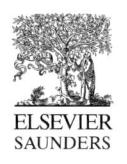

The Genetic Information Nondiscrimination Act: Why Your Personal Genetics are Still Vulnerable to Discrimination

Louise M. Slaughter, MSPH

US House of Representatives, 2469 Rayburn House Office Building, Washington, DC 20515, USA

Genetic research remains one of the most promising scientific fields, offering great potential for early treatment and the prevention of numerous diseases. Nearly 14 years ago, the field of medicine was transformed by the discovery of the first genetic mutation linked to breast cancer. Since the sequencing of the human genome in 2003, the number of identified genetic markers for a wide variety of chronic health conditions has expanded at an extraordinary rate.

These discoveries have had a profound effect on the field of medicine and on society as a whole. Approximately 13 million Americans are affected by nearly 16,000 recognized genetic disorders. Indeed, every human possesses some potentially lethal genes [1].

As more genetic links to diseases have been identified, genetic tests have become commercially available, and genetic technology has become embedded firmly in the practice of medicine. For example, the medical community now recognizes that up to 30% of infant deaths are associated with known genetic disorders, 15% of cancers have an identifiable genetic hereditary component, and 10% of chronic diseases such as heart disease and diabetes are known to have a strong genetic component [1]. Although most lethal genetic mutations never manifest themselves, they may have serious implications for children of carriers.

Louise McIntosh Slaughter is a microbiologist with a master's degree in public health. She has served as a member of the United States House of Representatives for 21 years and is the Chairwoman of the House Rules Committee. For the past 13 years, she has authored legislation to prevent discrimination of genetic information. In the 110th Congress, she is the coauthor of H.R. 493, the Genetics Information Nondiscrimination Act.

E-mail address: michelle.adams@mail.house.gov

As technology continues to advance, ethical, legal, and social challenges continue to present themselves. Consequently, the United States faces unprecedented questions about how it, as a nation, will allow genetic information to be handled and used. Almost 13 years ago, I introduced the first legislation in Congress to ban genetic discrimination in health insurance. It was a straightforward, noncontroversial proposal that would allow social policy to keep pace with rapidly expanding science. On that date in 1995, I could hardly have imagined that 6 years would pass before the House of Representatives held the first hearing on the issue and that it would be 12 years before the House took a vote on the Genetic Information Nondiscrimination Act (GINA). Finally in 2008, the Senate passed GINA unanimously and on May 21 the President signed this bill into law.

This legislation protects an individual's genetic information from employer and insurance discrimination, thereby encouraging Americans to take advantage of genetic testing to prevent and prepare for potential diseases. If GINA is not enacted now, Americans will continue to fear genetic testing, and scientific and medical progress will continue to be stalled.

Genetic testing: advantages and challenges

In 1991, Congress initiated the Human Genome Project as a collaborative effort with the Department of Health and Human Services and the Department of Energy for the purpose of decoding the human genetic sequence. Twelve years later, in April 2003, the first phase of the project, sequencing the human genome, was completed successfully. In 2004, the second phase of the project began, in which scientists continued to investigate the clinical applications of the sequenced genome [1]. By sequencing the human genetic code, scientists now have identified genetic markers for a variety of chronic health conditions, increasing the potential for early treatment and prevention of numerous diseases. Genetic tests are critical in providing information to diagnose and guide treatment decisions or predictive information about future risks.

The Johns Hopkins University Genetics and Public Policy Center defines genetic testing as "the laboratory analysis of DNA, RNA, or chromosomes. Testing can also involve analysis of proteins and metabolites that are the products of genes" [2]. Although there are few cures for genetic diseases, genetic testing does provide individuals information about their risk of developing a disease in the future [1]. There should not be assumed, however, that person testing positive for a genetic mutation will develop that disease. Genetic tests that reveal genetic mutations simply indicate risk. Individuals who test positive for a genetic mutation may remain asymptomatic over their entire lives.

More than 1000 genetic tests now are available clinically, and additional tests to determine future susceptibility to disease and responses to medication reach the market every day. Today, nearly 600 laboratories can provide genetic testing for more than 1100 diseases [1]. Without legal guarantees for job and insurance protection, however, individuals will forgo tests that could save their lives.

Genetic discrimination: how pervasive is it?

Some in Congress have called the GINA "a solution in search of a problem" and suggest that genetic discrimination occurs rarely, if ever. It is estimated, however, that all humans are genetically predisposed to between 5 and 50 serious disorders [3]. Because no human being has a perfect set of genes, every person is at risk for genetic discrimination. In fact, there are well-documented public instances of genetic discrimination; genetic issues are insinuating themselves into health care decisions and into many other aspects of Americans' lives.

The use of genetic information for a variety of purposes is more prevalent than critics contend. Throughout the country, advertisements for genetic tests for paternity can be seen in newspapers and on roadside billboards [3]. Other examples include an organization called "Dor Yeshorim" that offers genetic testing to Jewish youth. Hasidic youth can take a battery of genetic tests to determine whether they are carriers for any of 10 serious genetic disorders. Young men and women who are carriers for a given disorder may be discouraged from courting each other, because their children could be born with a fatal genetic disorder.

Genetic discrimination also is cited very frequently in the workplace. Congress and the Secretary's Advisory Committee on Genetics, Health, and Society have heard from several victims of such discrimination. For example, a North Carolinian woman was fired when her genetic tests revealed a risk for a lung disorder even though she had begun the treatments that would keep her healthy. In another instance, a social worker was fired despite outstanding performance reviews because of her employer's fears about her family history of Huntington's disease. There even was an instance in which an adoption agency refused to allow a woman at risk for Huntington's disease to adopt a child [4].

These examples are by no means uncommon. A 1996 study showed that a number of institutions, including health and life insurance companies, health care providers, adoption agencies, the military, and schools were reported to have engaged in genetic discrimination against asymptomatic individuals. Furthermore, a 2001 American Management Association survey of employer medical testing practices found that 1.3% of companies test new or current employees for sickle cell anemia, 0.4% test for Huntington's disease, and 20.1% ask about family medical history. When asked if they used these results in hiring, reassigning, retaining, or dismissing employees, 1% of employers indicated that they used data regarding sickle cell anemia, 0.8% used data regarding Huntington's disease, and 5.5% used data regarding family medical history [4].

When the Secretary's Advisory Committee on Genetics, Health, and Society met in 2004, many individuals presented personal testimonials of discrimination initiated by an insurance company or employer because of a genetic predisposition. In 2000, Jolene Hollar of Arizona was turned down by two life insurance companies because her family had a history of Huntington's disease. Mrs. Hollar herself had not been tested for the gene. One of the companies wrote, "Reconsideration would be available once the testing has been completed and you test negative to this gene" [5]. In the case of Terri Seargent, the repercussions of her genetic tests were more severe. Ms Seargent was tested and diagnosed with alpha-1 antitrypsin deficiency, which she could control with medication. Shortly following her diagnosis, she lost her job. Without employment, and having a pre-existing condition, she also lost her health, life, and disability insurance [1].

Notable examples also include a 2000 case in which the Burlington Northern Santa Fe Railroad performed genetic tests on employees without their knowledge or consent. The workers involved had applied for workers' compensation, and the tests were conducted to undermine their claims. One worker who refused to submit a blood sample for genetic testing was threatened with termination. Burlington Northern Santa Fe Railroad settled these cases in April 2001 for $2.2 million [1,6,7].

A few years earlier in 1998, the Lawrence Berkeley National Laboratory was found to have been performing tests for syphilis, pregnancy, and sickle cell anemia on employees without their knowledge or consent for years [1]. Throughout the 1970 s, many African Americans were denied jobs, educational opportunities, and insurance based on their carrier status for sickle cell anemia, even though a carrier lacks the two copies of a mutation necessary to develop sickle cell anemia [6].

Sadly, Ms Seargent's case, along with the cases at Burlington Northern Santa Fe Railroad, Lawrence Livermore Laboratories, and others provide excellent examples of why protections against discrimination are necessary both in the workplace and through health insurance companies.

Genetic discrimination: implications for America's public health and scientific research

Given the prevalence of genetic discrimination, many individuals are deciding against having genetic tests or participating in genetic research. Others are opting to take genetic tests under an assumed name or to pay out-of-pocket costs to obtain valuable information about their potential future health status and to avoid having that information used against them. In a letter to the National Institutes of Health, one person described how he and others were using "bogus" names and false addresses to get genetic testing so that they could acquire the necessary insurance without discrimination before becoming symptomatic with a disease [5].

The public shows an overwhelming desire to keep genetic information out of the hands of insurers and employers who might use it to undermine rather than advance the public's best interests. In a recent 2006 Cogent Research poll, 66% of respondents said they had concerns about how their genetic information would be stored and who would have access to it. Sixty-five percent said they were concerned about health insurance companies, and 54% were concerned with employers gaining unauthorized access [8].

The American people agree these protections should be guaranteed under federal law. In fact, 72% agreed that the government should establish laws and regulations to protect the privacy of individuals' genetic information. Eighty-five percent believe that without such legislation, employers would discriminate [8].

Fears about privacy do not resonate only with the public. Health care professionals also are hesitant to make genetic information available. In one survey, 108 of 159 genetic counselors indicated that they would not submit charges for a genetic test to their insurance companies, primarily because of fear of discrimination. Twenty-five percent responded that they would use an alias to obtain a genetic test to reduce the risk of discrimination and maximize confidentiality. Moreover, 60% indicated that they would not share the information with a colleague because of the need for privacy and fear of job discrimination [1].

Studies also have shown that, even if early detection of a particular genetic mutation may help avert premature morbidity and morality, Americans still are deciding to forego genetic testing altogether because of fears of discrimination. Hereditary nonpolyposis colorectal cancer (HNPCC) provides an instructive example. Six genes have been identified to determine if a person carries a mutation for HNPCC. HNPCC is the most common hereditary form of colon cancer, and it is estimated that 380,000 Americans carry an HNPCC mutation. Persons who have the mutation have a 90% lifetime risk of developing one of the cancers associated with HNPCC [9]. Between 1996 and 1999, people from families known to have the HNPCC mutations were asked to participate in a study that offered genetic testing for the mutation. Although there were other considerations for not participating in the study, 39% of those who declined genetic testing cited fears about losing health insurance as the reason [9]. The high fear factor led the authors of the study to conclude that without legal protection at the national level to address the public's fear of discrimination, a significant number of Americans will opt not to reap the benefits of advanced screening for cancer that would lead to healthier, longer lives [9].

This conclusion underscores a terrible reality—that the threat of genetic discrimination and the fear of being passed over for promotion, of being forced to pay more for health insurance, or even being denied coverage—is making men and women less likely to be tested and to take advantage of the potentially life-saving medical information.

Genetic discrimination: the need for federal legislation

Some argue that existing federal statutes already protect individuals from discrimination based on genetic information, but in fact no federal laws comprehensively and specifically provide protections for genetic information in employment and insurance settings. Several existing federal laws touch on the issues raised by the use of genetic information, including the Health Insurance Portability and Accountability Act (HIPAA), Executive Order 13145, the Americans with Disabilities Act, and Title VII of the Civil Rights Act of 1963. This patchwork of laws and interpretations is untested in the courts and does not address adequately the unique issues surrounding the specific use of genetic information. Furthermore, these laws leave many gaps in protection and fail to alleviate public fear of genetic testing. The ambiguity of current law has resulted in both actual and perceived acts of discrimination and leads to an inconsistent application of laws to deal with such grievances.

Recently, the Secretary's Advisory Committee on Genetics, Health, and Society at the Department of Health and Human Services conducted an analysis of the ability of current law to protect against genetic discrimination. The analysis found many gaps, and the Advisory Committee concluded, "current law does not adequately protect against discrimination based on genetic predisposition" [10]. After the release of its report, the Advisory Committee sent a letter to Secretary Michael Leavitt, urging him to exert influence to bring about the enactment of federal legislation [11]. At the June 2005 Secretary's Advisory Committee on Genetics, Health, and Society meeting, Agnes Masny, Chair of the Genetic Discrimination Task Force, again pointed out that current laws and court decisions have left substantial gaps in coverage. Consequently, they have failed to provide the safeguards necessary to protect genetic information [12]. Recognizing the importance of instituting legislative protections against genetic discrimination, 32 states have enacted genetic antidiscrimination provisions in employment laws, and 43 states have passed laws pertaining to the use of genetic information in health insurance (Michele Schoonmaker, Congressional Research Service, personal communication on Genetic Nondiscrimination Information, to Rosaline Cohen, et al., Feb. 16, 2005) [6]. Although it is commendable that states have recognized and acted on the public's desire for legal protections, these state laws vary widely in application and levels of protection. They also are limited in guaranteeing protection against insurer discrimination, because self-insured employee benefit plans generally are exempt from state laws under the Employee Retirement and Security Act (ERISA). Because state laws are diverse and inconsistent, companies operating in more than one state may experience substantial burdens when trying to comply with various laws [10]. Therefore there is a clear need for consistent legal protections at the federal level.

Strong, comprehensive legislation is needed to alleviate the public's fear about genetic information discrimination. Because more than 61.8% of Americans get their insurance through their employers [13], without job security, there are no guarantees of insurance protection. If a person is protected from insurers but not their employer, they could be fired and lose their insurance coverage anyway.

GINA provides protection against discrimination by both insurers and employers, because providing only partial protection against genetic discrimination still will deter people from genetic testing. As evidenced by Ms Seargent's case and the others noted earlier, what good is ensuring that insurers cannot discriminate if people can lose their jobs, and consequently their insurance coverage, because of the results of genetic testing? It is critical that the protections be extended to cover both insurers and employers.

The genetic information nondiscrimination act (P.L. 110–233)

P.L. 110–233, GINA [14], would provide critical protections against genetic discrimination for all Americans. GINA prohibits insurers from canceling, denying, refusing to renew, or changing the terms or premiums of coverage based on genetic information. It also would prohibit employers from making hiring, firing, promotion, and other employment-related decisions based on genetic factors. Title I of the bill deals with health insurers, and Title II deals with employers.

Title I—health insurers

Health insurers are most likely to use genetic information for discriminatory purposes before a person's enrollment. This is the time when insurance companies decide whether to offer an individual coverage and at what price. To prevent insurance companies from factoring genetic information into these decisions, GINA prohibits insurance companies from requesting, requiring, or purchasing genetic information about an individual before that individual's enrollment. Finally, recognizing that genetic information may be obtained incidentally, GINA does not penalize health insurance companies that inadvertently receive genetic information as long as the entity does not use the information to discriminate against an individual.

Title I applies to employer-sponsored group health plans, health insurance issuers in the group and individual markets, Medigap insurance, and state and local (non-federal) governmental plans.

ERISA currently prohibits a group health plan or health insurance issuer offering coverage in connection with a group health plan from discriminating against an individual, in the group, in setting eligibility, and premium or contribution amounts, and applying pre-existing condition exclusions to the policy based on the individual's genetic information. GINA expands protections by prohibiting a health insurance issuer offering health coverage in connection with a group health plan from adjusting premium or contribution amounts for an entire group on the basis of genetic information concerning an individual in the group or a family member of the individual. It also restricts an issuer's collection of genetic information.

Title I also prohibits an issuer of a Medicare supplemental policy from denying or conditioning the issuance of a policy, discriminating in the price of the policy, or applying pre-existing condition exclusions to the policy on the basis of genetic information.

The individual health insurance market is largely unregulated. GINA seeks to offer greater protections for individuals trying to obtain or already participating in an individual health insurance plan. As such, GINA prohibits health insurance issuers in the individual market from using genetic information about enrollees or their family members to adjust premium or contribution amounts. The legislation also prohibits using genetic information as a condition of eligibility for insurance coverage and applying pre-existing condition exclusions to the policy.

HIPAA standards already protect the use and disclosure of all individually identifiable health information, including genetic information. Under these standards, however, underwriting, a practice that is inherently discriminatory, is allowed. Because GINA deals only with genetic information that indicates a predisposition to a disease or disorder, the bill expressly bans the use or disclosure of genetic information for purposes of underwriting.

A critical component of this section is the methodology used to enforce protections. Title I is enforced through the use of an excise tax on group health plans that fail to comply with the rules. This enforcement mechanism is being used already under present law for violations of mental heath parity, existing antidiscrimination health law, and the rules relating to benefits for mothers and newborns.

Title I also builds on existing statutes (eg, ERISA) and generally uses the same mechanisms of enforcement. For group health plans and health insurance issuers in the individual and group markets, the appropriate Secretary may impose penalties of $100/day/person, with a minimum penalty of $2500 and up to $15,000 for multiple violations. The genetic privacy provisions are enforced by the Health and Human Services' Office of Civil Rights. The Secretary of Health and Human Services may impose civil monetary penalties beginning at $100/violation and increasing to $250,000 and 10 years in prison.

Title II—employers

In Title II, GINA explicitly prohibits the use of genetic information in employment decisions such as hiring, firing, job assignments, and promotions. This prohibition extends to employers, unions, employment agencies, and labor-management training programs. Employers, labor organizations, employment agencies, and joint labor-management committees are prohibited from requesting, requiring, or purchasing genetic information about an employee or family member, except in limited cases. Even in these limited cases, genetic information still could not be used or disclosed.

Title II of GINA is enforced through remedies outlined in Title VII of the Civil Rights Act of 1964. The bill provides the same compensatory and punitive damages available to prevailing plaintiffs under 42 U.S.C. 1981a, which are progressive with the size of the employer and are limited to cases of disparate treatment.

The genetic information nondiscrimination act: political influence and implications

Overview of the legislative process

The current political climate and the legislative process underscore why GINA took so long to be enacted into federal law. To understand why this bill had been held up for 13 years, one first must understand the legislative process.

Once a bill is introduced in either the House or Senate, it is referred to a committee, which has jurisdiction over the bill. The legislation may be referred to one committee that has exclusive jurisdiction or to a number of committees that may share jurisdiction over issues. Once referred, a committee typically holds a hearing on the bill before it schedules a mark-up. A mark-up of a bill is scheduled at the discretion of the Committee Chairman, and Members of Congress serving on the Committee are allowed the opportunity to offer amendments.

Once through this sometimes long and rigorous committee process, the bill then is available to be brought on the House or Senate floor for a vote. After floor passage, the bill is referred to the other legislative chamber. For example, a bill originating in the House is referred to the Senate upon passage on the House floor. The bill will go through a similar process in the Senate.

If the bill passes in both the House of Representatives and the Senate, but the versions passed by the two chambers are not identical, it must go to conference. Conferees from both the House and Senate reconcile any differences between the two versions of the bill. When conferees have come to an agreement on an identical version, both the House of Representatives and Senate must vote once again on the conferenced version of the bill.

Another option, which has been used more frequently in the 110th Congress, is to "ping-pong" the bill from one chamber to another. Under this scenario, one chamber passes a bill and then refers it to the other chamber. The other chamber amends the bill and sends the amended bill back to the originating chamber. This process can continue until both chambers pass an identical bill. By using this tactic, Congress avoids a conference, which sometimes can drag on for many months.

Only after an identical bill passes both chambers is it sent to the President. On receipt of the bill, the President may sign it into law or veto it. If a bill is vetoed, it must pass both chambers by a two-thirds majority for Congress to override the veto.

The US House of Representatives

Thirteen years ago, I introduced the first version of a genetics antidiscrimination bill. Since then, I have introduced a version of GINA each

Congress. On January 16, 2007, I introduced H.R. 493 with my Republican colleague, Congresswoman Judy Biggert of Illinois. Before passing the House the first time, we garnered 224 bipartisan cosponsors of the bill.

This bill then was referred to three House committees: the Education and Labor Committee, the Energy and Commerce Committee, and the Ways and Means Committee. Following the process described previously, the Education and Labor Subcommittee on Health, Employment, Labor, and Pensions held a hearing on GINA in January 2007. The bill then was marked up by the full Education and Labor Committee. Shortly thereafter, the Energy and Commerce Subcommittee on Health held a hearing, and the full Committee then marked up the bill. Similarly, the Ways and Means Subcommittee on Health also held a hearing on March 14, and 1 week later GINA was passed in the full Committee.

After easily winning approval by all three Committees of jurisdictions, GINA was brought to the House floor for consideration. On April 25, 2007, H.R. 493 passed overwhelmingly in the House of Representatives, by a vote of 420 to 3. Following passage in the House, the bill was referred to the Senate.

The US Senate

During both the 108th and 109th Congresses, the Senate passed GINA. Senators Olympia Snowe (R-ME), Edward Kennedy (D-MA), and many others have championed this bill in the Senate, and the bill had received strong backing from Bill First, then Senate Majority Leader [15]. In October 2003, the Senate passed this bill by a unanimous vote of 95 to 0. On February 17, 2005, the Senate again passed GINA by a vote of 98 to 0.

In early 2007, the Senate Health Education Labor and Pensions held a hearing and mark-up on the bill. In July, after months of meetings between the House and Senate, the Senate was ready to consider the House-passed version of GINA. Unfortunately, Sen. Coburn (R-OK), despite having supported GINA in 2005, put a hold on the bill, thereby preventing a Senate vote [16]. To override this hold, the Senate would have needed significant debate time and 60 votes in support of the bill. Instead, after nearly 10 months of negotiations, an agreement was reached with Senator Coburn. Shortly thereafter, the Senate passed the bill 95-0. The House took up the revised version which easily passed 414-1, and then sent it to the President.

The White House

For several years, the Bush Administration had come out strongly in support of GINA and issued Statements of Administration Policy to this effect when the bill passed in the Senate in the 108th and 109th Congresses and when H.R. 493 passed in the House of Representatives in 2007. In this statement, the President acknowledged that "the potential misuse of [genetic] information raises serious moral and legal issues." To address concerns about unwarranted use of genetic information, the President pledged to work with Congress on passage of this legislation [17].

The National Institutes of Health has echoed the White House's support. In fact, Dr. Francis S. Collins, director of the National Human Genome Research Institute at the National Institutes of Health, has played a key role in advancing protections for genetic information and has been urging Congress to pass this legislation since 1995 [15]. He testified about the need for GINA in front of both the Energy and Commerce and Ways and Means Committees in 2007. His testimony echoed a 2003 editorial in *Science*, in which Dr. Collins wrote, "[the] House needs to approve [GINA] as soon as possible." In this same editorial, Dr. Collins expressed the sentiment felt widely throughout the medical and scientific communities that genetic discrimination will "slow the pace of the scientific discovery that will yield crucial medical advances. [M]any people have already refused to participate in genetic research for fear of genetic discrimination." Dr. Collins argues that GINA is an "outstanding effort that successfully addresses the myriad concerns of the biomedical research and health communities." The editorial concludes with the compelling claim that without passage of this much-needed legislation, Americans cannot "fully reap the rewards of the investment already made in human genome research" [18].

Dr. Collins goes on to state that, "However, I really want to make it clear to the Congress that I hope they pass legislation that makes genetic discrimination illegal. In other words, if a person is willing to share his or her genetic information, it is important that that information not be exploited in improper ways—and Congress can pass good legislation to prevent that from happening. In other words, we want medical research to go forward without an individual fearing of personal discrimination" [19].

Supporters

Nearly 300 organizations have rallied in support of GINA. The Coalition for Genetic Fairness [20] consists of 141 organizations. Its mission is to promote legal protections for genetic information, and it has been outspoken in its support for GINA. Some of the most prominent medical and scientific organizations in the country support GINA, including the Personalized Medicine Coalition, the American Society of Human Genetics, the American Medical Association, the American Academy of Family Physicians, the American Academy of Pediatrics, the March of Dimes, the American Cancer Society, the American Heart Association, the National Association for the Advancement of Colored People, the Susan G. Komen Breast Cancer Foundation, and the United Cerebral Palsy Association and the pharmaceutical companies GlaxoSmithKline and Eli Lilly and Company.

Opponents

Despite widespread public support for GINA, the Genetic Information Nondiscrimination in Employment Coalition had actively opposed this bill.

On the Coalition's steering committee are the United States Chamber of Commerce, the Society for Human Resource Management, the National Association of Manufacturers, the HR Policy Association, and the College and University Professional Association for Human Resources. They opposed the bill on several grounds and argued that new federal legislation is not needed. The powerful United States Chamber of Commerce and National Association of Manufacturers had been especially outspoken against the bill.

The genetic information nondiscrimination act: refuting the opposition

Throughout the many years that GINA has been out there, and especially in the 110th Congress, the sponsors of the bill have made changes to the bill to address some of its opponents' concerns.

Time and again, supporters of stronger legal protections have refuted the opposition's contentions that such legislation is not necessary. Opponents argue there is no evidence that employers or insurers are engaging in discrimination based on genetic make-up, but many cases, including those described earlier, have emerged in which employers have indeed engaged in genetic discrimination or attempted to do so. In addition to the few cases listed previously, there might be many more that have not been documented.

It was vital that Congress not wait to act until hundreds or thousands of people have experienced genetic discrimination. Today, the opportunities for such discrimination are more limited, precisely because people are not taking tests for fear that this information will be used against them. They thereby are denying themselves valuable information that could be used to make important health care decisions and also are hindering the advancement of genetic technology.

Opponents of GINA also contended that genetic information can be useful in making some employment decisions. For example, they claimed that a health condition likely to cause seizures could properly be considered a threat to others if the employee were a bus driver or an airline pilot. As stated earlier, however, a positive test for a particular genetic mutation associated with an illness does not mean that the individual will develop that illness. To this day, scientists and geneticists have been unable to identify any existing genetic test that would guarantee that a person testing positive would develop a condition that would pose a significant danger to others. Rather, a genetic mutation confers only a higher risk of developing a disorder. Additionally, few such conditions develop suddenly or without warning in adulthood. Expecting human resources professionals to interpret a genetic test accurately is about as realistic as asking them to predict the weather for a particular city a year from that date.

Most genetic tests have no bearing whatsoever on an individual's ability to perform the duties of his or her job today. Therefore, employers should not be permitted to deny job opportunities to entire categories of workers on the possibility that someday a person might get sick.

There also are those who contended that it is too difficult for employers to comply with 50 different state laws but at the same time suggest that if Congress enacted legislation barring employment discrimination based on genetic information, it should include a safe harbor providing that employers in compliance with the federal standards cannot be liable under state or local laws banning such discrimination. True, a federal law can provide valuable uniformity, but it does not have to trample states' rights in the process.

At present, more than 30 states have passed laws dealing with some aspect of genetic discrimination, but they are a patchwork of different definitions, standards, and remedies. A federal "floor" provides a coherent national statement of policy while allowing states to pass additional protections for their residents if they so choose. This model is the one followed by civil rights laws, HIPAA, and numerous others. Congress has a long history of avoiding state pre-emption whenever possible in deference to states' rights. If a given state wishes to be more explicit or extensive in banning genetic discrimination, it should have that right.

Opponents of GINA had argued that a genetic discrimination law should "sunset," or expire automatically at a set date. Congress routinely uses its committee oversight and hearing processes to examine whether existing laws need to be updated or changed. A sunset provision, however, would have created a dangerous situation in which the law would lapse and genetic discrimination would become legal after a period of being banned. Furthermore, no major law protecting Americans' rights has ever contained a sunset provision, including the Americans with Disabilities Act, the Civil Rights Act of 1964, or the HIPAA. Most importantly, there was no reason why genetic discrimination should be banned only temporarily.

Another concern expressed by the opposition was that this legislation would encourage unnecessary and frivolous lawsuits, thereby inundating an already overburdened court system with expensive litigation [21]. Many legal analysts, however, have said that by deferring to current law, remedies remain uncertain and are likely to result in costly litigation [10]. GINA ensures a fair, balanced system of enforcement to discourage frivolous litigation. For example, the bill protects companies from being sued for the inadvertent acquisition of medical history or health information Additionally, the bill requires claimants to exhaust administrative state and federal Equal Employment Opportunity Commission procedures before seeking court damages or equitable relief and places a cap on all compensatory and punitive damages, even against the largest firms, at $300,000.

Opponents to the bill also tried to assert that a "business necessity" exemption was necessary in Title II that would allow employers to obtain and use genetic information about employees if they have a "reasonable basis." Business necessity is not well defined in current law. Although it is used in the context of the Americans with Disabilities Act, it is hard to conceive of a valid "business necessity" for discriminating against an employee with a genetic predisposition to a disease or disorder. In fact, one could imagine a scenario where an employer fires an individual who tests positive for the *BRAC-1* gene because it is a "business necessity," and indeed the business necessity could be the employer's not wanting to risk having to pay for future cancer treatment. Such a "business necessity" carve-out essentially would have gutted the protections of Title II.

Opponents of GINA also argued that a carve-out was necessary to limit liability for employers when the violation involves a group health plan. As the author of GINA, I contend that if an employer is in any way involved in a discriminatory act prohibited by Title II, that employer should be held liable under Title II remedies.

Opponents spent years putting up roadblocks and arguing semantics with the goal of preventing passage of this important legislation. In April 2004, an article in *Congress Daily AM* described the lack of action on this legislation as "a textbook case of obstruction by inertia" [22]. The article also identified the United States Chamber of Commerce as the primary interest group lobbying Congress not to take up this bill. The facts are clear, however: discrimination is occurring, the public is not seeking genetic testing for fear of discrimination, and the scientific community is suffering for lack of study participants.

Businesses that do not yet support this new law should do so for two key reasons. First, increased use of genetic information in the provision of health care will increase the effectiveness of health care and consequently reduce health care costs for employers over time. Second, the development and utilization of genetic information will result in a maturation of the personalized medicine market, with American companies in the molecular testing market predicted to generate $4.2 billion in revenues by 2006 (Michele Schoonmaker, Congressional Research Service, personal communication on genetic nondiscrimination information, to Rosaline Cohen, et al, February 16, 2005.). Without appropriate protections to encourage providers, the health care community, and the public to embrace genetic testing, the health care sector would be incapable of taking full advantage of the important opportunities resulting from the advances in genetic information and technology.

Ultimately, the true cost of failing to pass this legislation was the damage to America's public health.

Genetic information protection: the road ahead

The sequencing of the human genome is widely regarded as one of the greatest scientific advancements in human history. With this discovery, scientists have made significant progress in deciphering information likely to benefit the health and well being of people throughout this country and the world. Without adequate protections, however, fears of genetic discrimination have the potential to stifle valuable scientific research.

GINA will do more than stamp out a new form of discrimination. It will help the United States be a leader in a field of scientific research that holds as much promise as any other in history. I have worked 13 years to see these protections become law, and I am pleased that on May 21st this era came to an end. We must now look forward to the future.

References

[1] Schoonmaker M, Williams ED. Genetic testing: scientific background and nondiscrimination legislation. Congressional Research Service Report for Congress 3,4 (updated March 21, 2005).
[2] Johns Hopkins University Genetics and Public Policy Center. Reproductive genetic testing: what America thinks 4 (2004).
[3] Slaughter LM. Genetic non-discrimination: examining the implications for workers and employers. Statement at the hearing before the Subcommittee on Employer-Employee Relations of the House Education and the Workforce Committee, 108th Congress 87 (2004).
[4] Williams E, Sarata A, Redhead CS. Genetic discrimination: overview of the issue and proposed legislation. Congressional Research Service Report for Congress 10 (updated March 7, 2007).
[5] Public perspectives on genetic discrimination. Comments from the Secretary's Advisory Committee on Genetics, Health, and Society 29, 30 (2004). Available at: www4.od.nih.gov/oba/sacghs/reports/Public_Perspectives_GenDiscrim.pdf. Accessed July 1, 2008.
[6] A roadmap for the integration of genetics and genomics in society. Report on the study priorities of the Secretary's Advisory Committee on Genetics, Health, and Society 20 (2004). Available at: www4.od.nih.gov/oba/sacghs/reports/reports.html. Accessed July 1, 2008.
[7] The U.S. Equal Employment Opportunity Commission. EEOC settles ADA suit against BNSF for genetic bias (April 18, 2001). Available at: www.eeoc.gov/press/4-18-01.html. Accessed July 6, 2005.
[8] White C. Americans' attitudes towards genetic discrimination. Cogent Research 3–4, 2006.
[9] Hadley DW, Jenkins J, Dimond E, et al. Genetic counseling and testing in families with hereditary nonpolyposis colorectal cancer. Arch Intern Med 2003;163:573–82.
[10] Lanman RB. The Secretary's Advisory Committee on Genetics, Health, and Society. An analysis of the adequacy of current law in protecting against genetic discrimination in health insurance and employment 23 (May 2005). Available at: www4.od.nih.gov/oba/SACGHS.htm. Accessed July 1, 2008.
[11] Tuckson RV. Letter from the Chair of the Secretary's Advisory Committee on Genetics, Health, and Society to Michael O. Levitt, Secretary of Health and Human Services (May 3, 2005). Available at: www4.od.nih.gov/oba/sacghs/reports/letter_to_Sec_05_03_2005 pdf. Accessed July 1, 2008.
[12] Masny A. SACGHS efforts on genetic discrimination issue, slide 9 (June 15, 2005). Available at: www4.od.nih.gov/oba/SACGHS/meetings/June2005/Masny.pdf. Accessed July 1, 2008.
[13] Peterson CL. Health insurance coverage: characteristics of the insured and uninsured populations in 2003. Congressional Research Service Report for Congress 2 (last updated August 27, 2004).
[14] Genetic Information Nondiscrimination Act, H.R. 493, S. 358. 110th Cong., 1st Session. Available at: frwebgate.access.gpo.gov/cgi-bin/getdoc.cgi?dbname=110_cong_bills&docid=f:h493eh.txt.pdf and frwebgate.access.gpo.gov/cgi-bin/getdoc.cgi?dbname=110_cong_bills&docid=f:s358is.txt.pdf. Accessed February 1, 2008.
[15] Genetic discrimination bill clears Senate. House in no hurry to act. National Journal's Congress Daily. October 15, 2003.

[16] Roll call vote 11. Available at: http://www.senate.gov/legislative/LIS/roll_call_lists/roll_call_vote_cfm.cfm?congress=109&;session=1&vote=00011, February 17, 2005.
[17] Executive Office of the President, Office of Management and Budget. Statement of administration policy. H.R. 493—Genetic Information Nondiscrimination Act of 2007 (April 25, 2007). Available at: www.whitehouse.gov/omb/legislative/sap/110-1/hr493sap-h.pdf. Accessed July 1, 2008.
[18] Collins FS, Watson JD. Genetic discrimination: time to act. Science 2003;302:745.
[19] President Bush participates in roundtable on advances in cancer prevention at the National Institutes of Health, Bethesda, MD. Available at: www.whitehouse.gov/news/releases/2007/01/20070117-1.html, 2007. Accessed July 1, 2008.
[20] Coalition for Genetic Fairness. Available at: www.geneticfairness.org/members.html. Accessed July 11, 2005.
[21] Josten RB. Cause of action against employers based on claims of genetic discrimination. U.S. Chamber of Commerce letter to U.S. Senator Gregg (May 13, 2003). Available at: www.uschamber.com/issues/letters/2003/030513dna.htm. Accessed June 22, 2005.
[22] Genetic discrimination bill stalls in House. National Journal's CongressDaily April 20, 2004.

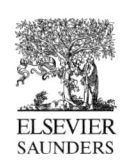

An Overview of the Role of Prophylactic Surgery in the Management of Individuals with a Hereditary Cancer Predisposition

Tawakalitu Oseni, MD[a], Ismail Jatoi, MD, PhD, FACS[b],*

[a]*Department of Surgical Oncology, Fox Chase Cancer Center, 333 Cottman Avenue, Philadelphia, PA 19111, USA*
[b]*Department of Surgery, National Naval Medical Center, The Uniformed Services University, 4301 Jones Bridge Road, Bethesda, MD 20889, USA*

Cancer is the second leading cause of death in the United States [1]. Over the last 20 years, the field of cancer genetics has grown exponentially, and the two-hit mutation model developed by Knudson [2] has served as a framework for studying human carcinogenesis. Several tumor suppressor genes have been identified, and the relevance of germline mutations to cancer development is understood better. One now can identify mutation carriers who are at increased risk for developing cancers and, in some instances, offer prophylactic surgery to reduce that risk. Before deciding on prophylactic surgery, however, individuals who have a genetic predisposition for cancer should consider nonsurgical management options. This article provides an overview for the role of prophylactic surgery for managing individuals who have a genetic predisposition for cancer, particularly those who have a predisposition for breast, colon, thyroid, and gastric cancers. It summarizes the role of prophylactic surgery in individuals who have a genetic predisposition for cancer, and other articles throughout this issue provide a more detailed review of these hereditary cancer syndromes.

The views or opinions expressed in this article are those of the authors and should not be construed as representing the official views of the Departments of the Army, Navy, or Defense.

* Corresponding author. Department of Surgery, The Uniformed Services University, 4301 Jones Bridge Road, Bethesda, MD 20889.
 E-mail address: ismail.jatoi@us.army.mil (I. Jatoi).

It long has been recognized that there is a hereditary component to certain cancers. In 1865, Broca described a case of hereditary breast cancer in relating the incidence of this disease in four generations of his wife's family [3]. In 1913, Aldrin Warthin [4] described a family, Family G, with a cluster of gastrointestinal (GI) and gynecologic malignancies that is similar to what is now reported in families with hereditary nonpolyposis colorectal cancer (HNPCC). Lynch and colleagues [5] described a series of 34 families with two or more relatives with breast cancer, establishing a hereditary link to some cases of breast cancer. Thus, epidemiologic studies confirmed that cancers cluster in certain families, and improved understanding of the hereditary basis for certain cancers [6]. In the past, high-risk patients were identified on the basis of family pedigree and clinical presentation, and these patients were managed with surveillance and then treated once disease developed. The expanding use of prophylactic surgery for managing individuals with a genetic predisposition for cancer is related directly to the explosion of information regarding the hereditary cancer syndromes. Once the genetic basis for a cancer syndrome is discovered and genetic testing becomes available, the clinical question becomes: If we can identify individuals who are increased risk for developing this disease, what can we do to prevent it? Molecular biology has allowed the identification of an array of mutations responsible for various hereditary cancer syndromes, and, in mutation carriers, prophylactic surgery might be considered as an option to avoid the potential morbidity and mortality associated with a cancer diagnosis.

Once a patient with a genetic predisposition for cancer has been identified, there are generally three management options: surveillance, chemoprevention, and prophylactic surgery. All options carry the potential for benefit and harm, and there are no randomized prospective trials that have assessed the impact of these options in mutation carriers. The suitability of these management options varies, depending on the particular hereditary cancer syndrome. For instance, in women who are at increased risk for developing ovarian cancer, the mortality rate associated with ovarian cancer and the lack of a reliable screening tool might make surveillance a less attractive option. For other cancers, chemoprevention might be an acceptable option, although chemopreventive agents may have adverse effects. Finally, prophylactic surgery should be considered, but only after its potential risks and benefits are discussed in detail.

You and colleagues [7] described five major criteria that should be met before the widespread use of prophylactic surgery is implemented for managing individuals with a genetic predisposition for cancer. Specifically, there should be a high penetrance (likelihood of developing cancer) associated with the mutation, a reliable genetic test to identify mutation carriers, an effective surgical procedure with low morbidity to remove the organ at risk, a suitable replacement for the function of the organ removed, and finally, a means to determine if the patient is disease-free over time.

Penetrance of disease

Ideally, individuals considered for prophylactic surgery should carry mutations with complete penetrance (100% chance of developing cancer). Mutations responsible for many of the hereditary cancer syndromes, however, generally have a high but incomplete penetrance. In the general population, the lifetime risk of breast and ovarian cancer is 12.7% and 1.4% respectively [8]. For BRCA1 and BRCA2 mutation carriers, however, the risk of breast cancer by age 80 is about 90% and 40%, respectively, and the corresponding risk for ovarian cancer is about 24% and 8% [9–11]. High-penetrance mutations also are associated with hereditary colon cancer syndromes. Almost 100% of individuals who carry the mutation for familial adenomatous polyposis (FAP) will develop colon cancer by age 50 [12], while those with hereditary nonpolyposis coli have a 70% to 82% lifetime risk of developing colon cancer [13]. Individuals who have the multiple endocrine neoplasia (MEN) 2 syndrome have almost a 100% risk of developing medullary thyroid cancer [14]. In individuals who carry the mutation for hereditary diffuse gastric cancer (HDGC) syndrome, the lifetime risk of gastric cancer is about 70% [15,16]. The cumulative risk of developing gastric cancer may vary between men and women, however, with a cumulative risk of gastric cancer by age 80 being 67% in men and 83% in women [17]. Although many mutations are associated with a high penetrance, complete penetrance never is observed. As a result, there always will be a certain number of mutation carriers who would not have developed cancer, but will be offered prophylactic surgery. Environmental and nongenetic factors may modify penetrance [18]. For example, in BRCA2 mutation carriers, pregnancy appears to increase breast cancer risk [19]. Age of menarche, spontaneous abortion, breast feeding, and oral contraceptive are additional factors that may modify penetrance in BRCA mutation carriers [18]. Modifying genes (genes which modify penetrance) also may alter cancer risk, and have been associated with hereditary breast and colon cancers [12,20,21]. In the future, these genes may help identify individuals who are at increased cancer risk and may benefit from prophylactic surgery.

Genetic testing

Genetic testing for cancer susceptibility is suitable if the test is associated with a high specificity and sensitivity. A genetic predisposition for hereditary cancer syndromes should be considered after careful assessment of clinical findings and family pedigree. In the early 1990s, linkage studies were undertaken to determine an individual's likelihood of having a genetic predisposition for hereditary cancer syndromes [22]. These studies paved the way for the discovery of mutations responsible for various hereditary cancer syndromes, thereby providing a more reliable means of identifying asymptomatic carriers. Despite the available technology, genetic testing for hereditary cancer syndromes remains a complex issue. Unlike other genetic diseases such as sickle cell anemia, hereditary cancer syndromes rarely are associated with a single gene mutation. In most cases, there are several mutations that may lead to a particular cancer, and commercial testing does not identify every mutation. Consider, for example, the case of hereditary breast cancer, often associated with mutations in the BRCA1 and BRCA2 tumor suppressor genes. Currently, genetic testing for BRCA1/2 mutations may identify up to 88% of all individuals who have a genetic predisposition for breast cancer, with false-negative results often attributed to other mutations, such as those in the p53, PTEN, STKll/LKB1, CDH1, and CHEK 2 genes [23,24]. Complete DNA sequencing may detect approximately 80% of all mutations in individuals who have FAP [25,26].

In some instances, there are only a limited number of gene mutations associated with a particular cancer, as evident in the association between the RET proto-oncogene and medullary thyroid cancer, and this simplifies genetic testing [3]. Although most genetic testing for cancer predisposition is highly reliable, it is not infallible, and interpretation of the results of these tests must be considered in light of these facts.

Approach to patient

Individuals who might potentially benefit from genetic testing should be selected carefully. A detailed family history should be obtained, and the patient's clinical history considered also. Before genetic testing, counseling is essential. The issues raised by genetic testing are complex and may have long-lasting implications for patients and their families. The implications of a positive, negative or inconclusive test should be discussed before testing. Studies have shown that patients handle the results of testing better if counseling occurs before testing [27–29]. In addition, the financial cost of testing should not be ignored, and concerns have been raised about the potential impact of genetic testing on overall health care costs [30]. Yet, very few studies have addressed these issues, and the impact of genetic testing and prophylactic surgery on health care costs in the United States is understood poorly. Cost analyses undertaken in countries with centralized (government-sponsored) health systems, however, indicate an overall positive benefit [31]. If one selects individuals who may benefit from genetic testing carefully, then this may improve the overall cost- effectiveness. The cost of genetic testing varies and may range from $200 to $3000 [32], but this does not include the cost of counseling, which is an essential component.

Many insurance companies indicate that they cover the cost of genetic testing, but others may not and are not required by law to do so [33]. If patients have to incur some of the cost of genetic testing, they are less likely to undergo testing. Also, given the cost of genetic testing services, these services are more likely to be used among patients in higher socioeconomic brackets [34]. Even though insurance companies generally cover the cost of genetic testing, some patients choose to bear the cost themselves. In a survey of genetic counselors, most indicated that they would not bill their insurance companies for fear of insurance discrimination [35]. A retrospective study examined reasons why women refused to undergo BRCA testing and found similar results. Of 78 women who declined testing, 48 cited concerns about discrimination [36]. There is clearly a widespread fear about the misuse of health care information by insurance companies, although this fear might not be justified [37]. Currently, many insurance companies do not seem to have standard protocols for dealing with patients who have hereditary cancer syndromes. Several years ago, Rodriguez-Bigas and colleagues [38] surveyed insurance companies regarding policies for insurance coverage in individuals who had at least a 50% chance of carrying a significant gene mutation. Most companies indicated that they did not use genetic test results in determining cost of insurance coverage, but only 7.7% of companies responded to the survey, making it difficult to draw any valid conclusions.

In addition to costs incurred from genetic testing, there are additional costs that must be considered if a patient is found to carry a mutation. These include the cost of surveillance, prophylactic surgery, or chemoprevention, should the patient choose any of these management options. As prophylactic surgery gains wider acceptance among mutation carriers, its financial burden on the health care system will have to be evaluated. In a survey of insurance coverage for prophylactic thyroidectomy in patients with familial thyroid cancer or a positive RET mutational analysis, most insurance companies indicated no standard policy. Of the private companies surveyed, 9% provided coverage, 12% provided no coverage, and 72% had no policy; government carriers had a similar pattern in coverage policy [39]. Another survey found similar results with respect to insurance coverage for prophylactic mastectomy or oophorectomy in patients who had BRCA mutations or those who had a strong family history of breast cancer [40]. In that survey, 481 medical directors from the American Association of Health Plans, Medicare, and Medicaid were queried, with a total of 150 respondents. Only 44% had a plan for coverage of prophylactic mastectomy in women who had a strong family history of breast cancer, and 38% had plans for coverage for women with BRCA mutations. Only 20% of those responding had a policy for coverage of prophylactic oophorectomy.

Several states have enacted laws that prohibit insurers' use of genetic information in pricing, issuing, or structuring of health insurance [41]. The enactment of these laws, however, does not seem to have allayed fears on this issue. As the use of genetic testing and prophylactic surgery increases, guidelines regarding insurance coverage and prevention of insurance discrimination will need to be developed. There is no doubt that, despite the availably of genetic testing, many high-risk individuals decide to forgo genetic testing. Although cost and fear of insurance discrimination might factor into their decision, the full reasons for this have not been well elucidated [42].

Timing of prophylactic surgery

There are several issues that should be considered when discussing the timing of prophylactic surgery. For example, alternative splicing of the APC gene may result in attenuated FAP, and these patients present with fewer polyps and at a later date than individuals who have classic FAP, which may influence the timing of prophylactic proctocolectomy. In MEN syndromes, mutations in the RET proto-oncogene generally result in the development of medullary thyroid cancer at a very early age, and thyroidectomy should be considered very early in life. Lastly, the timing of prophylactic surgery should be compatible with the life choices of the patient. Thus, women may choose to defer risk-reducing salpingo-oophorectomy (RRSO) until after childbearing.

Breast cancer

Genetics

Each year approximately 200,000 women in the United States develop breast cancer, with 5% to 10% of these cases occurring in women who have a genetic predisposition [43]. The most common of the hereditary breast cancer syndromes are caused by BRCA1 and BRCA2 mutations. The BRCA1 gene is located on chromosome 17, while BRCA2 is located on chromosome 13. Both are tumor suppressor genes, characterized in 1994 [44,45] and 1995 respectively [46,47].

BRCA-associated breast and ovarian cancer syndrome

The incidence of the BRCA1 and BRCA2 genes in the general population is 1 case in 150 to 800 individuals [48]. This incidence varies depending on geographic region and is higher in certain populations such as Ashkenazi Jews. Most of the studies done on hereditary breast cancer syndromes involve BRCA mutation carriers. Although both the BRCA1 and BRCA2 genes confer an increased risk of breast and ovarian cancer and often are considered together, there are significant differences between them, particularly with respect to phenotypic expression.

Surgical management

BRCA1 and BRCA2 mutation carriers have a high risk of developing breast cancer, but penetrance varies among different populations. In these mutation carriers, risk-reducing surgical options include bilateral prophylactic mastectomy (in women never diagnosed with breast cancer) and contralateral prophylactic mastectomy (in women already diagnosed with breast cancer). Both generally are performed with either immediate or delayed breast reconstruction. Lastly, prophylactic salpingo-oophorectomy should be considered in BRCA mutation carriers.

Risk-reducing salpingo-oophorectomy (RRSO) also appears to reduce breast cancer risk [49–51]. The magnitude of the risk reduction may vary, however, depending on the age at which this procedure is performed [52]. Rebbeck and colleagues studied 122 women who had BRCA1 mutations and found that these women experienced a significant reduction in the risk of breast cancer following RRSO [53]. These authors subsequently broadened their study to include a total of 551 women with BRCA1 and BRCA2 mutations, and found that RRSO reduced the risk of breast cancer by 53%. Furthermore, stage 1 ovarian cancers subsequently were diagnosed in only 2.3% of these women, and 0.8% received a diagnosis of serous peritoneal carcinoma within 3 years after RRSO. Thus, the risk of ovarian cancer was reduced by over 95% following RRSO [54]. In a more recent study, RRSO was associated with a significant risk reduction of BRCA2-associated breast cancers, and while there was a trend toward a reduced risk of breast cancers among BRCA1 mutation carriers, that risk reduction was not statistically significant [55]. Although RRSO in premenopausal BRCA mutation carriers reduces breast cancer risk, its consequences are not insignificant. The induction of menopause following RRSO may increase cardiovascular risk, osteoporosis, vaginal dryness, and sexual dysfunction. Additionally, it may result in cognitive changes. Hormone replacement therapy (HRT) has been used to treat menopausal symptoms associated with RRSO, but there are concerns that HRT may increase the risk of breast cancer and thereby decrease the utility of RRSO. Yet, in a Markov decision analysis model, RRSO in women between the ages of 30 and 40 was associated with a substantial increase in life expectancy, irrespective of HRT use [56].

In asymptomatic BRCA mutation carriers, bilateral prophylactic mastectomy (BPM) should be considered. Various studies have shown that BPM significantly decreases breast cancer risk, but there are no randomized prospective trials that have addressed this issue [57]. Meijers-Hejiboer and colleagues [58] conducted a prospective study of 139 women, and no breast cancers were seen in 76 women in the BPM group, while 8 out of 63 women in the surveillance group developed breast cancer. The mean length of follow-up in this study was only 3 years, however, making it difficult to assess the long-term benefit of BPM. Yet, additional studies that have included larger groups of women have found similar results [59]. In a large multicenter study looking at 483 women, BPM reduced the risk of breast cancer by 95% in women who also had an RRSO and by 90% in women who had intact ovaries [59]. Studies have shown that this benefit continues with longer follow-up, and several of these studies are summarized in Table 1 [60].

Women with BRCA1/2 mutations who develop breast cancer are also at increased risk of developing contralateral breast cancer, and estimates of this risk range from 20% to 42% [61–63]. In a retrospective study, Metcalfe and colleagues found that the incidence of contralateral breast cancer in BRCA mutation carriers was as high as 40% over a 10-year period, and

Table 1
Bilateral prophylactic mastectomy series in BRCA1 and BRCA2 carriers

Study	Number of patients	Number of patients with BRCA	Mean FU, years	Number of patients undergoing BPM	Number of BCs after BPM	Number of patients electing surveillance	Number of BCs during surveillance
Hartmann, et al [57]	214	26	13.4	26	0	NA	NA
Meijers-Heijboer, et al [58]	139	139	2.9	76	0	63	8
Rebbeck, et al [59]	483	483	6.4	105	2	378	184
Heemskerk-Gerritsen, et al [60]	358	236	4.5	177	1	NA	NA

Abbreviations: BC, breast cancer; BPM, bilateral prophylactic mastectomy; FU, follow up; NA, not applicable.

that risk was greater in BRCA1 mutation carriers than those who had BRCA2 mutations [64]. The risk of contralateral breast cancer was reduced if there was a history of oophorectomy or tamoxifen use. The dramatically increased risk of contralateral breast cancer in this population of women makes contralateral prophylactic mastectomy (CPM) an attractive option, and several studies have shown that CPM may reduce risk by about 90% [65]. BRCA1/2 mutation carriers who have a personal history of breast cancer are often particularly eager to discuss means of preventing development of a second primary. There are several factors, however, that may influence a woman's decision to proceed with CPM. Women who are younger at diagnosis, have opted for RRSO, and choose mastectomy (rather than breast-conserving therapy) as the surgical treatment for their initial breast cancer are more likely to opt for CPM [66]. Interestingly, Metcalfe and colleagues found that European and Israeli women were less likely to undergo CPM than North American women. This may reflect cultural differences or possibly differences in clinical practices between these countries.

There are several types of prophylactic mastectomy procedures available. Subcutaneous mastectomy is a nipple-sparing procedure that leaves some breast tissue behind. Skin-sparing mastectomy involves removal of almost all the breast tissue and nipple areola complex, but leaves most of the skin overlying the breast intact. Given that these procedures are prophylactic, axillary dissection generally is not indicated. The use of sentinel lymph node biopsy in these procedures might be considered, however, because some women occasionally are found to have occult cancers following prophylactic mastectomy. There have been reports that subcutaneous mastectomy is associated with an increased breast cancer risk, and skin-sparing mastectomy generally is considered the prophylactic procedure of choice [67]. Skin-sparing mastectomy facilitates breast reconstruction, which reduces the disfigurement associated with prophylactic mastectomy. In the past 20 years, the reconstructive options for patients undergoing mastectomy have increased. In addition to artificial breast implants, there are numerous tissue reconstruction options, including the traditional transverse rectus abdominis (TRAM) flap and the latissimus dorsi (LD) flap. Although the cosmetic results are improved, there might be a slightly increased risk of complications associated with reconstructive surgery, including an increased risk of infections and tissue necrosis.

Clearly, risk-reducing surgery is an important option to consider for managing patients who have hereditary breast cancer syndromes. Although there are no randomized controlled trials that have assessed its impact in mutation carriers, the studies outlined seem to indicate that prophylactic surgery is beneficial. Other management options (surveillance and chemoprevention), however, also should be discussed with the patient. Although prophylactic surgery reduces the risk of breast cancer, it does not eliminate it entirely. Women who undergo prophylactic surgery should continue to undergo surveillance.

Colon cancer

Genetics

It was not until the early 1990s that advances in molecular science made genetic testing for colon cancer syndromes possible. In 1993, the HNPCC locus was mapped to chromosome 2P [68]. In 1987, Bodmer and colleagues [69] localized the adenomatous polyposis coli (APC) gene to chromosome 5. This gene eventually was cloned in 1991 [70,71]. The details of the various mutations in the APC gene have been described, and these variations might be responsible for the variable phenotypic expression of FAP [72]. It is estimated that 20% of patients who have colorectal cancer have a genetic predisposition for this disease. Hereditary colon cancer can be divided into two main groups: those presenting with numerous polyps and those denoted by a lack of polyps.

Surgical management

Familial adenomatous polyposis

Familial adenomatous polyposis is the most common adenomatous syndrome. Classic FAP is associated with the development of multiple polyps (hundreds) at a very young age [73]. This syndrome also is associated with extracolonic manifestations, including upper GI polyps and cancers, congenital hypertrophy of the retinal pigment epithelium, desmoid tumors, thyroid tumors, hepatoblastomas in children, and other extracolonic malignancies [12,74]. Attenuated FAP is notable for a later age at presentation and fewer polyps. More recently, a non-APC gene-associated syndrome, MYH–familial polyposis syndrome, has been described [75,76]. As the lifetime risk of colon cancer in FAP approaches 100%, prophylactic surgery is recommended in these patients [7,77,78]. The prophylactic surgical options for FAP patients are subtotal colectomy with ileorectal anastomosis (IRA), proctocolectomy with ileal pouch anal anastomosis (IPAA), and finally proctocolectomy with permanent ileostomy. The timing of surgery remains ill-defined and may be influenced by the number of polyps [79]. Presentation remains too variable to give a definitive timing on surgery, but overall survival likely is improved if surgery is performed prophylactically [80,81]. In a review by Bertario and colleagues [80], patients without cancer at the time of surgery had a survival probability of 68% at 30 years compared with 41% at 10 years in those with cancer.

IPAA has become the preferred prophylactic surgical option in patients who have FAP. Although IRA eliminates the risk of cancer in the colon, there is still a risk of developing cancer in the rectum. Reports of this risk range from 4% to 8% at 10 years and 26% to 32% at 25 years [82,83]. Although IPAA lowers the risk of cancer in the rectum, it does not eliminate it entirely, because cancer still may occur at the transition zone [84]. In addition, there have been reports of polyps developing in the pouch [85]. No matter which prophylactic procedure is performed, lifelong surveillance is necessary and remains the only way to rule out disease over time.

The choice of procedure should be determined by the preferences of the patient and the quality of life (QOL) expected after surgery. Initial reports on the complications associated with IPAA include pelvic sepsis, high stool frequency, and fecal incontinence [86]. These complications have decreased with improvements in surgical technique, but there remains an increased perioperative morbidity associated with IPAA when compared with subtotal colectomy with IRA. A total proctocolectomy with permanent ileostomy is rarely necessary, and only in situations where a cancer is already present that involves the sphincter, poor baseline sphincter function, or when the frequency of daily stools might hamper a patient's lifestyle. In a review of 1895 patients evaluating surgical results and QOL after IPAA, pouch failure requiring pouch excision occurred in 4.1% of patients [87]. Incontinence, night seepage, and sexual dysfunction also were associated with this procedure.

Hereditary nonpolyposis colorectal cancer

HNPCC (Lynch syndrome) is an autosomal dominant disorder characterized by a predisposition to early onset colorectal cancer (primarily right-sided) and cancers of the endometrium, ovary, small intestine, hebatobiliary system, kidney, ureter, brain, skin, and pancreas [88,89]. The risk of rectal cancer, although low, is not negligible and has been estimated at 11% [90]. The penetrance of the HNPCC mutation is not as high as that of the FAP mutation, and HNPCC is associated with about an 80% lifetime risk of colorectal cancer [13,91]. Thus, surveillance with colonoscopy might be a more suitable management option in asymptomatic patients [92,93]. Prophylactic subtotal colectomy (with the rectum retained) and prophylactic proctocolectomy (removal of the entire colon to include the rectum) should also be considered as options for managing asymptomatic HNPCC patients, however, particularly those who are anxious or concerned about the safety of repeated colonoscopies. Given the choice between these two prophylactic surgical procedures, many patients may prefer subtotal colectomy with long-term surveillance of the rectum [74].

In HNPCC patients who go on to develop colon cancer (or an adenoma that cannot be resected endoscopically), the optimal extent of surgical resection has not been elucidated fully [94,95]. These patients are at increased risk for secondary colon cancers, so subtotal colectomy should be considered. Alternatively, some of these patients may choose a more limited segmental resection of the colon with frequent follow-up colonoscopies. Unfortunately, no studies have compared outcomes directly between these two surgical options. Nonetheless, it has been suggested that there might be a benefit to subtotal colectomy when compared with segmental resection. A Markov model evaluating the effect of subtotal colectomy versus segmental colectomy on life expectancy seemed to suggest that there was a benefit associated with subtotal colectomy, but this benefit decreased with age [96].

As mentioned previously, HNPCC patients are also at increased risk for the development of extracolonic malignancies, and much attention has focused on their increased risk for endometrial and ovarian cancers [80,95,97,98]. Thus, prophylactic hysterectomy and salpingo-oophorectomy often are recommended, as well as surveillance for other malignancies [92].

Multiple endocrine neoplasia type 2

Medullary thyroid cancer (MTC), although a less common form of thyroid cancer, has three main hereditary forms associated with MEN type 2: MEN 2A, MEN 2B, and familial medullary thyroid cancer (FMTC). MEN 2A is characterized by MTC, pheochromocytoma, and parathyroid hyperplasia. Hirschsprung's disease [99,100] and cutaneous lichen amyloidosis [101] also have been associated with MEN 2A infrequently. MEN 2B syndrome, while also characterized by MTC and pheochromocytoma, has neural gangliomas as an associated feature. All are characterized by an autosomal dominant inheritance pattern and, although highly penetrant, have variable expressivity. The development of pheochromocytoma and hyperparathyroidism in MEN 2A varies, with 42% to 50% of patients developing pheochromocytoma and 20% to 35% developing hyperparathyroidism [102]. Although hyperparathyroidism is not seen in MEN 2B, the incidence of pheochromocytoma is similar to that of MEN 2A. Almost 100% of all patients who have MEN 2A and 2B syndromes, however, will develop MTC in their lifetime.

Genetics

Multiple endocrine neoplasias type 2 are caused by germline mutations of the RET proto-oncogene. Initially, individuals with this syndrome were diagnosed by clinical history and family pedigree followed by linkage studies [22,103]. Linkage studies, although accurate, were tedious and required testing of at least two affected family members. The discovery that mutations in the RET proto-oncogene were associated with the MEN 2 syndrome, led to a reliable means of identifying carriers for this disease [104,105]. This genetic test has proved to be a highly sensitive means of identifying carriers for this disease [14,106]. The discovery that mutations in the RET proto-oncogene appear to cluster in certain specific regions of chromosome 10 helps explain the high sensitivity of this test [107]. Also, analysis of these mutations has revealed that genotype–phenotype correlations exist [108,109]. One of the most significant of these is the germline mutation in codon 918 of the RET proto-oncogene seen in MEN 2B. In these patients, MTC appears to present at a very early age, sometimes infancy, and appears more virulent.

Surgical management

Most patients who have MEN 2 will develop MTC during their lifetime, and prophylactic thyroidectomy should be considered at an early age. In patients who have MEN 2, MTC is usually multifocal and bilateral, and it can occur at an early age. Screening for MTC is accomplished by measuring baseline and stimulated calcitonin levels [110]. This is not an infallible method of identifying patients who have MTC, however. In a landmark study by Wells and colleagues [106], DNA analysis was used to identify individuals at risk for MEN 2A. Of those at risk, 13 children, (six with normal and seven with elevated calcitonin levels) underwent total thyroidectomy with central neck dissection and total parathyroidectomy with autotransplantation. All thyroid specimens in this study demonstrated C cell hyperplasia. All seven of the patients with elevated calcitonin levels had microscopic MTC, and two had macroscopic MTC. Of the six patients who had normal calcitonin levels, two had microscopic MTC, and one had macroscopic disease. Overall, 10 of the 13 patients had MTC, and lymph node dissection failed to identify nodal metastasis in all patients. An updated study by the same group, broadened to include 49 children with mutations in the RET proto-oncogene, produced similar results [111].

A larger study by Lips and colleagues [14] reported similar findings. In this study, DNA analysis was used to identify 61 of 80 carriers of the MEN 2A gene. Of these, 14 carriers who were children had normal calcitonin levels, and eight underwent total thyroidectomy. Small foci of MTC were seen in all eight specimens. Additional studies have shown consistently that despite normal calcitonin levels, prophylactic removal of the thyroid invariably shows either microscopic foci of MTC or C cell hyperplasia [112,113]. Given the high incidence of disease found in cases where surgery is performed in asymptomatic individuals, it might be said that surgical intervention is actually therapeutic and not prophylactic. Long-term follow-up studies have shown that asymptomatic carriers have a better chance of cure if surgery is performed at a very early age, preferably before 8 years of age [114]. The lack of chemopreventive options, combined with the poor chances of cure if disease is found, presents a strong argument for the use of prophylactic thyroidectomy in patients who test positive for the RET proto-oncogene. Experience appears to show that the sooner surgery is done the better. The low morbidity associated with total thyroidectomy (as well as the availability of Synthroid as replacement therapy) makes prophylactic surgery an even more attractive management option in these patients.

Hereditary diffuse gastric cancer

Genetics

Mutations in the CDH-1 (E-cadherin) gene are responsible for HDGC syndrome, initially described in Maori families [115–117]. HDGC is characterized by an autosomal dominant inheritance pattern with incomplete penetrance. Mutation carriers may develop gastric cancer at an early age, and women who carry this mutation also have a high incidence of invasive lobular breast cancer [17,118].

Prophylactic surgery

Prophylactic total gastrectomy with a Roux-en-Y esophagojejunostomy reconstruction often is recommended for individuals who carry the CDH-1 mutation [16]. Lewis and colleagues studied six asymptomatic carriers of the CDH-1 mutation who underwent prophylactic gastrectomy [119]. These individuals ranged from 22 to 40 years of age, and all were found to have occult foci of gastric cancer following detailed histologic assessment of the gastrectomy specimens. Similarly, Chun and colleagues [120] described five individuals from the same family with the CDH1 gene mutation who underwent prophylactic total gastrectomy with Roux-en-Y esophagojejunostomy, and occult gastric carcinoma again was found in all specimens. Chun and colleagues reported that all individuals in their study had undergone gastric endoscopy (with biopsies) before surgery, with no evidence of gastric cancer. Other series have reported similar results and these are summarized in Table 2. Thus, the situation with HDGC syndrome is similar to that of MEN 2 syndrome, in that asymptomatic individuals often are found to harbor occult cancer at the time of prophylactic surgery. There is considerable morbidity associated with total gastrectomy (eg, malnutrition and dumping syndrome), however, and patients should be made aware of this. Surveillance methods continue to evolve, and in a recent study, chromoendoscopy was found to facilitate the detection of early gastric carcinoma foci that were not visible with white light gastroscopy [123]. Although several authors recommend prophylactic gastrectomy at a young age in individuals who carry the mutation for HDGC, this should be done after other management options are discussed with the patient [15,78].

Summary

The ability to identify asymptomatic carriers of hereditary cancer syndromes through genetic testing has ushered in a new era in medicine. For all syndromes, management options fall into three categories: surveillance, chemoprevention, or prophylactic surgery. Deciding which option to follow

Table 2
Total gastrectomy series in CDH-1 mutation carriers

Study	Number of asymptomatic patients	Number with incidental gastric cancer	Age range of patients (years)
Lewis, et al [119]	6	6	22–40
Chun, et al [120]	5	5	37–47
Huntsman, et al [121]	5	5	22–40
Charlton, et al [122]	6	6	15–43

Table 3
Options for prophylactic surgical management of hereditary cancer syndromes

Hereditary cancer syndrome	Primary option	Secondary option
Hereditary breast and ovarian cancer syndrome (BRCA mutation carriers)	Bilateral mastectomy Prophylactic contralateral mastectomy in individuals already diagnosed with breast cancer Salpingo-oophorectomy	
FAP	Total proctocolectomy with ileal pouch anal anastomosis	Total proctocolectomy with permanent ileostomy
HNPCC	Subtotal colectomy with ileorectal anastomosis	
MEN type 2	Total thyroidectomy with or without central neck dissection	
HDGC	Total gastrectomy with Roux-en-Y esophagojejunostomy	

Abbreviations: FAP, familial adenomatous polyposis; HDGC, hereditary diffuse gastric cancer; HNPCC, hereditary nonpolyposis colon cancer; MEN, multiple endocrine neoplasias.

requires extensive counseling and discussions with the patient. Prophylactic surgery might be considered in three instances:

In those who undergo genetic testing and are found to carry a mutation
In individuals who test negative for a mutation but have a strong family history (testing does not cover all mutations)
In those who have a significant family history but do not undergo testing

Ideally, the latter should be a small group, and testing, if available, should be considered before risk-reducing surgery. The commonly accepted prophylactic surgical procedures for hereditary breast, colon, thyroid, and gastric cancers are outlined in Table 3. Prophylactic surgery is used increasingly for managing familial cancer syndromes and may reduce cancer risk significantly. Although there are no randomized prospective trials that have evaluated the efficacy of prophylactic surgery, current evidence indicates a benefit.

References

[1] American Cancer Society. Cancer facts and figures 2006. Available at: http://www.cancer.org/downloads/STT/CAFF2006PWSecured.pdf. Accessed March 20, 2008.
[2] Knudson AG Jr. Retinoblastoma: a prototypic hereditary neoplasm. Semin Oncol 1978; 5(1):57–60.
[3] Garber JE, Offit K. Hereditary cancer predisposition syndromes. J Clin Oncol 2005;23(2): 276–92.
[4] Warthin A. Heredity with reference to carcinoma. Arch Intern Med 1913;1:546–55.

[5] Lynch HT, et al. Hereditary factors in cancer. Study of two large Midwestern kindreds. Arch Intern Med 1966;117(2):206–12.
[6] Li FP. Molecular epidemiology studies of cancer in families. Br J Cancer 1993;68(2):217–9.
[7] You YN, Lakhani VT, Wells SA Jr. The role of prophylactic surgery in cancer prevention. World J Surg 2007;31(3):450–64.
[8] Ries LAG, Melbert D, Krapcho M, et al, editors. SEER Cancer Statistics Review, 1975-2005, National Cancer Institute. Bethesda, MD. Available at: http://seer.cancer.gov/csr/1975_2005/. Accessed March 20, 2008.
[9] Ford D, et al. Genetic heterogeneity and penetrance analysis of the BRCA1 and BRCA2 genes in breast cancer families. The Breast Cancer Linkage Consortium. Am J Hum Genet 1998;62(3):676–89.
[10] King MC, Marks JH, Mandell JB. Breast and ovarian cancer risks due to inherited mutations in BRCA1 and BRCA2. Science 2003;302(5645):643–6.
[11] Risch HA, et al. Population BRCA1 and BRCA2 mutation frequencies and cancer penetrances: a kin cohort study in Ontario, Canada. J Natl Cancer Inst 2006;98(23): 1694–706.
[12] Galiatsatos P, Foulkes WD. Familial adenomatous polyposis. Am J Gastroenterol 2006; 101(2):385–98.
[13] Annie Yu HJ, et al. Hereditary nonpolyposis colorectal cancer: preventive management. Cancer Treat Rev 2003;29(6):461–70.
[14] Lips C, et al. Clinical screening as compared with DNA analysis in families with multiple endocrine neoplasia type 2A. N Engl J Med 1994;331(13):828–35.
[15] Lynch HT, et al. Gastric cancer: new genetic developments. J Surg Oncol 2005;90(3):114–33 [discussion: 133].
[16] Caldas C, et al. Familial gastric cancer: overview and guidelines for management. J Med Genet 1999;36(12):873–80.
[17] Pharoah PD, Guilford P, Caldas C. Incidence of gastric cancer and breast cancer in CDH1 (E-cadherin) mutation carriers from hereditary diffuse gastric cancer families. Gastroenterology 2001;121(6):1348–53.
[18] Narod SA. Modifiers of risk of hereditary breast cancer. Oncogene 2006;25(43):5832–6.
[19] Cullinane CA, et al. Effect of pregnancy as a risk factor for breast cancer in BRCA1/BRCA2 mutation carriers. Int J Cancer 2005;117(6):988–91.
[20] Rebbeck TR, et al. Modification of BRCA1- and BRCA2-associated breast cancer risk by AIB1 genotype and reproductive history. Cancer Res 2001;61(14):5420–4.
[21] Runnebaum IB, et al. Progesterone receptor variant increases ovarian cancer risk in BRCA1 and BRCA2 mutation carriers who were never exposed to oral contraceptives. Pharmacogenetics 2001;11(7):635–8.
[22] Mathew CG, et al. Presymptomatic screening for multiple endocrine neoplasia type 2A with linked DNA markers. The MEN 2A International Collaborative Group. Lancet 1991; 337(8732):7–11.
[23] Available at: www.geneclinic.com. Accessed March 20, 2008.
[24] Walsh T, et al. Spectrum of mutations in BRCA1, BRCA2, CHEK2, and TP53 in families at high risk of breast cancer. JAMA 2006;295(12):1379–88.
[25] Rustgi AK. The genetics of hereditary colon cancer. Genes Dev 2007;21(20):2525–38.
[26] Barnetson RA, et al. Identification and survival of carriers of mutations in DNA mismatch-repair genes in colon cancer. N Engl J Med 2006;354(26):2751–63.
[27] American Society of Clinical Oncology policy statement update: genetic testing for cancer susceptibility. J Clin Oncol 2003;21(12):2397–406.
[28] Aktan-Collan K, et al. Psychological consequences of predictive genetic testing for hereditary non-polyposis colorectal cancer (HNPCC): a prospective follow-up study. Int J Cancer 2001;93(4):608–11.
[29] Jarvinen HJ. Genetic testing for polyposis: practical and ethical aspects. Gut 2003;52 (Suppl 2):ii19–22.

[30] Brown ML, Kessler LG. The use of gene tests to detect hereditary predisposition to cancer: economic considerations. J Natl Cancer Inst 1995;87(15):1131–6.
[31] Griffith GL, Edwards RT, Gray J. Cancer genetics services: a systematic review of the economic evidence and issues. Br J Cancer 2004;90(9):1697–703.
[32] Available at: http://www.ornl.gov/sci/techresources/Human_Genome/medicine/genetest.shtml. Accessed March 20, 2008.
[33] Johnson A. National conference of State Legislature. Genetics Brief Issue No VII June 2002. Available at: http://www.ncsl.org/programs/health/genetics/Geneticshealthins.pdf. Accessed March 20, 2008.
[34] Steel M, et al. Ethical, social and economic issues in familial breast cancer: a compilation of views from the E.C. Biomed II Demonstration Project. Dis Markers 1999;15(1–3):125–31.
[35] Matloff ET, et al. What would you do? Specialists' perspectives on cancer genetic testing, prophylactic surgery, and insurance discrimination. J Clin Oncol 2000;18(12):2484–92.
[36] Peterson EA, et al. Health insurance and discrimination concerns and BRCA1/2 testing in a clinic population. Cancer Epidemiol Biomarkers Prev 2002;11(1):79–87.
[37] Hall MA, Rich SS. Patients' fear of genetic discrimination by health insurers: the impact of legal protections. Genet Med 2000;2(4):214–21.
[38] Rodriguez-Bigas MA, et al. Health, life, and disability insurance and hereditary nonpolyposis colorectal cancer. Am J Hum Genet 1998;62(3):736–7.
[39] Dackiw AP, Kuerer HM, Clark OH. Current national health insurance policies for thyroid cancer prophylactic surgery in the United States. World J Surg 2002;26(8):903–6.
[40] Kuerer HM, et al. Current national health insurance coverage policies for breast and ovarian cancer prophylactic surgery. Ann Surg Oncol 2000;7(5):325–32.
[41] Hall MA. Legal rules and industry norms: the impact of laws restricting health insurers' use of genetic information. Jurimetrics 1999;40(1):93–122.
[42] Ramsoekh D, et al. The use of genetic testing in hereditary colorectal cancer syndromes: genetic testing in HNPCC, (A)FAP, and MAP. Clin Genet 2007;72(6):562–7.
[43] Pharoah PD, et al. Polygenic susceptibility to breast cancer and implications for prevention. Nat Genet 2002;31(1):33–6.
[44] Hall JM, et al. Linkage of early onset familial breast cancer to chromosome 17q21. Science 1990;250(4988):1684–9.
[45] Miki Y, et al. A strong candidate for the breast and ovarian cancer susceptibility gene BRCA1. Science 1994;266(5182):66–71.
[46] Wooster R, et al. Localization of a breast cancer susceptibility gene, BRCA2, to chromosome 13q12-13. Science 1994;265(5181):2088–90.
[47] Wooster R, et al. Identification of the breast cancer susceptibility gene BRCA2. Nature 1995;378(6559):789–92.
[48] Whittemore AS, Gong G, Itnyre J. Prevalence and contribution of BRCA1 mutations in breast cancer and ovarian cancer: results from three US population-based case–control studies of ovarian cancer. Am J Hum Genet 1997;60(3):496–504.
[49] Meijer WJ, van Lindert AC. Prophylactic oophorectomy. Eur J Obstet Gynecol Reprod Biol 1992;47(1):59–65.
[50] Parazzini F, et al. Hysterectomy, oophorectomy in premenopause, and risk of breast cancer. Obstet Gynecol 1997;90(3):453–6.
[51] Schairer C, et al. Breast cancer risk associated with gynecologic surgery and indications for such surgery. Int J Cancer 1997;70(2):150–4.
[52] Struewing JP, et al. Prophylactic oophorectomy in inherited breast/ovarian cancer families. J Natl Cancer Inst Monogr 1995;(17):33–5.
[53] Rebbeck TR, et al. Breast cancer risk after bilateral prophylactic oophorectomy in BRCA1 mutation carriers. J Natl Cancer Inst 1999;91(17):1475–9.
[54] Rebbeck TR. Prophylactic oophorectomy in BRCA1 and BRCA2 mutation carriers. Eur J Cancer 2002;38(Suppl 6):S15–7.

[55] Kauff ND, et al. Risk-Reducing Salpingo-Oophorectomy for the Prevention of BRCA1- and BRCA2-Associated Breast and Gynecologic Cancer: A Multicenter, Prospective Study. J Clin Oncol 2008;26(8):1331–7.
[56] Armstrong K, et al. Hormone replacement therapy and life expectancy after prophylactic oophorectomy in women with BRCA1/2 mutations: a decision analysis. J Clin Oncol 2004;22(6):1045–54.
[57] Hartmann LC, et al. Efficacy of bilateral prophylactic mastectomy in BRCA1 and BRCA2 gene mutation carriers. J Natl Cancer Inst 2001;93(21):1633–7.
[58] Meijers-Heijboer H, et al. Breast cancer after prophylactic bilateral mastectomy in women with a BRCA1 or BRCA2 mutation. N Engl J Med 2001;345(3):159–64.
[59] Rebbeck TR, et al. Bilateral prophylactic mastectomy reduces breast cancer risk in BRCA1 and BRCA2 mutation carriers: the PROSE study group. J Clin Oncol 2004; 22(6):1055–62.
[60] Heemskerk-Gerritsen BA, et al. Prophylactic mastectomy in BRCA1/2 mutation carriers and women at risk of hereditary breast cancer: long-term experiences at the Rotterdam Family Cancer Clinic. Ann Surg Oncol 2007;14(12):3335–44.
[61] Pierce LJ, et al. Ten-year multi-institutional results of breast-conserving surgery and radiotherapy in BRCA1/2-associated stage I/II breast cancer. J Clin Oncol 2006;24(16): 2437–43.
[62] Chappuis PO, et al. Germline BRCA1/2 mutations and p27(Kip1) protein levels independently predict outcome after breast cancer. J Clin Oncol 2000;18(24):4045–52.
[63] Haffty BG, et al. Outcome of conservatively managed early onset breast cancer by BRCA1/2 status. Lancet 2002;359(9316):1471–7.
[64] Metcalfe K, et al. Contralateral breast cancer in BRCA1 and BRCA2 mutation carriers. J Clin Oncol 2004;22(12):2328–35.
[65] van Sprundel TC, et al. Risk reduction of contralateral breast cancer and survival after contralateral prophylactic mastectomy in BRCA1 or BRCA2 mutation carriers. Br J Cancer 2005;93(3):287–92.
[66] Metcalfe KA, et al. Predictors of contralateral prophylactic mastectomy in women with a BRCA1 or BRCA2 mutation: the Hereditary Breast Cancer Clinical Study Group. J Clin Oncol 2008;26(7):1093–7.
[67] Horiguchi J, et al. Recurrence of breast cancer following local excision alone for ductal carcinoma in situ. Breast Cancer 2001;8(1):52–7.
[68] Peltomaki P, et al. Genetic mapping of a locus predisposing to human colorectal cancer. Science 1993;260(5109):810–2.
[69] Bodmer WF, et al. Localization of the gene for familial adenomatous polyposis on chromosome 5. Nature 1987;328(6131):614–6.
[70] Kinzler KW, et al. Identification of an amplified, highly expressed gene in a human glioma. Science 1987;236(4797):70–3.
[71] Groden J, et al. Identification and characterization of the familial adenomatous polyposis coli gene. Cell 1991;66(3):589–600.
[72] Spirio L, et al. Alleles of the APC gene: an attenuated form of familial polyposis. Cell 1993; 75(5):951–7.
[73] Campbell WJ, Spence RA, Parks TG. Familial adenomatous polyposis. Br J Surg 1994; 81(12):1722–33.
[74] Rodriguez-Bigas MA, Chang GJ, Skibber JM. Surgical implications of colorectal cancer genetics. Surg Oncol Clin N Am 2006;15(1):51–66, vi.
[75] Al-Tassan N, et al. Inherited variants of MYH associated with somatic G:C→T:A mutations in colorectal tumors. Nat Genet 2002;30(2):227–32.
[76] Sampson JR, et al. Autosomal recessive colorectal adenomatous polyposis due to inherited mutations of MYH. Lancet 2003;362(9377):39–41.
[77] Guillem JG, et al. ASCO/SSO review of current role of risk-reducing surgery in common hereditary cancer syndromes. J Clin Oncol 2006;24(28):4642–60.

[78] Bertagnolli MM. Surgical prevention of cancer. J Clin Oncol 2005;23(2):324–32.
[79] Debinski HS, et al. Colorectal polyp counts and cancer risk in familial adenomatous polyposis. Gastroenterology 1996;110(4):1028–30.
[80] Bertario L, et al. Causes of death and postsurgical survival in familial adenomatous polyposis: results from the Italian Registry. Italian Registry of Familial Polyposis Writing Committee. Semin Surg Oncol 1994;10(3):225–34.
[81] Church J, Simmang C. Practice parameters for the treatment of patients with dominantly inherited colorectal cancer (familial adenomatous polyposis and hereditary nonpolyposis colorectal cancer). Dis Colon Rectum 2003;46(8):1001–12.
[82] Vasen HF, et al. Molecular genetic tests as a guide to surgical management of familial adenomatous polyposis. Lancet 1996;348(9025):433–5.
[83] Bertario L, et al. Genotype and phenotype factors as determinants for rectal stump cancer in patients with familial adenomatous polyposis. Hereditary Colorectal Tumors Registry. Ann Surg 2000;231(4):538–43.
[84] Remzi FH, et al. Dysplasia of the anal transitional zone after ileal pouch–anal anastomosis: results of prospective evaluation after a minimum of ten years. Dis Colon Rectum 2003; 46(1):6–13.
[85] Parc YR, et al. Familial adenomatous polyposis: prevalence of adenomas in the ileal pouch after restorative proctocolectomy. Ann Surg 2001;233(3):360–4.
[86] Setti-Carraro P, et al. The first 10 years' experience of restorative proctocolectomy for ulcerative colitis. Gut 1994;35(8):1070–5.
[87] Delaney CP, et al. Prospective, age-related analysis of surgical results, functional outcome, and quality of life after ileal pouch-anal anastomosis. Ann Surg 2003;238(2):221–8.
[88] Watson P, Riley B. The tumor spectrum in the Lynch syndrome. Fam Cancer 2005;4(3): 245–8.
[89] Fitzgibbons RJ Jr, et al. Recognition and treatment of patients with hereditary nonpolyposis colon cancer (Lynch syndromes I and II). Ann Surg 1987;206(3):289–95.
[90] Rodriguez-Bigas MA, et al. Rectal cancer risk in hereditary nonpolyposis colorectal cancer after abdominal colectomy. International Collaborative Group on HNPCC. Ann Surg 1997;225(2):202–7.
[91] Guillem JG, et al. Gastrointestinal polyposis syndromes. Curr Probl Surg 1999;36(4): 217–323.
[92] Lindor NM, et al. Recommendations for the care of individuals with an inherited predisposition to Lynch syndrome: a systematic review. JAMA 2006;296(12):1507–17.
[93] Jarvinen HJ, et al. Controlled 15-year trial on screening for colorectal cancer in families with hereditary nonpolyposis colorectal cancer. Gastroenterology 2000;118(5): 829–34.
[94] Van Dalen R, et al. Patterns of surgery in patients belonging to Amsterdam-positive families. Dis Colon Rectum 2003;46(5):617–20.
[95] Lin KM, et al. Cumulative incidence of colorectal and extracolonic cancers in MLH1 and MSH2 mutation carriers of hereditary nonpolyposis colorectal cancer. J Gastrointest Surg 1998;2(1):67–71.
[96] de Vos tot Nederveen Cappel WH, et al. Decision analysis in the surgical treatment of colorectal cancer due to a mismatch repair gene defect. Gut 2003;52(12):1752–5.
[97] Vasen HF, et al. Cancer risk in families with hereditary nonpolyposis colorectal cancer diagnosed by mutation analysis. Gastroenterology 1996;110(4):1020–7.
[98] Lin KM, et al. Colorectal and extracolonic cancer variations in MLH1/MSH2 hereditary nonpolyposis colorectal cancer kindreds and the general population. Dis Colon Rectum 1998;41(4):428–33.
[99] Romeo G, et al. Point mutations affecting the tyrosine kinase domain of the RET protooncogene in Hirschsprung's disease. Nature 1994;367(6461):377–8.
[100] Cohen MS, et al. Gastrointestinal manifestations of multiple endocrine neoplasia type 2. Ann Surg 2002;235(5):648–54 [discussion: 654–5].

[101] Gagel RF, et al. Multiple endocrine neoplasia type 2a associated with cutaneous lichen amyloidosis. Ann Intern Med 1989;111(10):802–6.
[102] Brandi ML, et al. Guidelines for diagnosis and therapy of MEN type 1 and type 2. J Clin Endocrinol Metab 2001;86(12):5658–71.
[103] Simpson NE, et al. Assignment of multiple endocrine neoplasia type 2A to chromosome 10 by linkage. Nature 1987;328(6130):528–30.
[104] Donis-Keller H, et al. Mutations in the RET proto-oncogene are associated with MEN 2A and FMTC. Hum Mol Genet 1993;2(7):851–6.
[105] Mulligan LM, et al. Germ-line mutations of the RET proto-oncogene in multiple endocrine neoplasia type 2A. Nature 1993;363(6428):458–60.
[106] Wells SA Jr, et al. Predictive DNA testing and prophylactic thyroidectomy in patients at risk for multiple endocrine neoplasia type 2A. Ann Surg 1994;220(3):237–47 [discussion: 247–50].
[107] Eng C, et al. The relationship between specific RET proto-oncogene mutations and disease phenotype in multiple endocrine neoplasia type 2. International RET mutation consortium analysis. JAMA 1996;276(19):1575–9.
[108] Mulligan LM, et al. Specific mutations of the RET proto-oncogene are related to disease phenotype in MEN 2A and FMTC. Nat Genet 1994;6(1):70–4.
[109] Eng C, Mulligan LM. Mutations of the RET proto-oncogene in the multiple endocrine neoplasia type 2 syndromes, related sporadic tumours, and Hirschsprung disease. Hum Mutat 1997;9(2):97–109.
[110] Vasen HF, et al. Multiple endocrine neoplasia syndrome type 2: the value of screening and central registration. A study of 15 kindreds in The Netherlands. Am J Med 1987;83(5): 847–52.
[111] Skinner MA, et al. Medullary thyroid carcinoma in children with multiple endocrine neoplasia types 2A and 2B. J Pediatr Surg 1996;31(1):177–81 [discussion: 181–2].
[112] Frilling A, et al. Presymptomatic DNA screening in families with multiple endocrine neoplasia type 2 and familial medullary thyroid carcinoma. Surgery 1995;118(6): 1099–103 [discussion: 1103–4].
[113] Pacini F, et al. Early treatment of hereditary medullary thyroid carcinoma after attribution of multiple endocrine neoplasia type 2 gene carrier status by screening for ret gene mutations. Surgery 1995;118(6):1031–5.
[114] Skinner MA, et al. Prophylactic thyroidectomy in multiple endocrine neoplasia type 2A. N Engl J Med 2005;353(11):1105–13.
[115] Guilford P, et al. E-cadherin germline mutations in familial gastric cancer. Nature 1998; 392(6674):402–5.
[116] Gayther SA, et al. Identification of germline E-cadherin mutations in gastric cancer families of European origin. Cancer Res 1998;58(18):4086–9.
[117] Brooks-Wilson AR, et al. Germline E-cadherin mutations in hereditary diffuse gastric cancer: assessment of 42 new families and review of genetic screening criteria. J Med Genet 2004;41(7):508–17.
[118] Kaurah P, et al. Founder and recurrent CDH1 mutations in families with hereditary diffuse gastric cancer. JAMA 2007;297(21):2360–72.
[119] Lewis FR, et al. Prophylactic total gastrectomy for familial gastric cancer. Surgery 2001; 130(4):612–7 [discussion: 617–9].
[120] Chun YS, et al. Germline E-cadherin gene mutations: is prophylactic total gastrectomy indicated? Cancer 2001;92(1):181–7.
[121] Huntsman DG, et al. Early gastric cancer in young, asymptomatic carriers of germline E-cadherin mutations. N Engl J Med 2001;344(25):1904–9.
[122] Charlton A, et al. Hereditary diffuse gastric cancer: predominance of multiple foci of signet ring cell carcinoma in distal stomach and transitional zone. Gut 2004;53(6):814–20.
[123] Shaw D, et al. Chromoendoscopic surveillance in hereditary diffuse gastric cancer: an alternative to prophylactic gastrectomy? Gut 2005;54(4):461–8.

Hereditary Diffuse Gastric Cancer: Prophylactic Surgical Oncology Implications

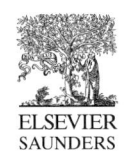

Henry T. Lynch, MD[a], Edibaldo Silva, MD, PhD[b],
Debrah Wirtzfeld, MD[c], Pamela Hebbard, MD[c],
Jane Lynch, BSN[a], David G. Huntsman, MD[d,e],*

[a]*Department of Preventive Medicine and Public Health, Creighton University School of Medicine, 2500 California Plaza, Omaha, NE 68178, USA*
[b]*Cancer Center, Creighton University Medical Center, 601 North 30th Street, Omaha, NE 68131, USA*
[c]*Memorial University of Newfoundland, PO Box 4200, St. John's, NL A1C 5S7, Canada*
[d]*University of British Columbia, Wesbrook Mall, Vancouver, BC V6T 2B5, Canada*
[e]*Department of Pathology, British Columbia Cancer Agency, 600 W 10th Avenue, Vancouver, BC V5Z 1L3, Canada*

Gastric cancer is the second most common cause of cancer death worldwide [1]. Its estimated incidence in the United States for 2008 is 21,500 with a mortality of 10,880 [2]. Gastric cancer is comprised of two major types [1,3]: (1) intestinal, which is the more common variant and which has a strong association with environmental factors, including cigarette smoking, dietary factors (particularly salted foods), and *Helicobacter pylori* [1], and (2) diffuse gastric cancer (DGC), which is less common than the intestinal type but is more likely to be attributed to host-factor effects [3].

This article was supported by revenue from Nebraska cigarette taxes awarded to Creighton University by the Nebraska Department of Health and Human Services. Its contents are solely the responsibility of the authors and do not necessarily represent the official views of the State of Nebraska or the Nebraska Department of Health and Human Services.

Support also was given by the National Institutes of Health through grant #1U01 CA 86389.

Dr. Lynch's work is funded in part through the Charles F. and Mary C. Heider Chair in Cancer Research, which he holds at Creighton University. Dr. Huntsman's work is funded by the Canadian Cancer Society.

* Corresponding author.
E-mail address: dhuntsma@bccancer.bc.ca (D.G. Huntsman).

Hereditary diffuse gastric cancer (HDGC) initially was described in 1964 in three Maori families from New Zealand [4]. It is an autosomal dominantly inherited syndrome attributed to mutations of the *E-cadherin* gene (*CDH1*, epithelial cadherin, OMIM#19,209), identified by Guilford and colleagues [5] in 1998 in members of these Maori families. Approximately 40% of well-defined HDGC families may be found to harbor this mutation [6]. Women carrying the mutation also have an increased lifetime risk of lobular carcinoma of the breast [7,8].

Knowledge of a patient's *CDH1* mutation carrier status provides a level of certainty of DGC expression limited only by its reduced penetrance, which is estimated to be in the range of 70% [6,9,10]. This reduced penetrance, along with the variable age of DGC onset, becomes a factor of extreme importance in patients' decision making when being counseled about the decision for prophylactic total gastrectomy [9].

The wide variability in age of onset within and among HDGC families may heavily influence the age at which prophylactic total gastrectomy should be given serious consideration. In the authors' experience, the average age of onset of HDGC has been 38 years, but it may range from 16 to 82 years [6]. Such variation in age of onset of DGC poses a challenge to genetic counselors and clinical geneticists when discussing genetic testing in concert with the timing of prophylactic total gastrectomy. Complex medical, ethical, psychologic, and medicolegal ramifications (eg, the level of the patient's understanding) influence decisions for both testing and surgery [11].

The identification of unaffected *CDH1* mutation carriers

The identification of families that have HDGC usually is prompted by a case of DGC occurring in an individual less than 50 years old. In 1999, the International Gastric Cancer Linkage Consortium proposed the following criteria for identifying families as candidates for *CDH1* genetic testing: "(1) two or more documented cases of diffuse gastric cancer in first/second degree relatives, with at least one diagnosed before the age of 50, or (2) three or more cases of documented diffuse gastric cancer in first/second degree relatives, independently of age of onset" [12]. An estimated mutation detection rate of 25% was suggested for such families [12]. The HDGC research program from the British Columbia Cancer Agency has modified the criteria to make them easier to use in environments in which obtaining pathologic confirmation on multiple families is difficult [6]. All criteria with an expected mutation detection rate are shown in Box 1.

The common criteria for identifying mutation-positive families are two or more cases of gastric cancer, with at least one case of DGC diagnosed before the age of 50 years [6,8,13,14]. The authors have found mutations in 46% (38/83) of families meeting these criteria (D. Huntsman, unpublished data, 2008). These mutations include nonsense, frame-shift, splicing, and missense

Box 1. Testing criteria

Modified testing criteria[a]
1. Family with two or more cases of gastric cancer, with at least one case of diffuse gastric cancer diagnosed before the age of 50 years (46%: 38/83)
2. Family with multiple cases of lobular carcinoma of the breast with or without diffuse gastric cancer in first- or second-degree relatives (23%: 3/13)
3. Isolated individual diagnosed with diffuse gastric cancer at age less than 35 years from a low-incidence population (10%: 3/31)

Potential additional criteria
4. Personal history but no family history of diffuse gastric cancer or lobular carcinoma of the breast (unknown)
5. Family with three or more cases of gastric cancer diagnosed at any age, one or more of which is a documented case of diffuse gastric cancer; no other criteria met (3%: 1/30)
6. Family with one or more cases of both diffuse gastric cancer and signet ring colon cancer (33%: 1/3)[b]

[a] Percentage of expected positive results based on the experience of the British Columbia Cancer Agency Hereditary Diffuse Gastric Cancer Program.
[b] This association is unproven.

mutations, and the authors currently are searching for nontraditional mutations that could account for some of the mutation-negative cases. Although these testing criteria are readily applicable to North America or northern Europe, they would lead to a much lower rate of mutation detection if used in populations with a higher background incidence of gastric cancer. After the family history has been confirmed and pretest genetic counseling has been given, genetic testing can be undertaken. A blood sample from an affected member of a prospective kindred is the best substrate for index testing. If that sample is not available, testing an obligate carrier is a reasonable alternative. Often, because this disease is rapidly lethal, no living affected individuals are available for testing. The remaining options include testing DNA extracted from archival paraffin blocks from an affected family member or testing unaffected first-degree relatives. The former option is problematic, because the DNA quality often is not sufficient for easy screening of a whole gene. Such blocks can be used to confirm mutations identified in unaffected at-risk relatives.

After the ascertainment of the proband's DNA sample, primary screening can be accomplished by two different approaches, namely, mutation scanning with a method such as denaturing high-performance liquid chromatography (DHPLC) [13] or direct sequencing [15]. Because DHLPC can be used only as an initial screening method, samples that exhibit aberrant DHPLC chromatograms still must undergo direct sequencing to identify the exact mutation. Once a family mutation has been identified, it is simple to set up a mutation-specific assay to assess the mutation status of family members [6].

Inadequacies of screening for diffuse gastric cancer

The medical, pathologic, and surgical literature shows an extraordinarily high rate of metastasis of DGC with frequent mortality when symptoms appear [16,17]. Knowledge of HDGC's natural history has led to a recommendation for prophylactic total gastrectomy among *CDH1* germline mutation carriers to reduce the risk of cancer morbidity and mortality [18]. The major clinical problem involving patients who have HDGC who are *CDH1* mutation carriers, which mandates consideration of prophylactic total gastrectomy, is the lack of effective DGC screening to allow an early, life-saving diagnosis. This problem is a consequence of the submucosal expression of the signet cell cancer pathology in DGC, which severely limits the ability to detect DGC sufficiently early in its clinical pathologic course to provide life-saving benefit to the high-risk *CDH1* mutation carrier. Because of this screening deficit, surgical extirpation of the entire stomach before DGC metastasis takes place seems to be the only way to achieve potential curative benefit to the patient at this time.

Lewis and colleagues [17] were among the first investigators to recommend prophylactic total gastrectomy for patients who had HDGC and the *CDH1* mutation. This recommendation was based on the finding of occult DGC in the prophylactic gastrectomy samples of six asymptomatic members of two families: two men and four women, with ages ranging from 22 to 40 years [19]. The prophylactic surgical procedure involved total gastrectomy using an upper midline incision with reconstruction of the gastrointestinal tract via a Roux-en-Y esophagojejunostomy. The complete removal of all gastric mucosa was documented intraoperatively, and it was confirmed that only esophageal mucosa remained at the proximal specimen margin. Each of the *CDH1*-positive patients underwent 150 to 250 tissue-block examinations, and all showed microscopic foci of cancer, frequently at multiple sites. Importantly, the overlying normal gastric mucosa was identified. They concluded that "Familial gastric cancer is a new disease for which prophylactic surgery must be considered. The morbidity of this operation is much higher than that for other genetic diseases, but the alternative is a mortality risk of more than 80% at a young age."

Subsequently, Norton and colleagues [16] studied a large HDGC family that had the *CDH1* cancer-causing mutation. Six of the patients (two men and four women) with a mean age of 54 years (range, 51–57 years) were identified as *CDH1* mutation carriers. Each underwent comprehensive cancer screening that included stool occult blood testing, standard upper gastrointestinal endoscopy with random gastric biopsies, high-magnification endoscopy, endoscopic ultrasonography, CT, and positron-emission tomography (PET) scans for evaluation of the stomach for occult cancer. This screening was followed by "total gastrectomy with D-2 node dissection and Roux-en-y esophago-jejunostomy. The stomach and resected lymph nodes were evaluated pathologically."

> None of these individuals showed signs or symptoms of gastric cancer. Although preoperative gastric findings were normal in each patient, with normal gastric and adjacent lymph nodes at surgery.

Each patient (6 of 6, 100%) was found to have multiple foci of T1 invasive diffuse gastric adenocarcinoma (pure signet-ring cell type). No patient had lymph node or distant metastases. Each was staged as T1N0M0. Each patient recovered uneventfully without morbidity or mortality.

The presence of the mutation identified patients manifesting cancer before detectable symptoms or signs of HDGC. These six unaffected mutation carriers came from an extended family in which 11 first cousins underwent prophylactic gastrectomy. In this family, the decision to undergo prophylactic surgery was eased greatly for these cousins, each of whom harbored the *CDH1* mutation, because most of them had witnessed a parent die as a result of the progressive course of DGC. When told that there was an approximately 30% chance that they would not develop DGC, because of its reduced penetrance, this information temporarily influenced the decision making of some members of the cohort, as evidenced by such statements as, "If they can beat it, why can't I?" Others reasoned that this knowledge could help them delay making the decision to have surgery. Knowing, however, that they harbored the deleterious mutation, they knew that they had to resolve these cancer probabilities, which they clearly realized mathematically favored their eventual development of DGC. They also learned through the program's educational genetic counseling program and the family information service [20] that available DGC screening procedures were wholly inadequate [21].

The DGCs detected in these and other prophylactic gastrectomies almost invariably have been minute, with many measuring less than 1 mm in diameter [22]. Because the cancers are minute and underlie normal gastric mucosa, their invisibility to endoscopy is understandable. The rate of progression of the microscopic lesions to metastatic and thus potentially lethal DGC is not known, and it is possible that some of these early DGC lesions could be indolent. The natural history and biology of these lesions is an area of active study [23]. Even if some of the microscopic DGCs detected in these gastrectomies have little metastatic potential, this possibility should not affect decision making, because the penetrance for invasive, clinically relevant gastric cancer in mutation carriers is 70%.

An important positive aspect of this cohort's decision-making process was the psychologic support they provided one another and the family commitment to help each other [20]. A very strong sense of solidarity emerged among these cousins about the importance of prophylactic gastrectomy; this camaraderie pervaded the genetic counseling sessions dealing with these high-risk individuals [24].

Once armed with facts about the natural history of DGC, many family members told the researchers that, in essence, the only decision left to them was when the prophylactic gastrectomy should be performed. Knowing that their prognosis would become extremely grave once DGC symptoms became manifest, all 11 of these first cousins decided to undergo prophylactic surgery, most within a couple of years of receiving their positive *CDH1* mutation results [24]. Ten of the 11 manifested submucosal foci of DGC in their stomach specimens.

The newfoundland experience with prophylactic surgery in hereditary diffuse gastric cancer

Perhaps the largest single institution experience with total prophylactic gastrectomy has taken place in Newfoundland (D.P. Hebbard, unpublished data, 2008). Several of the families that had *CDH1* mutations in that Canadian province have been documented previously [6]. To date, 17 affected individuals from these families have opted for prophylactic total gastrectomy. Ten patients were men, and seven were women; the average age was 45 years.

Preoperative evaluation

The process of considering prophylactic total gastrectomy began with patients' assessment in a medical genetics clinic. After appropriate counseling and confirmatory genetic testing, patients wishing to consider prophylactic gastrectomy were referred to one of two fellowship-trained surgical oncologists. The risks and benefits of surgery were discussed in detail. Patients must understand the potential complications including hemorrhage, anastomotic leak and/or stricture, cardiopulmonary concerns, and the low, but present, risk of death that this procedure carries. With the assistance of a dietician, they were counseled on a postgastrectomy diet, expected weight loss, and potential metabolic consequences including vitamin B_{12}, iron, thiamine, and zinc deficiencies.

Preoperative medical work-up began with a detailed history and physical examination with attention to any medical comorbidities. All patients to date have been in good health. Patients then underwent esophagogastroduodenoscopy with at least 15 random biopsies of the antrum, incisura, fundus, and body, because no gross mucosal abnormalities had been noted. Delineation of the gastroesophageal junction and the presence/absence of hiatal herniation were noted also. Random biopsies revealed microscopic foci of adenocarcinoma in one patient. Fourteen patients had colonoscopy and preoperative abdominal CT scans; none had evidence of malignancy. Patients then were sent to the preadmission clinic for anesthesia consultation and routine preoperative laboratory tests.

Operative details

All patients were admitted to hospital on the day of surgery. The average surgical time was 244 minutes (range, 120–580 minutes). Estimated blood loss was 1000 mL (range, 400–3000 mL), with three patients requiring blood transfusion of one to two units of red blood cells. One patient had gastric mucosa that extended into the chest identified by frozen-section evaluation of the proximal gastric margin. This finding required conversion to a thoracoabdominal approach. One patient had an intraoperative complication requiring right hemicolectomy for a devascularized colon. Postoperatively, 15 patients went to the general surgical floor, and 2 went to the ICU.

Postoperative details

The median length of hospital stay was 13 days (mean, 25 days; range, 10–107 days). There were no perioperative deaths or cardiovascular complications.

There were two anastomotic leaks with intra-abdominal abscesses. Both patients required operative drainage for definitive treatment. Three other patients had subclinical anastomotic leaks found on routine gastrograffin swallow performed on or about postoperative day 7. All were treated conservatively by maintaining their status of nothing by mouth, with J-tube supplementation, for 5 to 15 additional days.

One patient was readmitted to hospital on postoperative day 19 with an intra-abdominal abscess from an infected hematoma. This patient was treated with percutaneous drainage of the abscess and antibiotics. He was discharged 6 days later.

One patient had a prolonged small bowel obstruction and returned to the operating room on postoperative day 21. An internal hernia was found and repaired.

Finally, three patients had pulmonary emboli despite prophylactic heparin. One of these patients also had splenic infarction secondary to splenic vein thrombosis. All these patients were from the same family. A standard hypercoagulopathy screen was negative, although a familial predisposition for clotting is suspected.

Discussion

When patients are completely asymptomatic, they may wonder whether it is wise to undergo prophylactic gastrectomy, particularly when they have been informed fully about the long-term sequelae of DGC. To variable degrees, patients' anxiety and apprehension may be alleviated by knowing family members who have adjusted to the morbidity of prophylactic gastrectomy. On the other hand, their concern may be heightened greatly by learning about patients who have not done as well following surgery.

The known reduced penetrance of the *CDH1* mutation creates a special problem when a patient is aware of one or more close relatives who are known to be carriers of the *CDH1* mutation but who as yet are not symptomatic and who, indeed, may be thriving in their 70s or 80s, having been completely spared of any evidence of DGC. Other family members who carry the *CDH1* mutation may wonder whether they also will remain cancer free because of the reduced penetrance of this mutation. They also may wonder about possible interactions with unknown environmental protective factors should they forego prophylactic gastrectomy. Clearly, these concerns require intensive empathetic counseling by the surgeon.

Genetic counseling

The first experience with genetic counseling for HDGC in concert with the *CDH1* mutation involved a family (Fig. 1) in which the proband (III-3 on Fig. 1) consulted the authors because three of his siblings had died of DGC within a timeframe of only 18 months [21]. He was intensely concerned. He became extremely well informed about the natural history of HDGC in general and in his family in particular. Following lengthy discussions about the option of prophylactic gastrectomy, he continued to undergo periodic gastroduodenoscopy screening by his gastroenterologist. Contact with him was maintained through telephone communication every 6 months over a period of 3 years, during which time he was reminded of the option of prophylactic gastrectomy. He slowly began considering this option, decided that this procedure was the appropriate choice for him, and underwent the procedure. His surgical specimen showed no visible evidence of cancer (Fig. 2), and he recovered uneventfully. The gastric pathology showed significant submucosal involvement of DGC, however (Fig. 3). There was no evidence of regional or distal spread of DGC postsurgically or in the 5 years following this procedure, and he continues to fare extremely well. Indeed, he became a strong spokesman for a repeat meeting with the family information service in the interest of educating, testing, making appropriate recommendations for prophylactic gastrectomy to members of his family, and the authors obliged. The first family member to follow this advice for prophylactic gastrectomy was the proband's nephew (IV-1 in Fig. 1), who upon gastrectomy did show microscopic foci of DGC in the absence of local or regional spread.

Because Gayther and colleagues [25] have found evidence of DGC in persons as young as 14 years, the authors tested a 16-year-old female family member who, unfortunately, turned out to be positive for the *CDH1*

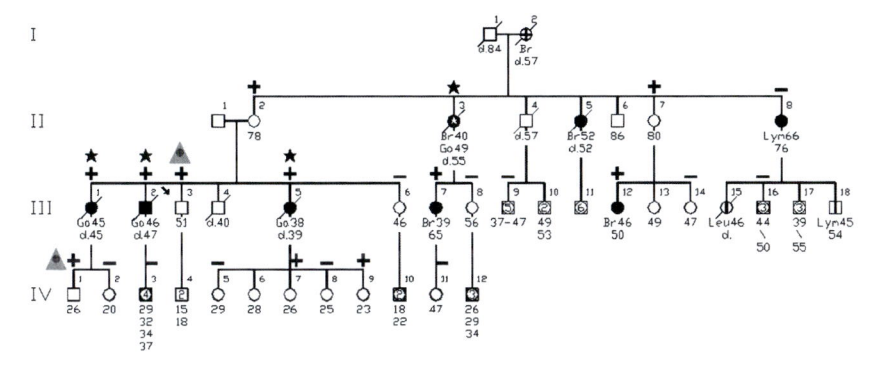

★ Diffuse Gastric Cancer
+ E-Cadherin Mutation Carriers
− Negative for E-Cadherin Mutation
▲ Prophylactic Gastrectomy
▲ Microscopic Foci of Early Diffuse Gastric Cancer

Fig. 1. Pedigree of family harboring a *CDH1* (E-cadherin) germline mutation. CSU, cancer site unknown; Lym, lymphoma; St, stomach cancer; Sk, skin cancer; Br, breast cancer. (*Updated from* Lynch H, Grady W, Suriano G, et al. Gastric cancer: new genetic developments. Journal of Surgical Oncology (Seminars) 2005;90(3):119; with permission.)

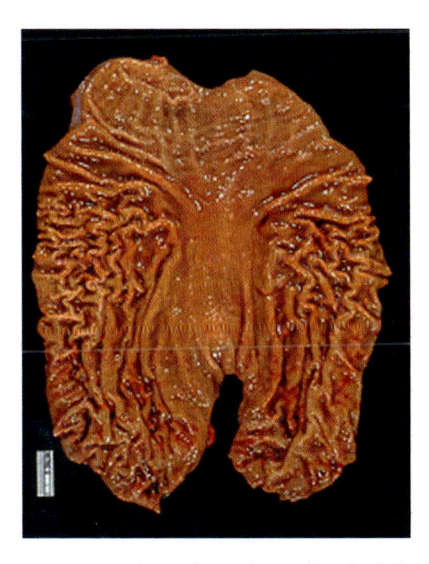

Fig. 2. Prophylactic gastrectomy specimen from the proband of the family shown in Fig. 1 showing no visible abnormalities in the gastric mucosa. (*From* Lynch H, Grady W, Suriano G, et al. Gastric cancer: new genetic developments. Journal of Surgical Oncology (Seminars) 2005;90(3):129; with permission.)

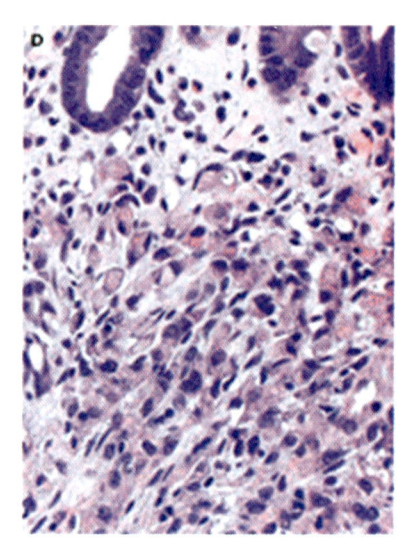

Fig. 3. Photomicrograph of a focus of occult diffuse gastric cancer (hematoxylin-eosin, original magnification ×100) from the specimen shown in Fig. 2. The cancer was stage 1A, and the gastrectomy was presumed curative. (*From* Lynch H, Grady W, Suriano G, et al. Gastric cancer: new genetic developments. Journal of Surgical Oncology (Seminars) 2005;90(3):128; with permission.)

mutation. She had a strong emotional response, cried uncontrollably, and expressed her concern about whether she ever would be able to have children; she immediately wanted to know more about prophylactic gastrectomy. The authors advised her that the penetrance of the mutation is not complete, but they also informed her that she still was a candidate for prophylactic gastrectomy and that this would be an option that she could consider, perhaps later in life after she had married and had children.

Another relative experienced severe stress and insomnia for at least a week before DNA test disclosure, fearing that she would test positive for the mutation. When told that she did not inherit the mutation, she was greatly relieved.

Prophylactic total gastrectomy: benefits and complications

Prophylactic surgical procedures carry a known risk of complications, but this risk should be weighed against the risk of performing the same surgery in the future on a patient who has become debilitated or compromised, particularly when the potential for curative intervention is negligible once the patient becomes symptomatic from the cancer. If the screening criteria are very sensitive, they can be used to proceed with prophylactic surgery in the healthy patient with acceptable morbidity and mortality. Of all the potential malignant disorders amenable to preventive screening and surgical prophylaxis, gastric cancer has emerged recently [26] as the one in which therapeutic intervention at the time of diagnosis in a symptomatic patient still is accompanied almost universally by a fatal outcome. Although they are less virulent cancers, a similar argument for early surgical prophylaxis can be made for ovarian cancer [27], medullary carcinoma of the thyroid [28], colon cancer in familial adenomatous polyposis (FAP), and Lynch syndrome [10,29,30], as well as breast cancer in *BRCA* mutation carriers [31–35]. All these have proportionately (as listed) increasing potential for survival through therapeutic advances, including adjuvant systemic therapy. (See [36] for a review.)

Of all these hereditary cancer disorders, perhaps none has yielded molecular screening methodology as sensitive as that for the *RET* mutation, which predisposes a carrier to the development of medullary thyroid cancer (MTC) in multiple endocrine neoplasia (MEN) kindreds [28]. With studies documenting a 93% incidence of MTC in *RET*-positive members of MEN kindreds, the decision to undergo a prophylactic, relatively low-risk procedure such as total thyroidectomy is less difficult. Reports show an increased survival advantage in *RET* mutation carriers undergoing prophylactic total thyroidectomy. Surgery performed well before age 8 years [28] allows the operation to be performed in a clinically normal neck, thus decreasing the morbidity associated with the operation in the affected patient, in whom the cancer may be fixed to vital structures (recurrent laryngeal nerve, trachea) in the operative field.

Recent advances in the molecular characterization of the *CDH1* germline mutation (E-cadherin, epithelial cadherin) and its association with the onset of HDGC is reminiscent of the *RET*/MTC experience [5,6,37,38]. *CDH1* germline mutations have a penetrance of approximately 70%, and the resulting HDGC phenotype for *CDH1* mutation carriers has almost 100% mortality when discovered in the symptomatic patient. As with ovarian cancer in the *BRCA* carrier, current screening modalities for HDGC in the *CDH1* mutation carrier are very poor. Given that, when the respective mutations are present, HDGC has a higher penetrance than ovarian cancer, that HDGC has a higher mortality when symptomatic, and that currently there is no reliable systemic chemotherapy for symptomatic HDGC patients, it stands to reason that curative surgical intervention should be adopted for the asymptomatic *CDH1* carrier.

Although, according to current understanding, the relationship between *CDH1* and HDGC is more complicated than that between *RET* and type 2 MEN, the syndromes raise similar questions regarding prophylactic surgery: (1) At what age should surgical intervention occur? (2) What is the associated mortality and morbidity of prophylactic total gastrectomy? (3) Are there any curative options for the patient who has a known *CDH1* mutation and symptomatic HDGC?

Similar questions also can be proposed for the management of colon cancer [30] and breast cancer [34,35] in known FAP or hereditary breast-ovarian cancer (HBOC) germline mutation carriers, but many additional effective adjuvant systemic therapies exist to treat these patients in the postoperative setting. For the symptomatic HDGC patient, such options are absent. What remains is a straightforward assessment of the risks and benefits of total gastrectomy and reconstruction, which has a more serious mortality and morbidity profile than any of the prophylactic surgical procedures contemplated by a patient in a type 2 MEN, HBOC, or FAP cancer-prone pedigree.

Prophylactic total gastrectomy: surgical complications

In the absence of complications associated with all gastrointestinal elective surgical resections (eg, bleeding, infection, and anesthetic misadventures), the most significant complication of a prophylactic total gastrectomy results from a potential leak at the single critical anastomosis, the esophagojejunostomy. Randomized, controlled trials have shown that the incidence of an anastomotic leak, stenosis, morbidity, and length of hospitalization are not statistically different when a stapled versus a hand-sewn anastomosis is performed [39,40]. A recent report from Japan in patients who had cancer showed a leak rate of 0.5% (2/390) [41]. Overall, mortality in 14 controlled, randomized trials of gastric pouch reconstruction after total gastrectomy ranges from 0% to 22% [42]. Most of these trials show mortality figures less than 4%. The latter figure should be expected of any team of surgical oncologists and other specialists attending to the management of a patient who has HDGC.

Morbidity estimates for total gastrectomy interposition and reconstruction are more germane to this discussion, given the nearly 100% mortality of untreated HDGC patients. A 0% to 4% intraoperative mortality can be quoted, although 2% should be a more reasonable estimate for a trained surgical oncologist. This figure is not exaggerated, given that all the documented *CDH1* carriers are likely to be young and otherwise healthy candidates, unlike the physiologically and nutritionally compromised patient from the general population who has gastric cancer, from whom the previously quoted mortality and morbidity figures are derived.

In patients undergoing total gastrectomy with reconstruction for cancer, morbidity estimates of 60% are alarming [42]. It is likely that these numbers would be lower for younger, healthy asymptomatic *CDH1* mutation carriers treated by an experienced surgeon. Nevertheless, the scope of the problems responsible for the reported morbidity rates remains the same.

The surgical oncologist, genetic counselor, and nutrition team need to discuss all these factors, as well as the reported mortality data, with the patient in preoperative conferences. The morbidity of a total gastrectomy interposition and reconstruction and its impact on the quality of life (QOL) encompass several areas affecting mechanical and metabolic consequences of the operation. Without a stomach, a patient can expect a decrease in eating capacity at one sitting as well as increased transit time because of the absence of the pyloric sphincter. Although historically many bemoan the malnutrition seen after total gastrectomy interposition, it now is understood that the potential accompanying malnutrition can be corrected or prevented by a measured increase in daily caloric intake [43]. Other expected metabolic deficits thought to be derived from a decrease in vitamin B_{12} absorption, malabsorption of protein, and bacterial overgrowth resulting from the loss of parietal and chief cells of the stomach, seem to be less serious and can be corrected by modest lifestyle adjustments [44]. More significant QOL problems such as reflux, dumping, and weight loss are known to persist. Attempts to remedy these problems account for the large number of proposed reconstructive procedures performed to re-establish intestinal continuity after a prophylactic total gastrectomy. Many technical variations for interposition have been reported; none seems to be universally better than the traditional Roux-en-Y esophagojejunostomy in eliminating all of the QOL issues mentioned previously [45].

Nearly all the variations in reconstructive technique involve the use of a side-to-side stapled jejunal pouch in the manner of a Hunt-Lawrence interposition [45]. These approaches were adopted under the assumption that loss of the gastric reservoir is responsible for most of the postoperative problems with weight loss and malnutrition seen after total gastrectomy. Because nearly all the randomized trials comparing total gastrectomy with and without a pouch for interposition failed to account for simple variations in total caloric intake after surgery and relied primarily on the patients' perceptions of what they could eat before and after surgery, little can be concluded about the impact of the use of the pouch in restoring nutritional deficits. Because most of these randomized studies do not standardize the total caloric intake or other, more variable postoperative parameters such as exercise or level of physical activity, even less can be concluded reliably about the impact of subtle changes in pouch length, length of the Roux-en-Y limb, and inclusion or exclusion of the duodenum from the reconstructed alimentary limb. Two studies that did assess daily energy intake noted no advantage when patients had a pouch interposition versus a straight Roux-en-Y esophagojejunostomy [46,47]. This flaw may account for the observation that in these trials no significant differences were noted in QOL parameters or weight gain. Most of these studies suggest that pouch reconstruction may improve the ability of patients to eat in the immediate months after surgery. In most individuals the putative early benefit of the pouch becomes less apparent over time [42]. Recent data from Japan also suggest that a short, 15-cm pouch may be more effective than a 20-cm pouch in controlling other QOL measures such as esophageal reflux [48]. The same group concluded that a short J-pouch, although better at controlling reflux, did not fare any better than standard Roux-en-Y esophagojejunostomy in controlling dumping and other less common postprandial complaints. In most cases, and in agreement with current surgical approaches to minimizing bile reflux, a putative QOL benefit was seen in patients undergoing a short pouch interposition with the standard 40-cm distance between the esophagojejunostomy and the Roux-en-Y jejunojejunostomy. In patients undergoing a prophylactic gastrectomy for HDGC, it is important to note that the more elaborate the reconstruction, the more potential exists for surgical complications. Although these complications probably are lessened by the good performance status of these individuals, other complications may result from additional surgical misadventures resulting from the performance of an extended lymphadenectomy (D2 node dissection) in the setting of a prophylactic gastrectomy.

Sentinel node mapping

HDGC has a significant propensity for nodal metastases and carcinomatosis. In the prophylactic setting, however, these considerations may not warrant the additional surgical problems associated with a D2 lymphadenectomy. For example, the Dutch trial [26] of limited D1 lymphadenectomy versus extended radical D2 lymphadenectomy as described by the Japanese [49] showed that D2 lymphadectomy led to marked increase in surgical morbidity and a threefold increase in operative mortality (1.7%–5.9%) with no improvement in survival.

Sentinel node mapping may seem an ideal alternative for the staging of nodal disease and an alternative to a D2 lymphadenectomy in the setting of a prophylactic total gastrectomy. It has been described using radiotracer with gamma probe localization in patients found to have T1N0 or T2N0 gastric cancer on preoperative staging [50,51]. The incidence of metastases was much higher in sentinel nodes than in non–sentinel nodes (nonradioactive nodes). A sentinel node was found in 95.2% of the cases, and metastases were documented in 7.8% of these patients. Non–sentinel node metastases were seen in only 0.3% of the patients [50]. A similar report by Hayashi [51] using blue dye and radionucleotide tracer in comparably staged patients demonstrated that a sentinel node could be identified in nearly 100% of the patients. The study included only 31 patients, compared with the 145 patients in the previously mentioned report by Kitagawa [50]. The use of two tracers is complementary: some nodes appear blue, whereas others may appear to be radioactive or hot. Similar observations have been made in the use of sentinel node mapping for breast cancer and melanoma: the use of two tracers has shown exquisite sensitivity in identifying micrometastases to otherwise normal-appearing nodes initially examined by routine hematoxylin and eosin but subsequently examined by step sections and reverse-transcription polymerase chain reaction (RT-PCR) technology. Thus, all nodes that are hot or blue are considered, by definition, to be sentinel nodes [52]. Perhaps the combined use of radiotracer and blue dye is the reason Hayashi [51] found lymph node metastases in 7 of the 31 patients studied (20%) who had T1N0 or T2N0 gastric cancer, compared with the 7.8% rate of positive sentinel nodes in Kitagawa's [50] report of 145 patients of similar stage.

In these series, T1 lesions were the smallest targets for radiotracer injection. In the prophylactic setting a clear lesion often is not evident. Endoscopic ultrasonography or other sensitive radiologic approaches such as PET-CT may localize early abnormalities in the gastric wall and provide a target area. Alternatively, before the application of signal node mapping technology in this setting, concordance studies with injection of the radiotracer and blue dye may be necessary to delineate the potential drainage routes of tumors arising in different parts of the stomach. Similar studies in patients who had breast cancer disclosed that the lymphatic drainage of the entire breast ultimately led to the same sentinel nodes, regardless of the location of the primary cancer or the site of the radiotracer or vital blue dye injection [53,54].

The potential need for any lymphadenectomy more extensive than a D1 procedure can be inferred from the Japanese data documenting the frequency of nodal metastases in early gastric cancer treated with D2 procedures. The frequency of nodal metastases in patients who have gastric cancer limited to the gastric mucosa is 5%, whereas 16% of patients who have submucosal involvement have nodal metastases [51]. Therefore, in the setting of a prophylactic gastrectomy for HDGC, the finding of nodal metastases by sentinel node mapping would convert a preventive procedure into a therapeutic procedure in a small number of cases, if nodal disease could be ascertained intraoperatively. Otherwise, the rationale outlined previously suggests that a D1 lymphadenectomy would suffice in this scenario. Obviously, should intraoperative sentinel node assessment, the standard of care in breast cancer management today, not be available for gastric cancer patients, then the standard of care for the patient who has a known *CDH1* mutation who elects to undergo a prophylactic gastrectomy should be a D1 lymphadenectomy. It would provide the putative therapeutic advantage of a lymphadenectomy without incurring the additional complications with a D2 lymphadenectomy as described by the Dutch trial [26]. Patients who have positive nodes would be eligible for postoperative adjuvant chemoradiation as described by Macdonald [55] or for participation in clinical trials.

Recently, detection of subclinical carcinomatosis in patients who have DGC was reported by Kodera and colleagues [56], who used peritoneal washings. Using RT-PCR probes to detect carcinoembryonic antigen mRNA in the washings, 80% of patients were found to have disseminated disease in the peritoneal cavity [56]. Asymptomatic patients undergoing a prophylactic gastrectomy for HDGC are very unlikely to have positive peritoneal washings, however. Even if they did, the finding would be analogous to that of positive peritoneal washings in pancreatic cancer [52,57]. In that situation, despite positive cytology, patients who were resectable underwent a pancreaticoduodenectomy with curative intent. The presence of positive peritoneal washings in these patients was found to be a surrogate for early recurrence and marked these patients as candidates for aggressive adjuvant systemic therapy. Similar findings in prophylactic gastrectomy could make these patients eligible for clinical trials.

In the typical patient from a HDGC pedigree who is found to be *CDH1* positive, management of the risk of gastric cancer is pressing. As mentioned, the average age of onset in studied pedigrees is 38 years; however, afflicted *CDH1* carriers from age 14 years to 82 years have been described [6]. Significantly, penetrance estimates reported for HDGC suggest that the risk of symptomatic HDGC arising in any individual carrier is 1% by age 20 years [10]. The risk increases with advancing age and may be inferred from the age of the youngest affected member of a known HDGC pedigree.

Guilford and colleagues [37] suggest that, once a known carrier is identified, a prophylactic total gastrectomy should be performed if the individual is older than 20 years. At this age and beyond, the 1% quoted mortality for the operation is exceeded by the risk of development of the fatal HDGC phenotype.

Lobular carcinoma of the breast in families that have hereditary diffuse gastric cancer

In female known *CDH1* carriers, the risk of DGC should be addressed first. These women, however, remain at risk for developing invasive lobular carcinoma of the breast [7,8]. Although penetrance estimates vary, current estimates as high as 39% to 52% have been reported [6]. Unfortunately, patient screening in this setting may be hindered by the limitations that plague screening modalities in the HBOC syndrome [34]. Invasive lobular carcinoma frequently is missed by routine mammographic surveillance. Patients who have very large tumors (even older women, whose breast density should be favorable for screening) can present with normal mammograms. These lesions can be spotted more readily with MRI [58]. In patients under age 40 years who have mammographic examinations of poor informative value, screening with MRI is preferable. Conversely, worrisome breast cancer pedigrees in which an affected surviving patient is afflicted with a lobular carcinoma of the breast should be tested for the *CDH1* mutation if they test negative for a *BRCA* mutation. As in the case of any hereditary breast cancer syndrome, negative test results in unaffected family members is only informative if there is a known cancer associated mutation in the family. When such negative results are received, a woman's breast cancer risk would drop to the population based risk levels and surveillance and screening should follow population based guidelines not the enhanced screening recommended for germline *CDH1* mutation carriers. In *CDH1*-afflicted pedigrees, prophylactic bilateral mastectomy, risk-reduction strategies using tamoxifen, or surveillance every 6 months with MRI alternating with breast ultrasonography may be reasonable approaches, depending on the age of the patient, after the more virulent HDGC risk is addressed. Management strategies and algorithms for care of the patient from a high-risk pedigree who has a recently diagnosed breast cancer have been reported recently by the authors' group [33–35]. Their algorithm for management of these patients has been endorsed as a practical and effective approach for patients who have breast cancer and who are at risk for carrying a germline mutation for breast cancer [59].

Future directions

Although prophylactic gastrectomy may be the most prudent option today for unaffected adult mutation carriers, it is likely that improvements in endoscopic and imaging modalities will make other options available for their children [60,61]. In addition, through the study of the early gastric cancers that have been detected in prophylactic gastrectomy specimens, biomarkers suitable for early detection may be identified [23].

The current knowledge of molecular and genetic diagnostics calls for the addition of HDGC to the roster of malignant familial syndromes in which early counseling and preventive surgical intervention should become the standard of care.

References

[1] Alberts SR, Cervantes A, van De Velde CJ. Gastric cancer: epidemiology, pathology and treatment. Ann Oncol 2003;14(Suppl 2):ii31–6.
[2] Jemal A, Siegel R, Ward E, et al. Cancer statistics, 2008. CA Cancer J Clin 2008;58:71–96.
[3] Lauren P. The two histological main types of gastric carcinoma: diffuse and so-called intestinal-type carcinoma: an attempt at a histo-clinical classification. Acta Pathol Microbiol Scand 1965;64:31–49.
[4] Jones EG. Familial gastric cancer. N Z Med J 1964;63:287–96.
[5] Guilford P, Hopkins J, Harraway J, et al. E-cadherin germline mutations in familial gastric cancer. Nature 1998;392:402–5.
[6] Kaurah P, MacMillan A, Boyd N, et al. Founder and recurrent CDH1 mutations in families with hereditary diffuse gastric cancer. JAMA 2007;297:2360–72.
[7] Keller G, Vogelsang H, Becker I, et al. Diffuse type gastric and lobular breast carcinoma in a familial gastric cancer patient with an E-cadherin germline mutation. Am J Pathol 1999; 155:337–42.
[8] Schrader KA, Masciari S, Boyd N, et al. Hereditary diffuse gastric cancer: association with lobular breast cancer. Fam Cancer 2008;7:73–82.
[9] Suriano G, Oliveira C, Ferreira P, et al. Identification of CDH1 germline missense mutations associated with functional inactivation of the E-cadherin protein in young gastric cancer probands. Hum Mol Genet 2003;12:575–82.
[10] Pharoah PDP, Guilford P, Caldas C, et al. Incidence of gastric cancer and breast cancer in CDH1 (E-cadherin) mutation carriers from hereditary diffuse gastric cancer families. Gastroenterology 2001;121:1348–53.
[11] MacDonald DJ, Lessick M. Hereditary cancers in children and ethical and psychosocial implications. J Pediatr Nurs 2000;15:217–25.
[12] Caldas C, Carneiro F, Lynch HT, et al. Familial gastric cancer: overview and guidelines for management. J Med Genet 1999;36:873–80.
[13] Suriano G, Yew S, Ferreira P, et al. Characterization of a recurrent germ line mutation of the E-cadherin gene: implications for genetic testing and clinical management. Clin Cancer Res 2005;11:5401–9.

[14] Brooks-Wilson AR, Kaurah P, Suriano G, et al. Germline E-cadherin mutations in hereditary diffuse gastric cancer: assessment of 42 new families and review of genetic screening criteria. J Med Genet 2004;41:508–17.
[15] Mullins F, Dietz L, Lay M, et al. Identification of an intronic single nucleotide polymorphism leading to allele dropout during validation of a CDH1 sequencing assay: implications for designing polymerase chain reaction-based assays. Genet Med 2007;9:752–60.
[16] Norton JA, Ham CM, Van Dam J, et al. CDH1 truncating mutations in the E-cadherin gene: an indication for total gastrectomy to treat hereditary diffuse gastric cancer. Ann Surg 2007; 245:873–9.
[17] Lewis FR, Mellinger JD, Hayashi A, et al. Prophylactic total gastrectomy for familial gastric cancer. Surgery 2001;130:612–7.
[18] Bacani JT, Soares M, Zwingerman R, et al. CDH1/E-cadherin germline mutations in early onset gastric cancer. J Med Genet 2006;43:867–72.
[19] Huntsman DG, Carneiro F, Lewis FR, et al. Early gastric cancer in young, asymptomatic carriers of germ-line E-cadherin mutations. N Engl J Med 2001;344:1904–9.
[20] Lynch HT. Family Information Service and hereditary cancer. Cancer 2001;91:625–8.
[21] Lynch HT, Grady W, Lynch JF, et al. E-cadherin mutation-based genetic counseling and hereditary diffuse gastric carcinoma. Cancer Genet Cytogenet 2000;122:1–6.
[22] Carneiro F, Huntsman DG, Smyrk TC, et al. Model of the early development of diffuse gastric cancer in E-cadherin mutation carriers and its implications for patient screening. J Pathol 2004;203:681–7.
[23] Humar B, Fukuzawa R, Blair V, et al. Destabilized adhesion in the gastric proliferative zone and c-Src kinase activation mark the development of early diffuse gastric cancer. Cancer Res 2007;67:2480–9.
[24] Lynch HT, Kaurah P, Wirtzfeld D, et al. Hereditary diffuse gastric cancer: diagnosis, genetic counseling, and prophylactic total gastrectomy. Cancer 2008;112:2655–63.
[25] Gayther SA, Gorringe KL, Ramus SJ, et al. Identification of germ-line E-cadherin mutations in gastric cancer families of European origin. Cancer Res 1998;58:4086–9.
[26] Hartgrink HH, van De Velde CJ, Putter H, et al. Extended lymph node dissection for gastric cancer: who may benefit? Final results of the randomized Dutch gastric cancer group trial. J Clin Oncol 2004;22:2069–77.
[27] Rebbeck TR, Lynch HT, Neuhausen SL, et al. Prophylactic oophorectomy in carriers of BRCA1 or BRCA2 mutations. N Engl J Med 2002;346:1616–22.
[28] National Cancer Institute. Genetics of medullary thyroid cancer (PDQ): health professional version. Available at: http://www.cancer.gov/cancertopics/pdq/genetics/medullarythyroid/HealthProfessional/allpages. Accessed March 11, 2008.
[29] Schmeler KM, Lynch HT, Chen L-M, et al. Prophylactic surgery to reduce the risk of gynecologic cancers in the Lynch syndrome. N Engl J Med 2006;354:261–9.
[30] Lynch HT. Is there a role for prophylactic subtotal colectomy among hereditary nonpolyposis colorectal cancer germline mutation carriers? Dis Colon Rectum 1996;39:109–10.
[31] Hartmann LC, Sellers TA, Schaid DJ, et al. Efficacy of bilateral prophylactic mastectomy in BRCA1 and BRCA2 gene mutation carriers. J Natl Cancer Inst 2001;93:1633–7.
[32] Rebbeck TR, Levin AM, Eisen A, et al. Breast cancer risk after bilateral prophylactic oophorectomy in BRCA1 mutation carriers. J Natl Cancer Inst 1999;91:1475–9.
[33] Lynch HT, Silva E, Snyder C, et al. Hereditary breast cancer: part I. Diagnosing hereditary breast cancer syndromes. Breast J 2008;14:3–13.
[34] Silva E, Gatalica Z, Snyder C, et al. Hereditary breast cancer: part II. Management of hereditary breast cancer: implications of molecular genetics and pathology. Breast J 2008;14: 14–24.
[35] Silva E. Genetic counseling and clinical management of newly diagnosed breast cancer patients at genetic risk for BRCA germline mutations: perspective of a surgical oncologist. Fam Cancer 2008;7:91–5.

[36] Guillem JG, Wood WC, Moley JF, et al. ASCO/SSO review of current role of risk-reducing surgery in common hereditary cancer syndromes. J Clin Oncol 2006;24:4642–60.
[37] Guilford P, Blair V, More H, et al. A short guide to hereditary diffuse gastric cancer. Hereditary Cancer in Clinical Practice 2007;5:183–94.
[38] Lynch HT, Grady W, Suriano G, et al. Gastric cancer: new genetic developments. J Surg Oncol 2005;90:114–33.
[39] Seufert RM, Schmidt-Matthiesen A, Beyer A. Total gastrectomy and oesophagojejunostomy–a prospective randomized trial of hand-sutured versus mechanically stapled anastomoses. Br J Surg 1990;77:50–2.
[40] Fujimoto S, Takahashi M, Endoh F, et al. Stapled or manual suturing in esophagojejunostomy after total gastrectomy: a comparison of outcome in 379 patients. Am J Surg 1991;162:256–9.
[41] Hyodo M, Hosoya Y, Hirashima Y, et al. Minimum leakage rate (0.5%) of stapled esophagojejunostomy with sacrifice of a small part of the jejunum after total gastrectomy in 390 consecutive patients. Dig Surg 2007;24:169–72.
[42] Lehnert T, Buhl K. Techniques of reconstruction after total gastrectomy for cancer. Br J Surg 2004;91:528–39.
[43] Braga M, Zuliani W, Foppa L, et al. Food intake and nutritional status after total gastrectomy: results of a nutritional follow-up. Br J Surg 1988;75:477–80.
[44] Buhl K, Lehnert T, Schlag P, et al. Reconstruction after gastrectomy and quality of life. World J Surg 1995;19:558–64.
[45] Sharma D. Choice of digestive tract reconstructive procedure following total gastrectomy: a critical reappraisal. Indian J Surg 2004;66:270–6.
[46] Liedman B, Bosaeus I, Hugosson I, et al. Long-term beneficial effects of a gastric reservoir on weight control after total gastrectomy: a study of potential mechanisms. Br J Surg 1998;85:542–7.
[47] Bozzetti F, Bonfanti G, Castellani R, et al. Comparing reconstruction with Roux-en-Y to a pouch following total gastrectomy. J Am Coll Surg 1996;183:243–8.
[48] Tanaka T, Fujiwara Y, Nakagawa K, et al. Reflux esophagitis after total gastrectomy with jejunal pouch reconstruction: comparison of long and short pouches. Am J Gastroenterol 1997;92:821–4.
[49] Kajitani T. Japanese Research Society for the Study of Gastric Cancer. The general rules for Gastric Cancer Study in Surgery and Pathology. Jpn J Surg 1981;11:127–45.
[50] Kitagawa Y, Fujii H, Mukai M, et al. Radio-guided sentinel node detection for gastric cancer. Br J Surg 2002;89:604–8.
[51] Hayashi H, Ochiai T, Mori M, et al. Sentinel lymph node mapping for gastric cancer using a dual procedure with dye- and gamma probe-guided techniques. J Am Coll Surg 2003;196:68–74.
[52] Beitsch PD, Clifford E, Whitworth P, et al. Improved lymphatic mapping technique for breast cancer. Breast J 2001;7:219–23.
[53] Chagpar A, Martin RC III, Chao C, et al. Validation of subareolar and periareolar injection techniques for breast sentinel lymph node biopsy. Arch Surg 2004;139:614–8.
[54] McMasters KM, Wong SL, Martin RC II, et al. Dermal injection of radioactive colloid is superior to peritumoral injection for breast cancer sentinel lymph node biopsy: results of a multiinstitutional study. Ann Surg 2001;233:676–87.
[55] Macdonald JS. Role of post-operative chemoradiation in resected gastric cancer. J Surg Oncol 2005;90:166–70.
[56] Kodera Y, Nakanishi H, Ito S, et al. Detection of disseminated cancer cells in linitis plastica-type gastric carcinoma. Jpn J Clin Oncol 2004;34:525–31.
[57] Yachida S, Fukushima N, Sakamoto M, et al. Implications of peritoneal washing cytology in patients with potentially resectable pancreatic cancer. Br J Surg 2002;89:573–8.
[58] Francis A, England DW, Rowlands DC, et al. The diagnosis of invasive lobular breast carcinoma. Does MRI have a role? Breast 2001;10:38–40.

[59] Chung MA, Cady B. Re: genetic counseling and management of newly diagnosed breast cancer patients at genetic risk for BRCA germline mutations. Breast J 2006;12:282–3.
[60] van Kouwen MC, Drenth JP, Oyen WJ, et al. [18F]Fluoro-2-deoxy-D-glucose positron emission tomography detects gastric carcinoma in an early stage in an asymptomatic E-cadherin mutation carrier. Clin Cancer Res 2004;10:6456–9.
[61] Shaw D, Blair V, Framp A, et al. Chromoendoscopic surveillance in hereditary diffuse gastric cancer: an alternative to prophylactic gastrectomy? Gut 2005;54:461–8.

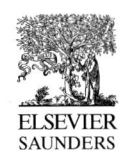

Hamartomatous Polyposis Syndromes

Daniel Calva, MD[a], James R. Howe, MD[b],*

[a]University of Iowa, Roy J. and Lucille A. Carver College of Medicine, 200 Hawkins Drive, Iowa City, IA 52242-2600, USA
[b]Division of Surgical Oncology and Endocrine Surgery, University of Iowa, Roy J. and Lucille A. Carver, College of Medicine, 200 Hawkins Drive, Iowa City, IA 52242-2600, USA

The hamartomatous polyposis syndromes are a fascinating group of disorders that share two characteristics: polyps of the gastrointestinal (GI) tract that appear relatively benign and an increased risk of cancer. These syndromes include juvenile polyposis syndrome (JPS), Peutz-Jeghers syndrome (PJS), Bannayan-Riley-Ruvalcaba syndrome (BRRS), Cowden syndrome (CS), Cronkhite-Canada syndrome (CCS), and hereditary mixed polyposis syndrome (HMPS). The progression of these polyps to cancer is not well understood and represents a different mechanism than that seen in adenomatous polyposis. This mechanism has been dubbed the landscaper effect, where changes predominantly affecting the lamina propria may lead to epithelial cancers [1]. In this article, we discuss the clinical features of these hamartomatous polyposis syndromes, their histopathologic characteristics, risk of cancer, genetics, and screening recommendations.

Juvenile polyposis syndrome

History

In 1939, Diamond [2] described a 30-month-old child with a prolapsed polyp that Diamond felt was of congenital origin. The child primarily had constipation and bright red blood per rectum, with a pedunculated and sessile polyp on proctoscopy. Ravitch [3] described a 10-month-old child who on autopsy was found to have multiple GI polyps, from the stomach to the anus. The child's symptoms were bloody diarrhea, failure to gain weight, cachexia, recurrent rectal prolapse, intussusception, and severe anemia. In

---

* Corresponding author. Department of Surgery, University of Iowa Hospitals and Clinics, 200 Hawkins Drive, Iowa City, IA 52242-1086.
  E-mail address: james-howe@uiowa.edu (J.R. Howe).

1957, Horrilleno and colleagues [4] performed a review of the literature on children with rectal and colonic polyps, and concluded that most polyps contained mucus-filled glands, with retention cysts, abundant connective tissue, and a chronic cellular infiltration of eosinophils. They introduced the term *hamartomatous polyp* based upon these observations. In 1964, McColl and colleagues [5] coined the term *juvenile polyposis* (JP) after careful analysis of the syndrome, and concluded that JP was a different entity than adenomatous polyposis coli. In 1970, Sachatello and colleagues [6] described a JP family with affected members in three generations with disease involving the stomach, small bowel, large bowel, and rectum. In 1975, Stemper and colleagues [7] reported a family with 10 members affected with JP. Individuals had juvenile polyps of the stomach, small bowel, colon, and rectum. Several also developed colon cancer or gastric cancer. One had pancreatic cancer.

Clinical features

In 1974, Sachatello and colleagues [8] defined the criteria for the diagnosis of JP. According to this definition, JP can be diagnosed when any one of the following conditions is fulfilled: (1) 10 juvenile polyps in the colorectum; (2) juvenile polyps throughout the GI tract; or (3) any number of juvenile polyps with a family history of juvenile polyposis. The criteria were later revised by Jass and colleagues [9], who decreased the requisite number of polyps from 10 to 5 to make the diagnosis of JP. Sachatello and colleagues [10] also proposed a classification of JP into (1) juvenile polyposis coli, where the only site of disease is the colon (Fig. 1); (2) JP of infancy, a subtype that carries a poor prognosis because of a very early age of onset, severe hypoalbuminemia, and failure to thrive; and (3) generalized JP, where individuals have juvenile polyps of both the upper and lower GI tract. Veale and colleagues [11] reviewed 145 cases of JP and found an average age onset of 6 years, with familial cases presenting at a later age (9.5 years) and sporadic cases younger (4.5 years). The most common symptom was rectal bleeding, prolapse, mucus per rectum, diarrhea, and abdominal pain. They found an equal incidence between males and females.

In 1986, Grosfeld and colleagues [12] described the differences between multiple versus solitary juvenile polyps in children. Patients with multiple polyps have considerable mucus secretion presenting with more severe hypokalemia, and protein-losing enteropathy, leading to hypoalbuminemia and hypoprotenimia. In addition, they have more severe anemia from blood loss compared with those having solitary juvenile polyps. Jass [13] stated that solitary juvenile polyps (as opposed to JPS) usually present in childhood, with a peak incidence at age 4 to 5 years, and were mainly located in the colon or rectum, with the most common symptom being rectal bleeding. The polyps have a tendency to autoamputate or prolapse. In JPS, he found that most cases were sporadic (66%), while family history of the disease was less frequent (33%). In 1995, Desai [14] reported that 85% of JP patients presented

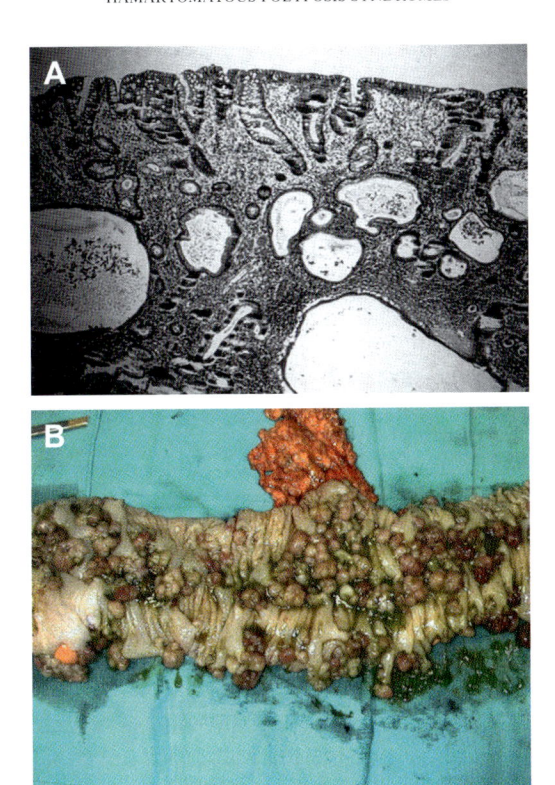

Fig. 1. (*A*) A typical juvenile polyp with the three classic histologic features that define a hamartomatous polyp: (1) dilated cystic glands that retain mucus and are lined by tall columnar epithelium, (2) a markedly expanded lamina propria, and (3) diffuse chronic infiltration of inflammatory cells. (*B*) Gross picture of the colon in a JP patient that is carpeted with juvenile polyps (*From* Merg A, Lynch HT, Lynch JF, et al. Hereditary colorectal cancer—part II. Curr Probl Surg 2005;42:267; with permission).

in the first or second decade of life, and 98% of patients had colorectal polyps relatively evenly distributed throughout the colon. Meanwhile, 14% had involvement of the stomach, 2% of the duodenum, and 7% of the jejunum or ileum. Coburn and colleagues [15] found that the mean age at diagnosis was 18.5 years, that 50% of patients had a family history of JP, and 15% had extracolonic anomalies. Anemia, rectal bleeding, prolapse, enteropathy, and intussusception were the most common symptoms.

Associated anomalies

The extracolonic anomalies described in JP patients include macrocephaly, hypertelorism, amyotonia congenita, extra toes on the foot, Meckel's diverticulum with umbilical fistula, mild communicating hydrocephalus, malrotation of the small bowel, undescended testes, mesenteric lymphangioma, malrotation of the cecum, and acute porphyria

[5,11,14]. Bussey and colleagues [16] estimated that 20% of JP patients suffered from congenital anomalies. Coburn and colleagues [15] performed a large review of JP patients, and found multiple thoracic anomalies, which included atrial septal defects, arteriovenous malformations of the lung, pulmonary stenosis, tetralogy of Fallot, coarctation of the aorta, patent ductus arteriosus, and subvalvular aortic stenosis. Central nervous system defects included macrocephaly, hydrocephalus, and spina bifida. In the GI system, Meckel's diverticulum, gastric and duodenal diverticuli, and malrotation were observed. Urogenital anomalies included undescended testes, unilateral renal agenesis, bifid uterus and vagina, and abnormal ureteropelvic insertion. Other abnormalities included osteoma, lymphangioma, pectus excavatum, hereditary telangiectasia, familial congenital lymphedema, hypertelorism, thyroglossal duct cyst, and amyotonia congenita. Jass [13] stated that congenital defects were more common in sporadic cases, compared with familial JP.

Histopathology

Horrilleno and colleagues [4] described juvenile polyps as having proliferation of mucus glands with formation of cystic structures in abundant connective tissue, with a background of chronic cellular infiltration of eosinophils. Morson [17] described the juvenile polyp as a hamartoma, with alteration of the layers above the muscularis mucosa. The stroma of the polyp has tubules lined by columnar epithelium and many goblet cells, with atrophy of the lining epithelium in the tubules, showing cystic dilation and retention of mucus. The epithelium, which covers the entire surface of the polyp, has no signs of hyperplasia, hyperchromatism, or increased mitotic activity. He also noted that ulceration, infection, and autoinfarction were evident in some of the polyps, which could be the reason for infiltration of inflammatory cells (see Fig. 1).

Jass [13] reported that 20% of polyps are multilobated or papillary. However, 80% had typical features, with the lamina propria thinned out and the epithelial cells possibly showing some evidence of dysplasia. Solitary polyps generally have a smooth, spherical, red head, with a narrow stalk. The surface of solitary polyps has cysts filled with mucin, with no muscularis mucosa in the expanded layer, and the epithelium is normal and has no evidence of excess mitotic activity. There is also a strong component of infiltration of inflammatory cells in the lamina propria. Subramony and colleagues [18] described juvenile polyps greater than 3 cm as being mostly pedunculated, with epithelium showing mild to moderate dysplasia resembling adenomas. The largest polyp they described had adenocarcinoma in the stalk of the polyp. In addition, they found that gastric polyps in JP patients had histologic features identical to hyperplastic polyps. However, the surrounding gastric mucosa showed a diffuse process consistent with chronic gastritis.

Cancer predisposition

Colorectal cancer

In 1975, Stemper and colleagues [7] described the Iowa JP kindred, which consisted of 56 members at the time. There were 15 affected members, and 11 had GI malignancies (5 colon, 2 stomach, 2 duodenum, 1 pancreatic, and 1 unknown GI cancer). At that time, the investigators did not infer the malignant potential of juvenile polyps, although it was evident that cancer was common within the three successive generations of this family. Goodman and colleagues [19] described the spectrum of changes in JP polyps in a 23-year-old male with sporadic JP who had rectal cancer. They found typical juvenile polyps, juvenile polyps with focal adenomatous changes, adenomas, and adenocarcinoma. They concluded that there must be a sequence of events that leads to adenocarcinoma formation within the juvenile polyp. Other investigators supported the notion of a pathologic sequence of events and that the polyps in JP patients had malignant potential [20–23].

Jones and colleagues [24] found an intramucosal carcinoma arising from a typical juvenile polyp in a 24-year-old JP patient who only had four juvenile polyps in the rectum. They concluded that individuals with solitary polyps are also at risk for malignancy. However, after an extensive review of the clinical and pathologic characteristics of juvenile polyps, Jass and colleagues [9] concluded that patients with JP are at risk for developing malignancies, but patients with solitary juvenile polyps are not. Bentley and colleagues [25] found that the subgroup of patients with JP at the greatest risk of malignancy were those with typical juvenile polyps and adenomatous features. In 1990, Jass [13] quantified the risk of developing cancer, and concluded that, in patients with solitary polyps, the risks are minimal, but for patients with JP, the cumulative risk is greater than 50%. Giardiello and colleagues [26] reported that the mean age of diagnosis of colorectal neoplasia was 37 years for both sporadic and familial JP, and found that the risk for neoplasia was approximately the same for both familial and sporadic JP. Howe and colleagues [27] updated the records of the Iowa JP kindred in 1998, which now consisted of 117 individuals, with 29 affected members. Eleven had been diagnosed with colon cancer, 4 with gastric cancer, 1 with cancer of the duodenum/ampulla, and 1 with pancreatic cancer. They concluded that the overall risk for colorectal cancer in this family was 38%, and of upper GI cancer was 21%, with 55% overall risk for GI malignancies.

Gastric cancer

Watanabe and colleagues [28] described a family that consisted of two siblings with JP localized mainly to the upper GI tract. The mother had passed away from gastric cancer at 37 years of age. Both siblings underwent a total gastrectomy. Although their stomachs were found to be diffusely involved with typical juvenile polyps, the siblings showed no evidence of dysplasia or cancer. Yoshida and colleagues [29] reported on a 31-year-old JP patient diagnosed with a well-differentiated gastric adenocarcinoma, and concluded that JP patients are also at risk for gastric cancer. Sassatelli and colleagues [30] reported a 16-year-old JP patient with diffuse polyposis of the stomach, who later developed an infiltrating adenocarcinoma from one of the JP polyps in the stomach at the age of 21. Howe and colleagues [27] reported that 6 of 29 affected patients in the Iowa kindred had upper GI malignancies (4 in the stomach), and that the overall risk of developing upper GI cancer in affected members of the family was 21%.

Pancreatic cancer

Stemper and colleagues [7] reported the first JP patient with pancreatic adenocarcinoma in 1975. In 1989, Walpole and Cullity [31] described another JP patient presenting with epigastric mass at age 19. Exploration revealed a poorly differentiated adenocarcinoma, which had replaced the majority of the pancreas, and metastasis to the left lung.

Management

The standard methods used to screen and survey JP patients are colonoscopy and esophagogastroduodenoscopy (EGD). Although capsule endoscopy has the potential for evaluation of the entire GI tract, its usefulness is primarily for evaluation of the small bowel. Howe and colleagues [32] published general guidelines (Fig. 2), which stated that, in patients at risk for JP, screening should begin with a thorough history and physical to evaluate for JP (rectal bleeding, prolapse, anemia, constipation, obstruction, diarrhea, abdominal discomfort), and this should be done soon after birth. EGD and colonoscopy, however, should be done at the age of onset of symptoms or, in asymptomatic patients at risk, at 15 years of age. If screening reveals no polyps, it should be repeated every 3 years. If polyps are found, they should be removed endoscopically, if possible. Then, the procedure should be repeated yearly until no polyps are seen, at which point screening should be repeated every 3 years. Individuals who do not have the mutation found in the family should undergo baseline screening at age 15 and, if screening is negative, this should be repeated every 10 years (instead of every 3 years) until the age of 45. If no polyps are ever found, screening should then be done as one would do for the normal population. However, if a genetic mutation is found in an individual at risk, that person should continue to be screened every 3 years or, if polyps are found, yearly. If the individual or the family does not have a genetic mutation found in one of the two known JP genes, then screening should follow the same guidelines as those for patients at risk for JP.

Grosfeld and colleagues [12] felt that subtotal colectomy with ileorectal anastomosis was the procedure of choice in selected JP patients, with

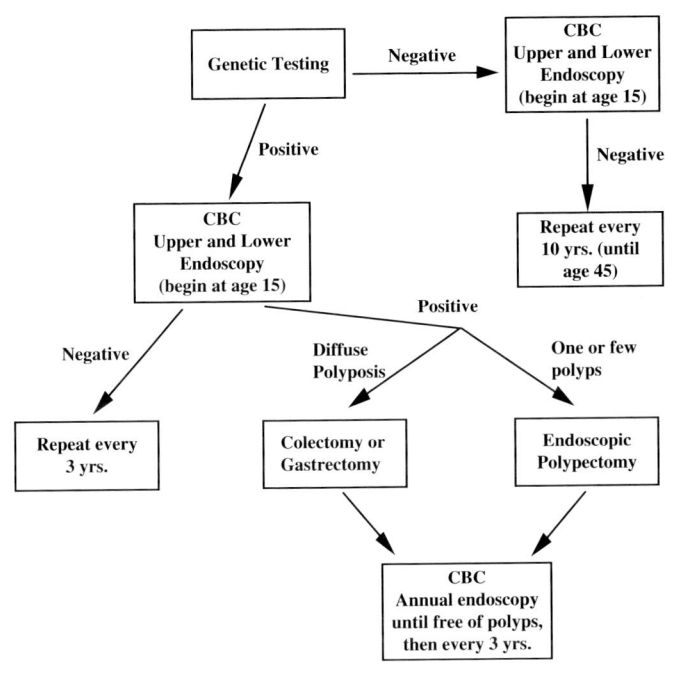

Fig. 2. Algorithm for the surveillance and management of JP patients, incorporating genetic testing. CBC, complete blood cell count. (*From* Howe JR, Ringold JC, Hughes J, et al. Direct genetic testing for Smad4 mutations in patients at risk for juvenile polyposis. Surgery 1999;126;162; with permission.)

indications for the procedure being children with anemia from chronic bleeding, hypoproteinemia, failure to thrive, and nonreducible intussusception. Jarvinen and colleagues [33] recommended prophylactic colectomy with ileorectal anastomosis for (1) children with JP who have severe or repeated bleeding (leading to failure to thrive or death), and (2) adults with JP because of the greater than 50% lifetime risk for cancer. They felt that the optimal age for surgery was 20 to 25 years of age, since the risk for cancer is greater than the risk of surgery. Subtotal colectomy was also favored by Howe and colleagues [32], who stressed that the rectum needs to be screened with flexible sigmoidoscopy every 1 to 3 years because of the risk of recurrence in the rectal remnant. However, they felt that surgery should be reserved for those patients with large numbers of polyps, significant anemia, or other complications of JP. Most patients can have repeated colonoscopic removal of polyps rather than colectomy, especially if the polyp burden is low. Many investigators have published their experiences with a high rate of recurrence of polyps after various surgical procedures [8,23,34–36]. This has led Scott-Conner and colleagues [36] to recommend total colectomy with J pouch ileoanal anastomosis as their procedure of choice. Some believe that the frequency and urgency of bowel movements and the reduced continence associated with this procedure may be less desirable than the required surveillance for recurrent polyps in the rectosigmoid [32].

Patients with generalized JP should undergo close surveillance of the upper GI tract because of the high risk of malignancy [19,29,32,33,36–38]. Howe and colleagues [32] recommend screening the upper GI tract by EGD starting at the age 15 for asymptomatic individuals at risk, or as soon as signs or symptoms develop. Screening should be repeated every 3 years and, if polyps are present, every year to make sure no dysplastic polyps are present. Polyps of the stomach tend to be diffuse and difficult to remove endoscopically. Therefore, total or subtotal gastrectomy should be performed for bleeding, gastric outlet obstruction, dysplasia, adenomatous changes, or adenocarcinoma. Particularly close surveillance should be directed toward patients with *SMAD4* mutations, since they are at greater risk for developing gastric cancer [39,40].

Genetics

Based upon observations in the Iowa kindred, Stemper and colleagues [7] suggested that JP had an autosomal-dominant mode of inheritance with a high degree of penetrance. In 1978, Bussey, Veale, and Morson [16] speculated that in 25% of JP cases there must be an inherited defect in a gene, while in the other 75% of JP patients a de novo mutation or environmental factor promoted disease.

In 1998, Howe and colleagues [41] performed genetic linkage analysis on affected members of the Iowa kindred, and found linkage to chromosome 18q21. This region contained the tumor suppressor genes *DCC* and *SMAD4/DPC4*. They then searched for germline mutations in both genes by direct sequencing, and identified a 4–base pair (bp) deletion in exon 9 of *SMAD4* in all affected members of the kindred, and mutations in four other JP kindreds [42]. Soon thereafter, these findings were confirmed in other JP families [43–45]. In 2001, Howe and colleagues [46] performed genetic linkage analysis in four unrelated JP families without *SMAD4* or the phosphatase and tensin homolog gene (*PTEN*) mutations, and found linkage to markers on chromosome 10q22–23. Mutations were found in all affected members of each family in the bone morphogenetic protein receptor type IA gene (*BMPR1A*). These findings were later confirmed by other investigators [39,47,48]. The overall prevalence of germline mutations is 20% for *SMAD4* and 20% for *BMPR1A* in JP probands [49], which has been validated in other large studies of JP patients [50,51].

SMAD4 is a protein that functions as the common intracellular mediator of the transforming growth factor β (TGF-β), bone morphogenetic protein (BMP), and activin signaling pathways. The BMP signaling pathway has a wide range of actions, including regulation of cell proliferation, differentiation, survival, and apoptosis. BMPR1A is a transmembrane protein, which is a type I receptor. TGF-β superfamily ligands (TGF-β, bone morphogenetic proteins, activins, and inhibins) bind to serine/threonine kinsase type 2 receptors that then bind to and phosphorylate the serine and threonine domains of the type I receptors. These then phosphorylate intracellular SMAD proteins (SMAD2 and 3 in the TGF-β pathway, and SMAD1, 5, and 8 in the BMP pathway), which then form heteromers with SMAD4. The complexes recruit DNA binding proteins as they migrate into the nucleus. Here, they bind directly to DNA sequences and regulate the transcription of various genes [52,53].

Counseling

Because two genes have been identified for JP, individuals at risk can be tested for mutations before the onset of symptoms. In 1999, Howe and colleagues [32] suggested that screening individuals at risk within a JP family for a known genetic mutation would allow clinicians to make the diagnosis at an earlier age, and would lead to closer endoscopic screening and follow-up. Individuals without the mutation would need less frequent endoscopic screening and perhaps only endoscopy after age 50 as in the normal population. Therefore, genetic testing can help to define the recommended interval for screening and surveillance and, it is hoped, prevent malignancy by early polypectomy and heightened surveillance.

Peutz-Jeghers syndrome

History

In 1896, Hutchinson [54] described healthy twin sisters who, at the age of 9, developed pigmentation around the mouth, lips, and oral mucous membranes. One of the sisters died at age 20 from intussusception. In 1921, Peutz [55] described a family with 10 affected members within three generations. Seven of the affected members had pigmentation of the lips, mouth, and oral mucosa, and also had polyps confined to the small intestine. Two of these family members also had nasal polyps, and 1 had bladder polyps. One of the patients underwent resection of a portion of the jejunum secondary to intussusception, and adenomatous polyps were described in the specimen. In 1949, Jeghers and colleagues [56] reviewed the literature on patients with pigmentation of the mouth, lips, and oral cavity that was associated with intestinal polyposis, and found 10 cases. They came to the conclusion that the syndrome consists of two distinctive clinical features: (1) the melanin deposition around the mouth, oral mucosa, and lips (Fig. 3), and (2) polyposis of the small intestine. They concluded that the syndrome had an autosomal-dominant pattern of inheritance. In 1954, the term *Peutz-Jeghers syndrome* (PJS) was coined by Bruwer and colleagues [57].

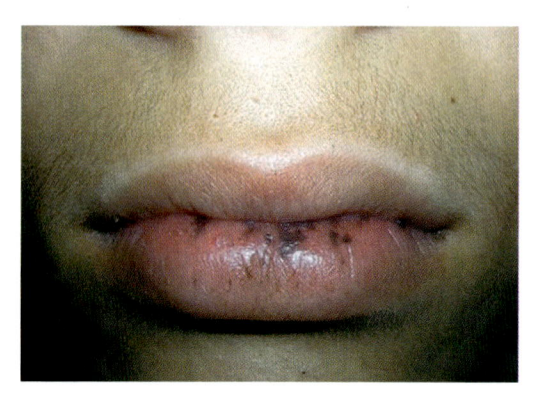

Fig. 3. Oral melanosis in a patient with Peutz-Jeghers syndrome. (*From* Cureton E, Kim S. Images in clinical medicine. Peutz-Jeghers syndrome. N Engl J Med 2007;357:e9; with permission. Copyright © 2007, Massachusetts Medical Society.)

Clinical features

In 1962, Bartholomew and colleagues [58] defined PJS as mucocutaneous melanosis and small bowel polyposis. The pigmentation may develop at any age. However, it most commonly manifests in infancy and early childhood. The melanosis occurs almost universally on the lips (>95%), with the buccal mucosa being the second most common site (83%) (see Fig. 3). Less frequent locations are the hands, feet, and areas around the mouth and nose. This pigmentation tends to fade with age. In terms of the polyposis, lesions vary in size from microadenomas within the intestinal wall to polyps several centimeters in size. Most of the polyps are found in the jejunum, ileum, and, to a lesser extent, the rectum, colon, stomach, and duodenum. The number of polyps varies from solitary polyps to hundreds of polyps where the intestine is virtually carpeted. There is no difference in prevalence between males and females, or in specific races or ethnic groups, and the average age of diagnosis is 24.3 years. The most common presenting symptoms are recurrent episodes of abdominal pain as a result of intussusception, anemia secondary to occult GI bleeding, melena, and hematochezia. Hematemesis was also reported in patients with gastric or duodenal polyposis, and prolapse of rectal polyps may also occur.

In 1999, Westerman and Wilson [59] performed a review of the literature on PJS, and stated that the polyps tend to be either several millimeters and sessile, or several centimeters and pedunculated. They can be solitary, or can occur in clusters, at times carpeting the entire GI surface. These polyps can lead to intussusception most commonly in the small bowel, but two cases have been described of the colon. Another common presentation is bleeding from the polyps, which occurs in 81% of patients, and tends to present as hematochezia or hematemesis in 10% of patients with polyps in the duodenum or stomach. It can also present as occult bleeding with anemia. Sixty percent of patients present by their early 20s, and 33% present in the first decade of life.

Associated anomalies

In 1957, Dormandy and colleagues [60] reviewed the PJS cases described up to that time, and concluded that bladder, renal pelvis, bronchial, and nasal polyps are associated with PJS. Skeletal anomalies include clubbed foot, scoliosis, and bony tumors, as well as ovarian lesions, such as cysts, cystadenomas, and malignant tumors. Polyps in the nasal cavity may present as epixtasis or symptoms of sinus obstruction. Ureteral polyps were described in one patient with hematuria and frequency [61]. Polyps in the gallbladder have also been reported, although histologically these were considered adenomatous polyps, while polyps removed from the ileum were hamartomatous [62]. Polyps of the biliary tract were described in two patients, both with signs and symptoms of obstructive jaundice [63,64].

Histopathology

Areas of pigmentation consist of melanin in the subepithelial regions both within the cells and around them, without any abnormal pathology at the microscopic level. Acanthosis with prominent melanin in the basal layers may also be seen. Polyps in the small intestine are made of columnar, goblet, and Paneth cells. Within the stroma are arborizing strands of smooth muscle, which represent the muscularis mucosa branching in various directions. This is the major difference from juvenile polyps, where there is no muscularis mucosa in the lamina propria (Fig. 4). There is no nuclear atypia or proliferation. Gastric polyps are also hamartomas and contain all the cell types found in the gastric mucosa. The duodenal polyps have Brunner's glands. Colonic polyps, however, have a more adenomatous appearance and, therefore, should be regarded as potentially malignant [58]. Farmer and colleagues [65] described polyps as having minor variations depending upon the location in which they are found. Polyps in the small intestine have goblet cells that form the typical tubular glands within the stroma, and there are cryptlike formations resembling the crypts of Lieberkuhn. The epithelial component of gastric polyps resembles the pyloric or gastric mucosa with less prominent smooth muscle.

Cancer predisposition

Colorectal

Although many investigators have described the incidence of colorectal cancer in patients with the PJS, most have been case reports and descriptions of kindreds that do not provide a full risk analysis [66–68]. Konishi and colleagues [69] reviewed all cancer cases reported in PJS patients and found 20 colorectal cancers in 103 patients (12 in Japan and 8 in the Western literature). The mean age of diagnosis was 48 years of age. Giardiello and colleagues [70] found similar results when they reviewed all PJS papers from 1966 to 1998 for reports of cancer. They found an 84-fold relative risk of developing colon cancer (Fig. 5) and cumulative risk of 39% of

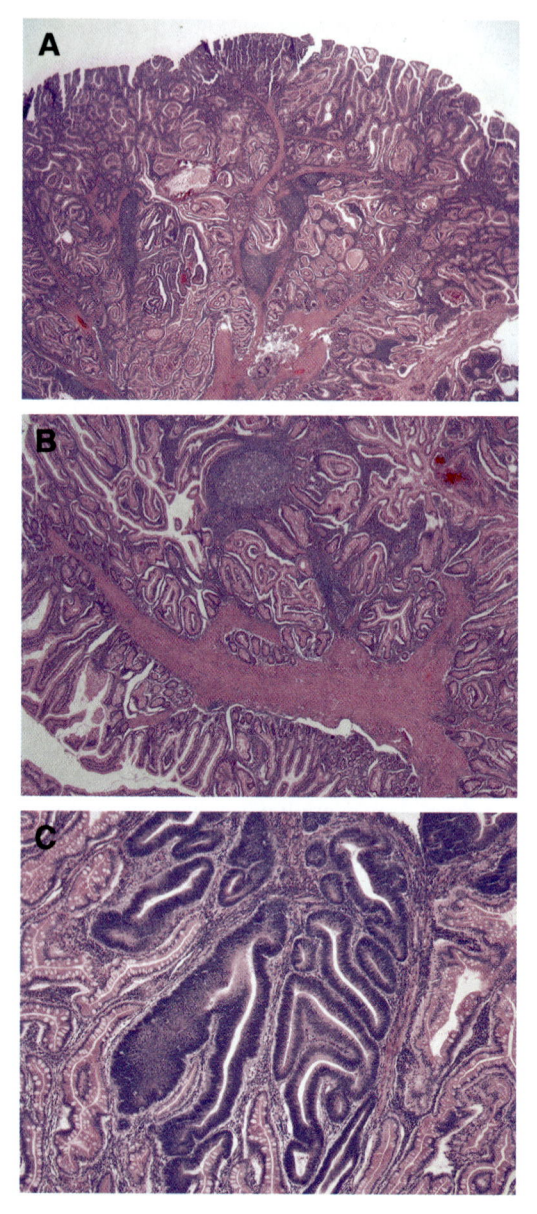

Fig. 4. Polyp from a Peutz-Jegher syndrome patient. (*A*) Note the arborizing smooth muscle that branches into the stroma to where the absorptive epithelium, goblet, and Paneth cells are located. (*B*) One can see the smooth muscle fibers that make up a large part of the stroma, originating from the muscularis mucosae. (*C*) An area with low-grade dysplasia can be seen. (*From* Burkart AL, Sheridan T, Lewin M, et al. Do sporadic Peutz-Jeghers polyps exist? Experience of a large teaching hospital. Am J Surg Pathol 2007;31:1209; with permission.)

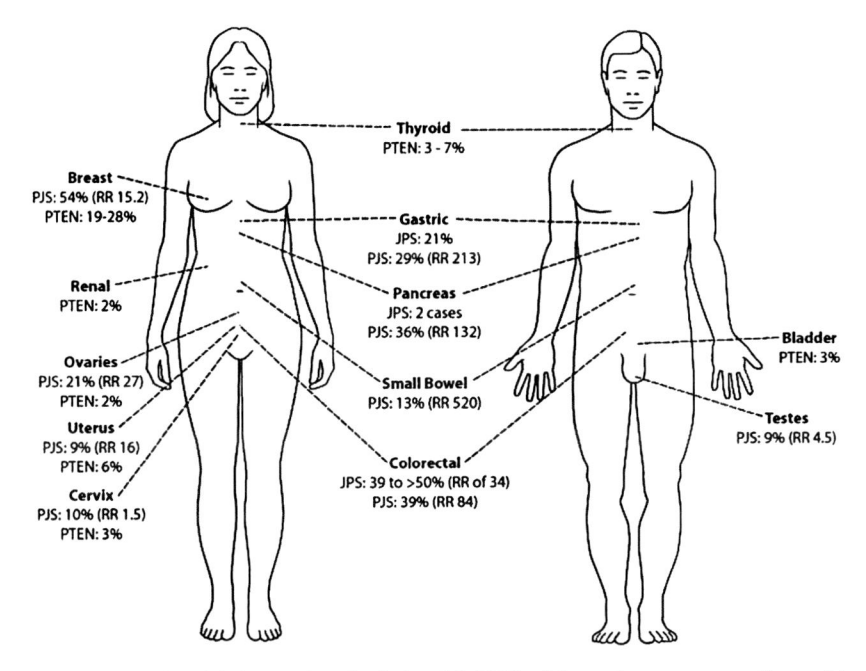

Fig. 5. Cumulative risk (percent) and relative risk (RR) of the various organs predisposed to the development of cancer in JPS, PJS, and *PTEN* hamartoma-tumor syndromes (*Data from* [27,70–73]).

developing colon cancer between ages of 15 to 64, with a mean age of diagnosis of 46 years. There was no statistically significant difference in the incidence of colon cancer between males and females.

Gastric and small bowel

The malignant potential of gastric and duodenal polyps was originally described in 1967 by Payson and Moumgis when they reported a 21-year old with a 2-year history of hematochezia, with weight loss, poor appetite, and fatigue. He developed hematemesis and on workup was found to have jejunal intussusception, multiple polyps throughout the colon, stomach, duodenum, and jejunum. A large hard mass was found in the antrum and a subtotal gastrectomy with omentectomy was performed, in addition to small bowel resection for the intussusception. On pathology, the patient had gastric adenocarcinoma with multiple positive nodes and multiple polyps in the stomach. The rest of the small and large bowel polyps did not show any evidence of malignancy. A review of the literature at that time showed six other cases of upper GI cancers associated with PJS, and investigators concluded that polyps in the stomach and duodenum must be considered as having malignant potential, and should not be dismissed as being benign [74]. The malignant potential of PJS polyps in the small bowel and stomach has been well established and described by many investigators [75–78]. Foley, McGarrity, and Abt [79] did a clinicopathologic survey of the largest PJS kindred, the Harrisburg family, which was originally described by Jeghers in 1949. In their survey, they reported one member who died at the age of 40 from metastatic gastric carcinoma. Another member, at the age of 27 underwent an antrectomy, partial duodenectomy, and gastrojejunostomy for duodenal polyps, and was found to have a focus of adenomatous elements with dysplasia in the duodenum. He ended up having a pancreaticoduodenectomy and, 14 months later, died from a malignant pleural effusion. Giardiello and colleagues [70] found a 93% overall cumulative risk for the development of cancer in PJS patients (15.2-fold relative risk [RR]), with the cumulative risk for gastric cancer being 29% (RR 213), and of the small intestine 13% (RR 520). It should be noted that this study only looked at familial cases of PJS. Therefore, the risk in patients with sporadic PJS has not been as well studied.

Reproductive organs

The association of PJS and a functional ovarian tumor was made by Christian and colleagues [80] in 1964 when they described a 4-year-old girl with precocious puberty. At the age of 3, she developed vaginal spotting, and then heavier bleeding similar to menses. Her mother had pigmentation of her lips, but no evidence or symptoms of GI polyposis, and the rest of the family history was unremarkable. The girl underwent an exploratory laparotomy and was found to have multiple polyps of the small intestine, stomach, and duodenum, and a mass on the left ovary that turned out to be a granulosa-theca cell tumor. Other investigators have described ovarian tumors in patients with PJS [66,81,82], and Scully and colleagues [83] concluded that up to 5% of females with PJS develop an unusual tumor of the ovary, called ovarian sex cord tumor with annular tubules, which are microscopic and tend to be bilateral and multifocal. Functional tumors of the testes (leading to feminizing characteristics) have also been described in boys with PJS. Most of these tumors are Sertoli cell tumors, which arise from the same embryonic cells [84–86]. Cases of well-differentiated adenocarcinoma, infiltrating ductal carcinoma, and papillary carcinoma from the breast have also been described in women with PJS [75,76]. Giardiello and colleagues [70] found that PJS patients have an absolute risk for cancer of the breast of 54% (RR 15.2), the ovaries 21% (RR 27), the cervix 10% (RR 1.5), and the uterus and testes of 9% (RR 16 and 4.5, respectively).

Pancreatic and gallbladder cancer

In 1986, Bowlby and colleagues [87] described a 14-year-old boy with sporadic PJS found to have a retroperitoneal mass with a nonfunctioning left kidney. Autopsy revealed that the mass replaced the body and tail of the pancreas and was a pancreatic adenocarcinoma. Giardiello and colleagues [70] found six cases of pancreatic cancer in the literature, and concluded that PJS patients have a 132-fold increased risk of developing pancreatic cancer (36% cumulative risk). Wada and colleagues [88] described a 39-year-old woman with PJS who was found to have two polyps in the gallbladder, with cholelithiasis and choledocholithiasis on endoscopic retrograde cholangiopancreatography. Cholecystectomy and common bile duct exploration revealed a well-differentiated adenocarcinoma of the gallbladder arising from the mucosa close to the largest polyp.

Management

In 2006, Giardiello and Trimbath published a review of PJS in which they recommended screening from birth of all first-degree relatives of PJS patients. Screening should be directed to identifying melanosis and ruling out testicular or ovarian tumors that might cause precocious puberty. Asymptomatic first-degree relatives who do not show any clinical signs of the disease should be offered genetic testing for mutations in the serine/threonine kinase 11 gene (*STK11/LKB1*) starting at the age of 8. Asymptomatic individuals at risk, without knowledge of the mutation status, should undergo careful screening with upper endoscopy, colonoscopy, and small bowel follow-through at the ages of 12, 18, and 24. Another strategy is to have just the small bowel follow-through every 2 years until the age of 25. In addition, the patient at risk should be advised to follow the same screening guidelines as those for affected individuals to make sure no other organ systems are involved. If a mutation is found in *STK11/LKB1*, then colonoscopies every 2 to 3 years should be done starting at the age of 18 or with symptoms. Upper endoscopy should start at the age of 8 and be repeated every 2 years if any polyps are found, which should be removed endoscopically. Endoscopic ultrasound to look at the pancreas should be done every 1 to 2 years starting at the age of 25 to 30. Males should have careful testicular examination starting at birth, with ultrasounds every 2 years until the age of 12. Females should have regular breast self-examinations starting at the age of 18, and annual mammograms or MRI as an alternative, with physician-directed breast examinations starting at the age of 25, or at the age when the first relative was diagnosed with the PJS if earlier than age 25. Pelvic examination with annual Pap smears should start at the age of 21 to rule out cervical cancer, with transvaginal ultrasound and serum CA-125 done annually at the age of 25 to rule out cancer of the uterus and ovaries [89].

Soares and colleagues [90] performed capsule endoscopy in two groups of PJS patients. Group A consisted of 14 patients who were known to have polyps in the small bowel and who had undergone small bowel surgical procedures. Group B consisted of 6 first-degree relatives who had GI symptoms but no polyps found by prior endoscopic evaluations. No member of group B had undergone any related surgical procedures. Capsule endoscopy identified multiple polyps in all patients from group A, but none from group B. Seven patients of group A had polyps larger than 1 cm, and 5 of these patients underwent enteroscopy to remove the polyps. At the time of enteroscopy, 20 more polyps, missed by capsule endoscopy, were identified in all 5 patients. There were no complications from the procedure, and all the capsules were expelled within 24 hours. The investigators concluded that capsule endoscopy is a safe and well-tolerated method for evaluating the small intestine in PJS patients. However, polyps were missed by this method.

Plum and colleagues studied double-balloon endoscopy in patients with PJS. This technique features an endoscope and a sliding tube with two balloons, one attached to the distal end of the scope and the other attached to a transparent tube, which slides over the endoscope. When the two balloons are inflated, they can trap the small intestine and allow the scope to be advanced until the whole small bowel is visualized. Plum and colleagues [91] performed the procedure on 16 patients with the diagnosis of PJS between the years 2003 and 2006. A total of 47 procedures were done, 39 were via the oral approach, and 8 by the anal approach. A total of 178 polyps were documented, mostly in the jejunum, and 47 endoscopic polypectomies were performed. Thirty-seven polyps were larger than 1 cm with the largest being 5 cm, and 10 were removed due to an abnormal gross appearance. No evidence of malignancy was found in any of these polyps on pathologic evaluation. Investigators reported four complications, one perforation, one episode of hypoxia associated with a large dose of propofol, and two episodes of bleeding with a drop in hemoglobin. They concluded that double-balloon endoscopy is not only a safe, effective, and well-tolerated method of screening, but it allows the clinician to evaluate and treat polyps that might cause intussusception, small bowel obstruction, or hemorrhage, or be suspicious for malignancy. Polyps can also be tattooed so their exact location in the small bowel can be determined at surgery.

Westerman and Wilson [59] stated that most cases of intussusception resolve on their own, but when paralytic ileus evolves, or the obstruction does not resolve within a few hours, laparotomy is required. Surgery should be conservative because resection of additional small bowel might be required in the future. Surgery should focus on removing responsible polyps that caused the intussusception, as well as the diseased small bowel. The small bowel should be cleared of all large polyps by enterotomy at the same time. Giardiello and Trimbath [89] recommended polypectomy of polyps larger than 1 cm in the stomach and colon if encountered during surveillance. In the small intestine, surgery was recommended for polyps that are rapidly enlarging (noted by serial exams with endoscopy or upper GI series) or that are larger than 1 cm. If the patient becomes symptomatic and requires a laparotomy, an attempt to clear the small intestine of polyps should be made at the same time, which can be done by enterotomy if the polyps are large, usually with the aid of intraoperative endoscopy.

Genetics

PJS can be either familial or sporadic, and it is transmitted in an autosomal-dominant fashion [58,92]. In 1997, Hemminki and colleagues [93] studied 12 families with PJS by comparative genomic hybridization (CGH), loss of heterozygosity (LOH) in polyps, and linkage analysis. They found that 6 out of 16 polyps had had a subtle loss of chromosome 19p on CGH, which was confirmed by LOH of markers on 19p. To verify that the region deleted from 19p was the area containing the PJS gene, linkage analysis was performed. Investigators found a logarithmic odds (LOD) score of 7.00 with the marker *D19S886* at theta equal to 0.00. Their results showed that PJS is a genetically homogeneous syndrome with a very high penetrance. Based upon LOH in polyps, they hypothesized that the gene responsible was a tumor-suppressor gene. Mehenni and colleagues [94] confirmed these findings in six different PJS families (with 39 affected and 48 unaffected individuals), localizing the PJS locus to chromosome 19p13.3, with a multipoint LOD score of 7.51 at theta equal to 0.045.

In 1998, Hemminki and colleagues [95] performed a search for the predisposing gene in the PJS by constructing a cosmid contig across the putative PJS gene region from markers *D19S886* to *D19S883*. Transcripts from this region were identified using various methods, and 27 transcripts were further screened for mutations by reverse transcription followed by polymerase chain reaction from lymphoblastoid cell lines from 12 affected individuals with PJS. The *LKB1* gene, which encodes for a 433-amino-acid serine threonine kinase, was chosen for further screening. Five PJS patients were found to have deletions of *LKB1* (188 bp, 29 bp, 2 bp, and 1 bp in length leading to frameshifts, and another 174 bp in-frame with loss of 58 amino acids), and 5 had substitutions (4 nonsense, 1 missense). Another had a 1-bp insertion and frameshift, and 1 individual had no mutations found. Jenne and colleagues [96] independently found the PJS gene in a PJS kindred with 5 affected individuals within three generations, which they called *STK11*. Volikos and colleagues [97] reported that approximately 80% of PJS patients have mutations in the *LKB1/STK11* gene. Sixty-three percent (48 of 76) of patients had mutations by direct sequencing, another 14% (11 of 28) had larger deletions (5 whole gene deletions, 2 with the promoter and exon 1 deleted, and 1 with exon 8 deleted) found by the multiple ligation probe-dependent amplification technique. The *LKB1/STK11* product localizes to both the nucleus and cytoplasm, has been found to interact with p53 and some SMAD4 complexes, and is involved in cell polarity, chromatin remodeling, cell cycle arrest, and Wnt signaling [98].

Counseling

Eighty percent of PJS patients will have *LKB1* mutations, of which 60% are identified by sequencing and another 20% by multiple ligation probe-dependent amplification [97]. PJS patients need to be educated as to the resources available for genetic testing, which can be very helpful, although the diagnosis can be made clinically in most cases when there is a positive family history. A positive *LKB1* mutation test confirms the need for careful screening and follow-up, while a negative test spares individuals from unnecessary screening procedures [99]. Patients need to be educated on the natural history of the disease, the high incidence of the various cancers, possible complications, and the signs and symptoms of different polyps and cancers associated with PJS. They need to learn about the recommended screening procedures and be set up with physicians who will carry out appropriate long-term follow-up.

Hereditary mixed polyposis syndrome

History

In 1971, Kaschula [100] described an 11-year-old girl with profuse diarrhea mixed with blood and mucus and no associated anomalies. She was found to have polyps throughout the colon and small bowel. A total colectomy with ileorectal anastomosis was done, and the polyps were found to have both adenomatous and juvenile features, but no link was made to a new syndrome. In 1987, Sarles and colleagues [101] described a father and son having multiple polyps throughout the colon that on pathologic examination were adenomas and metaplastic polyps in the father, and adenomas, metaplastic polyps, and juvenile polyps in the son. The investigators proposed a new syndrome they called mixed familial polyposis based on this description.

Clinical features

In 1997, Whitelaw and colleagues coined the term *hereditary mixed polyposis syndrome* (HMPS), although they stated that it is not entirely clear weather this was a new syndrome or a variant of JPS. They performed an extensive evaluation of St. Mark's family 96 (SM96), which had been followed for over 40 years. The family had over 20 members in the second generation, 64 in the third generation, 102 in the fourth generation, and 42 members in the fifth generation. Family members are located throughout the world, and 42 (18 women and 24 men) had either colorectal cancer or polyps. The polyps in the family were tubular adenomas, villous adenomas, flat adenomas, hyperplastic polyps, and atypical juvenile polyps. All atypical juvenile polyps had mixed histologic elements with overlapping adenomatous and hyperplastic features. HMPS patients develop polyps only in the colon and rectum and, on initial colonoscopy, they tend to usually have fewer than 15 polyps. Patients had a median age at presentation of 40 years. The most common symptoms were bright blood per rectum; altered bowel habits, such as blood in the stool or diarrhea; abdominal pain; and, on rare occasions, bowel obstruction. On laboratory examination, signs of anemia were common. They found that 1 member had an epidermoid cyst removed from his face, and another had a lipoma overlying the left scapula, but otherwise no other extracolonic anomalies were found [102].

In 2003, Rozen and colleagues [103] published clinical data on members of a large family in Israel with HMPS. These patients are relatives of the SM96 family, which originated from Lithuania. There are 37 members in the family, and 17 are affected with either colorectal cancer or polyps, which ranged from juvenile, hyperplastic, or mixed juvenile or hyperplastic polyps with adenomatous features, to serrated and tubular adenomas. Cao and colleagues [104] found the mean age of presentation to be 32.4 years. In their study they published data on two families from Singapore, and found that the patients had polyps that ranged from hyperplastic, adenomatous, juvenile, or mixed hyperplastic or juvenile with adenomatous elements. They also concluded that there are no extracolonic anomalies associated with HMPS.

Histopathology

According to Whitelaw and colleagues [102], polyps show evidence of mixed elements, such as tubular, villous, and sessile adenomas, and atypical juvenile polyps with adenomatous or hyperplastic features. HMPS patients also tend to develop inflammatory and metaplastic polyps [105]. Rozen and colleagues [103] described mixed hyperplastic-adenomatous polyps, as the adenomatous part of the polyp has crypts lined by dysplastic epithelium, and the hyperplastic part shows crypts with stellate lumens lined by nondysplastic epithelium. In the mixed juvenile-adenomatous polyp, adenomatous areas were composed of serrated crypts, while the juvenile parts had dilated nondysplastic crypts.

Cancer predisposition

Sarles and colleagues [101] felt that in all cases with mixed polyposis, especially with adenomatous features, there was a risk of malignancy. Jeevaratnam and colleagues [106] described a three-generation family with 6 members having colonic adenocarcinoma and evidence of hyperplastic polyps. The grandmother in the family underwent surgical resection for colon cancer. She had 10 children, 5 of them with colon adenocarcinoma and evidence of mixed hyperplastic polyps with adenomatous changes. Three of these individuals had poorly differentiated adenocarcinoma, and passed away from metastatic disease. The other 2 were found to have moderately differentiated adenocarcinoma. Two grandchildren from affected parents were also found to have hyperplastic polyps on colonoscopy. Jeevaratnam and colleagues [106] suggested that cancer arises from within hyperplastic or mixed polyps that develop foci of dysplasia, or from adenomas that might also be present in the GI tract. Whitelaw and colleagues [102] also felt that HMPS carries a risk for the development of colorectal cancer.

They found that in family SM96, 13 individuals had colorectal cancer, with a median age at diagnosis of 47 years. In addition, they reported 2 female members with breast cancer, but no evidence of colonic polyps, and 1 member, a nonsmoker with bronchial carcinoma, who had not been screened for polyps at the time of the study. Rozen and colleagues [103] also described a branch of this family in Israel that had 5 members with colorectal cancer.

In 1999, Tomlinson and colleagues [107] reported an Ashkenazi family, named St. Mark's family 1311 (SM1311), whose members had the predisposition to develop colorectal adenomas and carcinomas. The kindred was composed of four generations, in which 12 members developed colorectal cancer, 1 member had pancreatic cancer, and another had renal cancer. Affected members had tubulovillous, villous, and serrated adenomas throughout the colon and rectum. Cao and colleagues [104] reported 6 members with colorectal cancer in the two families from Singapore (3 from each family). One member of family 2 was also diagnosed with papillary thyroid carcinoma at the age of 40.

Management

Because of the risk of malignancy, Sarles and colleagues [101] recommend annual colonoscopy for screening patients with mixed polyposis. Whitelaw and colleagues [102] recommend colonoscopy every 2 years for surveillance because they found in family SM96 one individual who developed 12 tubular adenomas in a 2-year period. They felt that sigmoidoscopic surveillance played no role in HPMS since over half of the cancers in family SM96 were proximal to the midtransverse colon. Rozen and colleagues [103] also recommend careful screening and polypectomy to prevent the development of colorectal cancer. Sarles and colleagues [101] propose that, when surgical management is needed, total colectomy is justified with patients who are found to have adenomas on colonoscopy, or when there is a family history that increased the risk of malignancy.

Genetics

Jeevaratnam and colleagues [106] examined a three-generation kindred with HMPS, and suggested that the disorder could be caused by a mutation in a mismatch repair gene and, furthermore, that the germline mutation seems to be inherited in an autosomal-dominant pattern. Since then, other investigators have concurred that HMPS appears to be a distinct syndrome and is inherited in an autosomal-dominant fashion [102,104,105]. In 1996, Thomas and colleagues performed linkage analysis on the SM96 family. Linkage excluded *APC, hMSH2, MLH1, TP53, DCC,* and other loci involved in HNPCC [102,105,107]. The maximum multipoint LOD score was 3.93, found between markers *D6S301* and *D6S283* located on chromosome 6q. Karyotype analysis combined with fluorescence in situ hybridization analysis revealed no inversion or other gross rearrangements on chromosome 6 [105]. In 1999, Tomlinson and colleagues [107] performed linkage analysis in family SM1311, where members had the predisposition to develop colorectal adenomas and carcinomas. They had previously found no mutations of the *APC* gene nor of any other known genes that cause colon cancer. They found a LOD score of 3.06 with *D15S118*, which mapped a new colorectal cancer susceptibility gene to chromosome 15q14–q22, which they called colorectal adenoma and carcinoma (*CRAC1*). Won Sang Park and colleagues [108] performed high-density LOH with markers spanning chromosome 15q15–q22 in family SM1311, and found a deletion mapping to 15q21.1, where the tumor suppressor gene *THBS1* was thought to be the most likely candidate gene.

In 2003, Jaeger and colleagues [109] reassessed family SM96. They felt that the linkage done earlier by Thomas and colleagues might not be correct because a member of the family who did not have the disease haplotype, had developed multiple colorectal adenomas. Updating the affection status of individuals, and performing a genome-wide linkage analysis, chromosome 6 was excluded, and a maximum 2-point LOD score of 3.98 and a multipoint LOD score of 4.67 was found on chromosome 15q13–q21. In addition, Jaeger and colleagues compared haplotypes at the *CRAC1* locus found by Tomlinson and colleagues in 1999 to that in SM96 and discovered that they shared the same alleles between markers *D15S1031–D15S118*. Furthermore, Jaeger and colleagues examined another Ashkenazi family believed to have HMPS (SM2952), and typing of markers *D15S1031–D15S118* at 15q13–q14 showed that all affected members shared the *HMPS/CRAC1* haplotype. Therefore, using data from the three families, 2-point and multipoint LOD scores were 5.31 and 7.19 respectively [109]. However, Peng and colleagues [110], using the markers *D15S1031–D15S118* for the *HMPS/CRAC1* haplotype, did not find linkage in the two HMPS families from Singapore. Later, Cao and colleagues [104] updated the affection status of families 1 and 2 from Singapore and found linkage with a multipoint LOD score of 4.60 between *D10S1696* and *D10S1739* on chromosome 10q23. They also found the same haplotype from markers on 10q23.1 to 10q23.32 segregated with disease in the two families. This area was then screened for mutations by sequencing all coding exons in the *PTEN, MINPP1, PCSH21,* and *BMPR1A* genes, and an 11-bp deletion was found in the proband of family 2 in exon 2 of *BMPR1A*, which resulted in a frame shift. There were no mutations identified in these genes in affected members of family 1, however.

Counseling

Physicians should provide genetic counseling and, if a hamartomatous polyposis syndrome or another polyposis syndrome is suspected, genetic testing. Because the gene responsible for HMPS has not been clearly identified, these patients should be managed accordingly and perhaps should be considered for sequencing of JP genes (*SMAD4* and *BMPR1A*) and perhaps HNPCC genes. If the family is large enough, linkage studies using markers from chromosome 15q13–21 should be considered. Although some evidence suggests that medical management with aspirin or cyclooxygenase-2 inhibitors significantly inhibit sporadic colorectal adenoma recurrences and reduce the risk for colorectal cancer [111], careful screening via colonoscopy, either annually or every 2 years, and surveillance of all polyps found via polypectomy is the most effective method to date to prevent advanced cancers from developing. When colorectal cancer has been identified, more aggressive surgical management is indicated, and either a subtotal or total colectomy should be the procedure of choice.

PTEN hamartoma tumor syndrome: Cowden syndrome and Bannayan-Riley-Ruvalbaba syndrome

History

In 1960, Riley and Smith [112] described a mother and her four (of seven) children with macrocephaly and pseudopapilledema. The father of the children did not exhibit any of these traits. Riley and Smith concluded that this syndrome was due to a mutation in a single autosomal gene. In 1962, Lloyd and Dennis [113] described a 20-year-old female with a lesion of her right breast that was ulcerated and draining. She had mild mental retardation, poor fine motor movements, microstomia, macrocephaly, and multiple hyperkeratotic papillomata over her lips. She underwent bilateral modified simple mastectomies, and pathology demonstrated adenocarcinoma of the right breast. Biopsy from a thyroid mass was consistent with an adenoma. They concluded that the spectrum of findings might be genetically linked, and coined the disease entity as *Cowden syndrome*, named after the patient, Rachel Cowden. In 1971, Bannayan [114] described a 3-year-old girl with macrocephaly and numerous subcutaneous lesions that ranged from lipolymphangio-hemangiomas to vascular hamartomas. She underwent resection of multiple masses in the thoracic cavity, which all grossly appeared to be adipose tissue. At autopsy, the entire central nervous system was enlarged, with prominent gyri, but no dilation of the ventricles. The thoracic and abdominal cavities had multiple fatty tumors. The entire subserosa of the GI tract had sessile and pedunculated fatty tumors. Bannayan felt that this syndrome was related to the one reported by Riley and Smith, since both lipomatosis and hemangiomatosis are hamartomatous malformations. In 1980, Ruvalcaba, Myhre, and Smith [115] described two patients with macrocephaly, mental retardation, pigmented spotting of the glans penis and shaft, and multiple polyps of the GI tract. Histologically, the polyps were consistent with hamartomas, and they felt that this syndrome differed from PJS. The cases described by Bannayan, Riley, Ruvalcaba, Myhre, and Smith would be come known as the Bannayan-Riley-Ruvalcaba syndrome (BRRS) in 1992 when Gorlin and colleagues coined the term, and later would be linked to mutations in the *PTEN* gene, which also causes CS.

Many physicians and researchers now consider BRRS and CS to be a single entity, with a phenotypic spectrum caused by mutations of the *PTEN* gene, now referred to as the *PTEN* hamartoma tumor syndrome [116–119].

Clinical features

Sogol and colleagues [120] reviewed all cases of CS up to the year 1978, and found that, out of the 40 cases described, thyroid disease occurred in 68% (27 of 40) of CS patients, with the most common thyroid lesion being goiter, which occurred in 45% of patients. Sixty-six percent of these patients underwent total thyroidectomy. Thyroid cancer was found in only 7.5% of patients with CS (2 patients had follicular carcinoma, and 1 had a mixed papillary-follicular carcinoma). They also found that 55% (22 of 40) of women had breast disease. However, they did not specify the various types of breast pathology. In contrast, Starink and colleagues found that 68% of CS patients had thyroid disease, with only 3% having follicular carcinoma, and 70% of patients had breast disease, with 52% having fibrocystic changes, and 28% ductal adenocarcinoma. Furthermore, 100% of the patients had mucocutaneous lesions, which included facial trichilemmomas (Fig. 6), acral keratoses, oral papillomas and fibromas, skin tags, scrotal tongue, arteriovenous malformations, and lipomas [73]. Carlson and colleagues [121] described involvement of the GI system with a review of the literature revealing that 27% of CS patients had hamartomatous polyps in the colorectum. In contrast, Starink and colleagues [73] reported that 43% of patients had involvement of the GI tract, with 22% of patients having hamartomatous polyps in the upper GI tract, and 29% in the colorectum.

Albrecht and colleagues [122] suggested that Lhermitte-Duclos disease (LDD), where individuals have cerebellar hamartomas (gangliocytomas) and mental dullness, is associated or closely linked to CS. In 1991, they published two cases with both CS and LDD and, on review of the literature, they found 52 other cases of patients diagnosed with LDD who also had clinical signs of CS. They concluded that patients with LDD might have a broader diagnosis of CS. The two patients they described had, in addition to classical clinical signs of CS, vertigo, headaches, visual changes, and ataxia, all due to hydrocephalus secondary to enlarged and thickened cerebellar tonsils, with cerebellar biopsies consistent with LDD. Since then, other investigators have included LDD in the diagnosis of CS [123,124]. The International Cowden Consortium Diagnostic Criteria are divided into three categories: (1) pathognomonic criteria, in which individuals are diagnosed with CS if they have facial trichilemmomas, keratosis of the palms or plantar surfaces, oral papillomatous lesions, and mucosal lesions (there must be six or more of these lesions, and three or more must be trichilemmomas); (2) major criteria, which include LDD, macrocephaly, breast cancer, and thyroid cancer (especially papillary thyroid cancer); and (3) minor criteria, which include

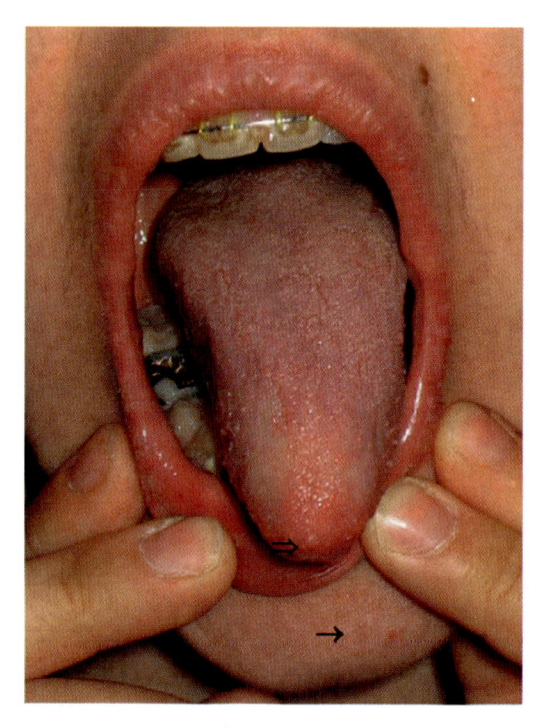

Fig. 6. Some of the pathognomonic features of CS, which are facial trichilemmoma (*solid black arrow*), papillomatosis of the tongue (*open arrow*), and acral keratoses. (*From* Jornayvaz FR, Philippe J. Mucocutaneous papillomatous papules in Cowden's syndrome. Clin Exp Dermatol 2008;33:151; with permission).

multinodular goiter, mental retardation, gastrointestinal hamartomas, fibrocystic disease of the breast, lipomas, fibromas, and genitourinary tumors or malformations. If the individual does not have any of the pathognomonic criteria, then, to make the diagnosis of CS, there must be two major criteria (where one is either LDD or macrocephaly), one major and three minor criteria, or four minor criteria (Box 1) [125].

Gorlin and colleagues [126], upon review of the literature for BRRS, reported that the macrocephaly with a normal ventricular system is common to all BRRS patients. Sixty percent have downslanting of the palpebral fissures, 15% have strabismus or amlyopia, 35% have Schwalbe lines, and most have birth weight above the mean and body length above the 97th percentile. Fifty percent of patients have hypotonia, mild mental retardation, gross motor delay, and speech delay. The motor delay is, for the most part, transient, and improves with time, but 60% of patients have irreversible myopathic disease. Fifty percent of patients have speckling of the glans penis and shaft, cutaneous angiolipomas, lymphangiomyomas, angiokeratomas, joint hyperextensibility, pectus excavatum, scoliosis, and accelerated growth of the metacarpals and of the first and second phalanges.

Box 1. Diagnostic criteria for Cowden syndrome

Pathognomonic criteria
  Six facial papules (three must be trichilemmomas)
  Facial papules and oral mucosal papillomatosus
  Oral papillomatosus and acral keratoses
  Six palmoplantar keratoses
Major criteria
  Breast cancer
  Thyroid cancer (follicular)
  Macrocephaly (>97%)
  Lhermitte-Duclos disease
Minor criteria
  Thyroid lesions (adenoma/goiter)
  Mental retardation
  GI hamartomas
  Lipomas
  Fibromas
  Genitourinary tumors

Data from Eng C. Will the real Cowden syndrome please stand up: revised diagnostic criteria. J Med Genet 2000;37:828.

Seventy-five percent of patients have subcutaneous lipomas, 10% have hemangiomas and café-au-lait spots of the trunk and lower extremities. Forty-five percent of patients have hamartomatous polyps, which are limited to the ileum and colon and can lead to rectal bleeding and intussusception. In 1999, Marsh and colleagues [118] noted that BRRS and CS have several clinical features in common: Hashimoto's thyroiditis, vascular malformations, and mental retardation. However, BRRS patients develop pigmented macules of the glans penis and shaft, and delayed motor development, which are not seen in CS patients. Lipomatosis is rarely seen in patients with CS, but is common in BRRS.

Associated anomalies
  Starink and colleagues [73] reviewed the CS patients in 1986, and found that 7% of males had bilateral gynecomastia, 3% of males had hydroceles, 20% of females had menstrual irregularities, 19% had ovarian cysts, 5% had leiomyomas of the uterus, and 6% had cysts in the uterus. Macrocephaly was found in 21% of patients, adenoid facies (long, thin face with malar hypoplasia; high-arched palate, which is seen alone in 14% of patients; and a narrow maxillary arch) in 8%, pectus excavatum in 6%, and bone cysts in 4%. In terms of the neurologic system, 5% had neuromas

of cutaneous nerves, 3% had neurofibromas, 3% had meningiomas, and 2% had hearing loss. Some patients have eye involvement, with 3% of patients having cataracts, 2% having angioid streaks, 3% myopia, and 1% congenital blood vessel anomalies.

Histopathology

Brownstein and colleagues [127,128] described the cutaneous tumors as trichilemmomas, which are benign neoplasms arising from the outer root sheath of hair follicles. Histologically, these are made up of keratinized, palisading cells in the periphery, which are surrounded by a vitreous, thick basement membrane, rich in glycogen. These tumors tend to occur around the mouth, nose, and ears. The acral keratoses found on the palms are hyperkeratotic, and are colored or brownish lesions. Oral lesions, which tend to be fibromas, are seen under the tongue, in the lips, on the mucous membranes, or on the palate. These lesions are benign, and are formed by a fibrovascular core covered by epithelial cells with no nuclear atypia [127].

Cancer predisposition

Colorectal

In 1985, Walton and colleagues [129] described a 36-year-old female with CS who was found to have breast cancer incidentally after bilateral prophylactic mastectomies. Her father, who was believed to have CS, died from metastatic colon cancer. This was the first individual with CS reported to have colon cancer. Starink and colleagues [73] found that out of 100 patients with CS, 2 females had adenocarcinoma of the cecum, and 1 male had adenocarcinoma of the colon. However, both patients who had cancer in the cecum did not have polyps throughout the colon. Therefore, investigators concluded, no meaningful association between colorectal cancer and CS could be made. In BRRS, colorectal cancer, and cancer of the small bowel have not been reported [118].

Thyroid and reproductive organs

In 1986, Starink and colleagues [73] reviewed 100 cases of CS and found that the most common organs affected with cancer are the thyroid and the female organs. Three percent had follicular thyroid cancers, 28% had breast adenocarcinoma, 6% had adenocarcinoma of the uterus, 3% had carcinoma of the cervix, 2% had carcinoma of the ovary, and 2% of females had transitional cell carcinoma of the renal pelvis. In addition, investigators found that 3% of males had transitional cell carcinoma of the bladder. In 1995, Hanssen and colleagues [72] reported that malignancies of the thyroid were present in 7% of patients, breast cancer was present in 19%, and there was a 45% risk of cancer of the reproductive organs (see Fig. 5).

In 2001, Frackenthal and colleagues [130] reported two males with CS who developed breast cancer. One patient had a sporadic case of CS diagnosed at the age of 31, and developed breast cancer at the age of 41. He was found to have a de novo mutation in *PTEN*. The second patient belonged to a three-generation CS family with six affected members. He developed breast cancer at the age of 43, and also had a *PTEN* mutation, which segregated with the disease in his family. Both of these patients died from breast cancer in their early 50s. Longy and colleagues [131] described a BRRS family with four affected individuals, in which the grandmother of the proband was diagnosed with adenocarcinoma of the breast and endometrium at age 53. This was the first report of cancer in a BRRS patient and the investigators concluded that it might be warranted to follow BRRS patients for the cancers screened for in CS. Marsh and colleagues [118] confirmed that breast cancer and fibroadenoma were also found in patients with BRRS or CS, or in patients with overlapping features. They found that patients with truncating mutations in *PTEN* were at higher risk of developing breast cancer or fibroadenomas.

Management

Walton and colleagues [129] felt that periodic contrast studies of the GI tract and colonoscopies should be done to screen CS patients for disease of the upper and lower GI tracts. Today, the method of choice for screening suspicious nodules of the thyroid gland is by performing thyroid ultrasound with fine needle aspiration, in addition to taking measurements of thyrotropin and free T4 levels, which should be obtained if one is suspicious of thyroid disease. Williard and colleagues [132] stated that female patients should perform monthly breast self-examinations, combined with physician breast examinations every 3 months, and mammography every 6 to 12 months with biopsies of any suspicious lesions.

Walton and colleagues [129] described a 36-year-old female with CS who had bilateral oophorectomy at the time of tubal ligation for reportedly incidentally found benign cysts. Colonoscopy was normal. She had facial trichilemmomas, multinodular goiter, and facial verruca vulgaris. Mammography showed fibrocystic breast disease bilaterally, but no suspicious areas for cancer. She elected to undergo total thyroidectomy and prophylactic bilateral simple mastectomy with immediate reconstruction. On pathologic examination, an unexpected small focus of infiltrating ductal carcinoma surrounded by epithelial dysplasia was identified in her right breast. She then had a right axillary dissection, and 1 out of 17 nodes was positive for metastatic disease. Investigators believe that serial mammography should start at the age of 30, with monthly breast self-examinations. They felt that females with CS should be offered prophylactic mastectomy around the fourth decade of life with counseling about the procedure and its indications. Williard and colleagues [132] described a 32-year-old female with a 2-month history of a painless mass in her right breast and nipple inversion. She was diagnosed earlier with fibrocystic breast disease, and had had several benign cysts removed from her breasts 10 years earlier. She was diagnosed with CS, and her family had a very high incidence of breast cancer. Her mother died of breast cancer at the age of 42, and she had two maternal aunts that had breast cancer before menopause. She was found to have bilateral intraductal and infiltrating ductal carcinoma, and had bilateral modified radical mastectomies, with 7 of 49 nodes on the left breast positive for metastatic disease, and 10 of 31 nodes on the right breast positive for metastatic disease. Williard and colleagues [131] felt that female patients with CS should be offered prophylactic bilateral total mastectomy in the third decade, or have monthly breast self-examinations and physician breast examinations every 3 months.

Genetics

Cowden syndrome is an autosomal-dominant inherited disorder [73,133,134], and Hanssen and colleagues [134] suggest that anticipation and imprinting through the female are also part of CS. In 1996, Nelen and colleagues [124] performed a linkage-based genome screen in 12 families with CS. They found linage to markers on the long arm of chromosome 10 with a maximum LOD score of 6.67 with the marker *D10S215*. In 1997, Liaw and colleagues [135] sequenced all coding exons of the *PTEN* gene from 10q22–3 in 5 CS families, of which 4 were linked to markers on 10q22–23. They found that 2 families had missense mutations in exon 5, a third family had a nonsense mutation in exon 7, and a fourth family had a different nonsense mutations in exon 7. Since then, other investigators have confirmed the involvement of *PTEN* in CS [136,137], and germline mutations have been found by sequencing in about 80% of cases [135,138]. PTEN is a dual-specificity tyrosine phosphatase with homology to the chicken protein tensin and bovine auxilin [139]. The phosphatase domain is where the active site is located and performs the enzymatic function, and the C2 domain allows PTEN to bind to the cell membrane where its substrate is located. PTEN dephosphorylates phosphatidylinositol (4,5)-bisphosphate, so that phospholipase C can hydrolyze the phosphodiester link and form inositol triphosphate and diacylglycerol, which are two important intracellular messengers. PTEN plays an important role in apoptosis, preventing uncontrolled cell growth, and possibly is also involved in cell migration and adhesion [140–143].

Also in 1997, Marsh and colleagues [144] examined two unrelated families with BRRS syndrome. One was found to have a germline missense mutation in exon 7, and the other a nonsense mutation in exon 6 of the *PTEN* gene. Both mutations segregated with affected members in each family, and were absent in unaffected members and in 100 control subjects. They concluded that BRRS and CS represent the clinical spectrum of the same disease. Marsh and colleagues [118] later examined 43 unrelated BRRS patients (32 had features of BRRS, and 11 had mixed features of CS and BRRS) for germline *PTEN* mutations by sequencing. Twenty-six of the 43 (60%) individuals had *PTEN* mutations, 17 of which were substitutions (10 missense, 7 nonsense), 5 were small deletions, 1 was a gross deletion of 10q23.3–q24.1, 3 were insertions, and 1 was a balanced translocation. All exons were involved except 1, 4, and 9, and the mutations segregated within affected members of each family (27 were familial cases and 16 were sporadic). Of the 17 BRRS cases that did not have any mutations found in *PTEN*, all retained hemizygosity when analyzed with various markers of the *PTEN* region, which eliminated the likelihood of gross gene deletions. From the 27 familial cases, 11 had clinical symptoms that overlapped between the two syndromes, and 10 of these families had mutations in *PTEN*. In 37 CS families, the findings were very similar, and there were no significant differences in the spectrum of mutations. Four nonsense mutations were common to both CS and BRRS (Q110X, R130X, R233X, and R335X). The balanced translocation and large deletion were only seen in BRRS patients, and no gross deletions were seen in CS. Longy and colleagues [131] confirmed that CS and BRRS syndrome are allelic diseases, and noted that in BRRS syndrome mutations occurred preferentially in exons 6 and 7, while in CS the spectrum of mutations occur in all exons except 1, 4, and 9.

Zhou and colleagues [143] evaluated 122 *PTEN* mutation negative cases of CS and BRRS, and found 3 with deletions, one involving the entire gene, exons, and one involving exons 1 through 5. They also found 9 cases with heterozygous germline promoter mutations. Sarquis and colleagues sequenced 85 subjects with the CS/BRRS phenotype or suggestive features (65 females and 20 males). Out of the 85 patients, 22 did not have *PTEN* mutations and 63 had *PTEN* mutations (43 with known pathogenic *PTEN* mutations, and 20 with variants). Of the 63 patients with *PTEN* mutations, 28 had mixed phenotypic features of both CS and BRRS, 26 had clear phenotypic features of CS, 1 of BRRS, and 8 could not be classified as either CS or BRRS. Investigators analyzed the full-length *PTEN* mRNA and found eight novel splice variants and reduced expression of full-length transcripts compared with controls. They found that five of the eight novel splice variants showed differential expression in individuals with CS/BRRS phenotype compared with controls, and differential expression correlated with the distinct phenotypes seen in the various groups (mixed CS/BRRS, CS, and BRRS) [145].

Counseling

Higginbottom and Schultz [146] feel that genetic counseling is important and could lead to early diagnosis. Liaw and colleagues [135,137] recommend that, because *PTEN* has been identified as the gene responsible for CS, individuals at risk should be tested to receive heightened cancer surveillance for tumors of the breast, thyroid, and GI tract.

Cronkhite-Canada syndrome

History

In 1955, Cronkhite and Canada [147] described two female patients—one 42 years old and the other 75 years old—presenting with several months of diarrhea, vomiting, nausea, and abdominal pain. Several weeks before symptoms, loss of hair of the eyebrows and axillary region; diffuse brown discoloration of the face, neck, and hands; and onychotrophia were noted. On laboratory examination, the only abnormality found was anemia. They had multiple large polyps in the stomach and duodenum, as well as small sessile and polypoid defects covering the entire colonic mucosa on barium examination. The mucosal pattern throughout seemed coarser than normal, especially in the jejunum. Biopsies of the gastric and colonic lesions showed histology consistent with benign adenomatous polyps. Both patients died, and an autopsy on one revealed pitting edema that extended from the feet to the costal margins. Epidermal bullae were noted over the hip area, and xanthomas were present bilaterally. The tongue was atrophic and the surface had a brown discoloration. The tip of the index finger was gangrenous and she had ascities, as well as a pleural and pericardial effusions. Gross examination of the GI tract showed a normal esophagus, but the gastric and duodenal mucosa was covered with polypoid lesions, and the architecture of the mucosa was distorted. The jejunum and ileum were not as heavily involved, but did have polyps, which were more sessile than in the stomach and duodenum. The large bowel and rectum were also carpeted with polyps. All polyps were consistent with simple adenomatous polyps without evidence of malignancy.

Clinical features

In 1966, Jarnum and Jensen [148] published their observation on the syndrome now recognized as Cronkhite-Canada syndrome (CCS). In addition to the features of generalized gastrointestinal polyposis (not affecting the esophagus), alopecia, dermal pigmentation, and atrophy of the nail beds, they found that severe protein-losing enteropathy with electrolyte disturbances (hypocalcemia, hypomagnesimia, and hypokalemia) was also part of the clinical syndrome. Another very important observation by Jarnum and Jensen was that, histologically, the polyps only showed cystic dilatation of glands with no areas of adenomatous epithelium. In 1972, Johnson [149] reported that the stomach and large bowel are not carpeted with adenomatous polyps as originally described, but with hamartomatous polyps, which confirmed the original description of Jarnum and Jensen in 1966. Multiple investigators have described all the above clinical characteristics, as well as the fact that this disease spares the esophagus [150–152].

In 1995, Goto and colleagues [153] proposed a classification of the CCS into five groups:

Type 1: patients complaining of diarrhea as the presenting symptom
Type 2: patients with disguesia (abnormal taste sensation)
Type 3: patients complaining of abnormal sensation in the mouth accompanied by thirst
Type 4: patients with abdominal symptoms other than diarrhea
Type 5: patients with alopecia as the main symptom

All patients must have gastrointestinal polyposis and hyperpigmentation to be diagnosed with CCS, which carries an unfavorable prognosis, with a 5-year mortality rate of 55%. Daniel and colleagues [154] described the potential for life-threatening gastrointestinal bleeding, intussusception, and rectal prolapse. Other complications have been described, such as portal vein thrombosis, high titers of antinuclear antibodies, and membranous glomerulonephritis [155].

Histopathology

Egawa and colleagues [151] identified nests of cancer cells in the gastric mucosa, which were predominantly poorly differentiated with tubular formation as well. The gastric specimen showed typical features of hamartomatous polyps. However, mild infiltration of inflammatory cells, massive submucosal edema (mostly located in the lamina propia), hyperplasia of the foveolar epithelium, and cystic dilation of the mucosal glands were also noted. No adenomatous changes were noted around the cancer cells, which suggested to them that the cancer originated from the gastric mucosa and not from the polyps. To validate this theory, they stained the tissue for Ki-67 and p53, which showed that only cancer cells had overexpression of these proteins, reinforcing the theory that only these cells have the ability to proliferate without cellular control, and had the mutated p53 protein. There were no intermediate changes in the surrounding tissue [151].

Cancer predisposition

Colorectal

Egawa and colleagues [151] reviewed the CCS literature and found that 9% of patients had colorectal cancer (34 of 374 patients), and 41% of these also had adenomas or adenomatous changes. In addition, there were multiple reports showing a clear transition from hamartomatous polyps to adenomatous polyps, with some of the adenomatous polyps having evidence of dysplasia and carcinoma. P53 accumulation was seen in the carcinomatous parts of the polyp, but not in the hamartomatous elements [151]. In 2005, Yashiro and colleagues [156] reviewed 31 cases of CCS and colorectal cancer reported in the literature, and found that 40% had serrated adenomas. They hypothesized that, not only were CCS patients with serrated adenomas at a higher risk of colorectal cancer, but that this was a precursor lesion.

Gastric

Egawa and colleagues [151] described a 52-year-old male with CCS and adenocarcinoma of the stomach arising from the gastric mucosa and not from polypoid lesions. Review of the literature revealed a 5% rate of gastric cancer, seen in 19 out of 374 cases. The mean age of diagnosis was 64 years of age, and 15 were males. Although it seems there is a high risk for gastric cancer, Egawa and colleagues felt it was hard to make a precise correlation, and that the risk of gastric cancer was low in CCS.

Management

Since there is no evidence to date of germline mutations predisposing to this condition, and most experts consider CCS a rare, sporadic, and acquired syndrome, there are no genetic tests for screening individuals that meet the diagnostic criteria [156]. However, due to the high risk of colorectal cancer, screening of the stomach, colon, and rectum by endoscopy should be performed. Biopsies aid in identifying dysplastic or adenomatous epithelium, which would lead to early surgical intervention [151,155]. Egawa and colleagues [151] recommend total gastrectomy in CCS patients diagnosed with gastric cancer to remove the malignant potential in the rest of the stomach, to prevent the high rate of anastomotic leak due to the edema, and to prevent protein loss from the gastric mucosa. As for addressing colorectal cancer, the procedure of choice is determined by the location of the lesion and, if the colon is carpeted with polyps, subtotal or total proctocolectomy would be indicated.

References

[1] Kinzler KW, Vogelstein B. Landscaping the cancer terrain. Science 1998;280:1036–7.
[2] Diamond M. Adenoma of the rectum in children: report of a case in a thirty month old girl. American Journal of Diseases in Children 1939;57:360–7.
[3] Ravitch MM. Polypoid adenomatosis of the entire gastrointestinal tract. Ann Surg 1948; 128:283–98.
[4] Horrilleno EG, Eckert C, Ackerman LV. Polyps of the rectum and colon in children. Cancer 1957;10:1210–20.
[5] McColl I, Bussey HJ, Veale AM, et al. Juvenile polyposis coli. Proceedings of the Royal Society of Medicine 1964;57:896–7.
[6] Sachatello CR, Pickren JW, Grace JT. Generalized juvenile gastrointestinal polyposis. Gastroenterology 1970;58:699–708.
[7] Stemper TJ, Kent TH, Summers RW. Juvenile polyposis and gastrointestinal carcinoma. Ann Intern Med 1975;83:639–46.
[8] Sachatello CR, Hahn IL, Carrington CB. Juvenile gastrointestinal polyposis in a female infant: report of a case and review of the literature of a recently recognized syndrome. Surgery 1974;75:107–14.

[9] Jass JR, Williams CB, Bussey HJR, et al. Juvenile polyposis-A precancerous condition. Histopathology 1988;13:619–30.
[10] Sachatello CR. Polypoid diseases of the gastrointestinal tract. J Ky Med Assoc 1972; 70:540–4.
[11] Veale AMO, McColl I, Bussey HJR, et al. Juvenile polyposis coli. J Med Genet 1966;3: 5–16.
[12] Grosfeld JL, West KW. Generalized juvenile polyposis coli. Arch Surg 1986;121:530–4.
[13] Jass JR. Pathology of polyposis syndromes with special reference to juvenile polyposis. In: Utsunomiya J, Lynch HT, editors. Hereditary colorectal cancer. Tokyo: Springer-Verlag; 1990. p. 343–50.
[14] Desai DC, Neale KF, Talbot IC, et al. Juvenile polyposis. Br J Surg 1995;82:14–7.
[15] Coburn MC, Pricolo VE, DeLuca FG, et al. Malignant potential in intestinal juvenile polyposis syndromes. Ann Surg Oncol 1995;2:386–91.
[16] Bussey HJ, Veale AM, Morson BC. Genetics of gastrointestinal polyposis. Gastroenterology 1978;74:1325–30.
[17] Morson BC. Some peculiarities in the histology of intestinal polyps. Dis Colon Rectum 1962;5:337–44.
[18] Subramony C, Scott-Conner CEH, Skelton D, et al. Familial juvenile polyposis. Study of a kindred: evolution of polyps and relationship to gastrointestinal carcinoma. Am J Clin Pathol 1994;102:91–7.
[19] Goodman ZD, Yardley JH, Milligan FD. Pathogenesis of colonic polyps in multiple juvenile polyposis. Cancer 1979;43:1906–13.
[20] Grigioni WF, Alampi G, Martinelli G, et al. Atypical juvenile polyposis. Histopathology 1981;5:361–76.
[21] Jarvinen HJ, Franssila KO. Familial juvenile polyposis coli: Increased risk of colorectal cancer. Gut 1984;25:792–800.
[22] Ramaswamy G, Elhosseiny AA, Tchertkoff V. Juvenile polyposis of the colon with atypical adenomatous changes and carcinoma in situ. Dis Colon Rectum 1984;27:393–8.
[23] Rozen P, Baratz M. Familial juvenile colonic polyposis with associated colon cancer. Cancer 1982;49:1500–3.
[24] Jones MA, Hebert JC, Trainer TD. Juvenile polyp with intramucosal carcinoma. Arch Pathol Lab Med 1987;111:200–1.
[25] Bentley E, Chandrasoma P, Radin R, et al. Generalized juvenile polyposis with carcinoma. Am J Gastroenterol 1989;84:1456–9.
[26] Giardiello FM, Hamilton SR, Kern SE, et al. Colorectal neoplasia in juvenile polyposis or juvenile polyps. Arch Dis Child 1991;66:971–5.
[27] Howe JR, Mitros FA, Summers RW. The risk of gastrointestinal carcinoma in familial juvenile polyposis. Ann Surg Oncol 1998;5:751–6.
[28] Watanabe A, Nagashima H, Motoi M, et al. Familial juvenile polyposis of the stomach. Gastroenterology 1979;77:148–51.
[29] Yoshida T, Haraguchi Y, Tanaka A, et al. A case of generalized juvenile gastrointestinal polyposis associated with gastric carcinoma. Endoscopy 1988;20:33–5.
[30] Sassatelli R, Bertoni G, Serra L, et al. Generalized juvenile polyposis with mixed pattern and gastric cancer. Gastroenterology 1993;104:910–5.
[31] Walpole IR, Cullity G. Juvenile polyposis: a case with early presentation and death attributable to adenocarcinoma of the pancreas. Am J Med Genet 1989;32:1–8.
[32] Howe JR, Ringold JC, Hughes J, et al. Direct genetic testing for *Smad4* mutations in patients at risk for juvenile polyposis. Surgery 1999;126:162–70.
[33] Jarvinen HJ. Juvenile gastrointestinal polyposis. Problems in General Surgery 1993;10: 749–57.
[34] Haggitt RC, Pitcock JA. Familial juvenile polyposis of the colon. Cancer 1970;26:1232–8.
[35] Pollack JL, Swinton NW. Congenital of the colon with extension to the small intestine and stomach. Lahey Clin Bull 1955;9:174–9.

[36] Scott-Conner CEH, Hausmann M, Hall TJ, et al. Familial juvenile polyposis: Patterns of recurrence and implications for surgical management. J Am Coll Surg 1995;181:407–13.
[37] Hofting I, Pott G, Schrameyer B, et al. Familiare juvenile polyposis mit vorwiegender magenbeteiligung. Zeitschrift fur Gastroenterologie 1993;31:480–3.
[38] Jarvinen H, Franssila KO. Familial juvenile polyposis coli; increased risk of colorectal cancer. Gut 1984;25(5):792–800.
[39] Friedl W, Uhlhaas S, Schulman K, et al. Juvenile polyposis: massive gastric polyposis is more common in MADH4 mutation carriers than in BMPR1A mutation carriers. Hum Genet 2002;111:108–11.
[40] Sayed MG, Ahmed AF, Ringold JC, et al. Germline SMAD4 or BMPR1A mutations and phenotype of juvenile polyposis. Ann Surg Oncol 2002;9:901–6.
[41] Howe JR, Ringold JC, Summers RW, et al. A gene for familial juvenile polyposis maps to chromosome 18q21.1. Am J Hum Genet 1998;62:1129–36.
[42] Howe JR, Roth S, Ringold JC, et al. Mutations in the *SMAD4/DPC4* gene in juvenile polyposis. Science 1998;280:1086–8.
[43] Friedl W, Kruse R, Uhlhaas S, et al. Frequent 4-bp deletion in exon 9 of the SMAD4/MADH4 gene in familial juvenile polyposis patients. Genes Chromosomes Cancer 1999; 25:403–6.
[44] Houlston R, Bevan S, Williams A, et al. Mutations in DPC4 (SMAD4) cause juvenile polyposis syndrome, but only account for a minority of cases. Hum Mol Genet 1998; 7:1907–12.
[45] Roth S, Sistonen P, Salovaara R, et al. SMAD genes in juvenile polyposis. Genes Chromosomes Cancer 1999;26:54–61.
[46] Howe JR, Bair JL, Sayed MG, et al. Germline mutations of the gene encoding bone morphogenetic protein receptor 1A in juvenile polyposis. Nat Genet 2001;28:184–7.
[47] Kim IJ, Park JH, Kang HC, et al. Identification of a novel BMPR1A germline mutation in a Korean juvenile polyposis patient without SMAD4 mutation. Clin Genet 2003;63: 126–30.
[48] Zhou XP, Woodford-Richens K, Lehtonen R, et al. Germline mutations in BMPR1A/ALK3 cause a subset of cases of juvenile polyposis syndrome and of Cowden and Bannayan-Riley-Ruvalcaba syndromes. Am J Hum Genet 2001;69:704–11.
[49] Howe JR, Sayed MG, Ahmed AF, et al. The prevalence of MADH4 and BMPR1A mutations in juvenile polyposis and absence of BMPR2, BMPR1B, and ACVR1 mutations. J Med Genet 2004;41:484–91.
[50] Aretz S, Stienen D, Uhlhaas S, et al. High proportion of large genomic deletions and a genotype phenotype update in 80 unrelated families with juvenile polyposis syndrome. J Med Genet 2007;44:702–9.
[51] Pyatt RE, Pilarski R, Prior TW. Mutation screening in juvenile polyposis syndrome. J Mol Diagn 2006;8:84–8.
[52] Heldin CH, Miyazono K, Ten Dijke P. TGF-β signaling from cell membrane to nucleus through SMAD proteins. Nature 1997;390:465–71.
[53] Massague J. TGFβ signaling: receptors, transducers, and mad proteins. Cell 1996;85: 947–50.
[54] Hutchinson J. Pigmentation of lips and mouth. Arch Surg 1896;7:290–8.
[55] Peutz JL. A very remarkable case of familial polyposis of mucous membrane of intestinal tract and accompanied by peculiar pigmentations of skin and mucous membrane. Nederlands Tijdschrift voor Geneeskunde 1921;10:134–46.
[56] Jeghers H, McKusick VA, Katz KH. Generalized intestinal polyposis and melanin spots of oral mucosa, lips, and digits. N Engl J Med 1949;241:993–1005, 1031–6.
[57] Bruwer A, Bargen JA, Kierland RR. Surface pigmentation and generalized intestinal polyposis; (Peutz-Jeghers syndrome). Mayo Clin Proc 1954;29:168–71.
[58] Bartholomew LG, More CE, Dahlin DC, et al. Intestinal polyposis associated with mucocutaneous pigmentation. Surg Gynecol Obstet 1962;115:1–11.

[59] Westerman AM, Wilson JH. Peutz-Jeghers syndrome: risks of a hereditary condition. Scand J Gastroenterol Suppl 1999;230:64–70.
[60] Dormandy TL. Gastrointestinal polyposis with mucocutaneous pigmentation (Peutz-Jeghers syndrome). N Engl J Med 1957;256:1141–6.
[61] Sommerhaug RG, Mason T. Peutz-Jeghers syndrome and ureteral polyposis. JAMA 1970; 211:120–2.
[62] Foster DR, Foster DB. Gall-bladder polyps in Peutz-Jeghers syndrome. Postgrad Med J 1980;56:373–6.
[63] Gentile AT, Bickler SW, Harrison MW, et al. Common bile duct obstruction related to intestinal polyposis in a child with Peutz-Jeghers syndrome. J Pediatr Surg 1994;29:1584–7.
[64] Parker MC, Knight M. Peutz-Jeghers syndrome causing obstructive jaundice due to polyp in common bile duct. J R Soc Med 1983;76:701–3.
[65] Farmer RG, Hawk WA, Turnbull RB Jr. The spectrum of the Peutz-Jeghers syndrome. Report of 3 cases. Am J Dig Dis 1963;8:953–61.
[66] Humphries AL Jr, Shepherd MH, Peters HJ. Peutz-Jeghers syndrome with colonic adenocarcinoma and ovarian tumors. JAMA 1966;197:296–8.
[67] Niimi K, Tomoda H, Furusawa M, et al. Peutz-Jeghers syndrome associated with adenocarcinoma of the cecum and focal carcinomas in hamartomatous polyps of the colon: a case report. Jpn J Surg 1991;21:220–3.
[68] Tweedie JH, McCann BG. Peutz-Jeghers syndrome and metastasising colonic adenocarcinoma. Gut 1984;25:1118–23.
[69] Konishi F, Wyse NE, Muto T, et al. Peutz-Jeghers polyposis associated with carcinoma of the digestive organs. Report of three cases and review of the literature. Dis Colon Rectum 1987;30:790–9.
[70] Giardiello FM, Brensinger JD, Tersmette AC, et al. Very high risk of cancer in familial Peutz-Jeghers syndrome. Gastroenterology 2000;119:1447–53.
[71] Brosens LA, van Hattem A, Hylind LM, et al. Risk of colorectal cancer in juvenile polyposis. Gut 2007;56:965–7.
[72] Hanssen AM, Fryns JP. Cowden syndrome. J Med Genet 1995;32:117–9.
[73] Starink TM, van der Veen JP, Arwert F, et al. The Cowden syndrome: a clinical and genetic study in 21 patients. Clin Genet 1986;29:222–33.
[74] Payson BA, Moumgis B. Metastasizing carcinoma of the stomach in Peutz-Jeghers syndrome. Ann Surg 1967;165:145–51.
[75] Burdick D, Prior JT. Peutz-Jeghers syndrome. A clinicopathologic study of a large family with a 27-year follow-up. Cancer 1982;50:2139–46.
[76] Lehur PA, Madarnas P, Devroede G, et al. Peutz-Jeghers syndrome. Association of duodenal and bilateral breast cancers in the same patient. Dig Dis Sci 1984;29:178–82.
[77] Lin JI, Caracta PF, Lindner A, et al. Peutz-Jeghers polyposis with metastasizing duodenal carcinoma. South Med J 1977;70.882–4.
[78] Matuchansky C, Babin P, Coutrot S, et al. Peutz-Jeghers syndrome with metastasizing carcinoma arising from a jejunal hamartoma. Gastroenterology 1979;77:1311–5
[79] Foley TR, McGarrity TJ, Abt AB. Peutz-Jeghers syndrome: a clinicopathologic survey of the "Harrisburg family" with a 49-year follow-up. Gastroenterology 1988;95:1535–40.
[80] Christian CD, McLoughlin TG, Cathcart ER, et al. Peutz-Jeghers syndrome associated with functioning ovarian tumor. JAMA 1964;190:935–8.
[81] Solh HM, Azoury RS, Najjar SS. Peutz-Jeghers syndrome associated with precocious puberty. J Pediatr 1983;103:593–5.
[82] Young RH, Welch WR, Dickersin GR, et al. Ovarian sex cord tumor with annular tubules: review of 74 cases including 27 with Peutz-Jeghers syndrome and four with adenoma malignum of the cervix. Cancer 1982;50:1384–402.
[83] Scully RE. Sex cord tumor with annular tubules a distinctive ovarian tumor of the Peutz-Jeghers syndrome. Cancer 1970;25:1107–21.

[84] Cantu JM, Rivera H, Ocampo-Campos R, et al. Peutz-Jeghers syndrome with feminizing sertoli cell tumor. Cancer 1980;46:223–8.
[85] Wilson DM, Pitts WC, Hintz RL, et al. Testicular tumors with Peutz-Jeghers syndrome. Cancer 1986;57:2238–40.
[86] Young S, Gooneratne S, Straus FH II, et al. Feminizing sertoli cell tumors in boys with Peutz-Jeghers syndrome. Am J Surg Pathol 1995;19:50–8.
[87] Bowlby LS. Pancreatic adenocarcinoma in an adolescent male with Peutz-Jeghers syndrome. Hum Pathol 1986;17:97–9.
[88] Wada K, Tanaka M, Yamaguchi K. Carcinoma and polyps of the gallbladder associated with Peutz-Jeghers syndrome. Dig Dis Sci 1987;32:943–6.
[89] Giardiello FM, Trimbath JD. Peutz-Jeghers syndrome and management recommendations. Clin Gastroenterol Hepatol 2006;4:408–15.
[90] Soares J, Lopes L, Vilas Boas G, et al. Wireless capsule endoscopy for evaluation of phenotypic expression of small-bowel polyps in patients with Peutz-Jeghers syndrome and in symptomatic first-degree relatives. Endoscopy 2004;36:1060–6.
[91] Plum N, May AD, Manner H, et al. [Peutz-Jeghers syndrome: endoscopic detection and treatment of small bowel polyps by double-balloon enteroscopy]. Z Gastroenterol 2007;45:1049–55 [in German].
[92] McAllister AJ, Hicken NF, Latimer RG, et al. Seventeen patients with Peutz-Jehgers syndrome in four generations. Am J Surg 1967;114:839–43.
[93] Hemminki A, Tomlinson I, Markie D, et al. Localization of a susceptibility locus for Peutz-Jeghers syndrome to 19p using comparative genomic hybridization and targeted linkage analysis. Nat Genet 1997;15:87–90.
[94] Mehenni H, Blouin J-L, Radhakrishna U, et al. Peutz-Jeghers syndrome: Confirmation of linkage to chromosome 19p13.3 and identification of a potential second locus, on 19q13.4. Am J Hum Genet 1997;61:1327–34.
[95] Hemminki A, Markie D, Tomlinson I, et al. A serine/threonine kinase gene defective in Peutz-Jeghers syndrome. Nature 1998;391:184–7.
[96] Jenne DE, Reimann H, Nezu JI, et al. Peutz-Jeghers syndrome is caused by mutations in a novel serine threonine kinase. Nat Genet 1998;18:38–43.
[97] Volikos E, Robinson J, Aittomaki K, et al. LKB1 exonic and whole gene deletions are a common cause of Peutz-Jeghers syndrome. J Med Genet 2006;43:e18.
[98] Marignani PA. LKB1, the multitasking tumour suppressor kinase. J Clin Pathol 2005;58:15–9.
[99] McGarrity TJ, Kulin HE, Zaino RJ. Peutz-Jeghers syndrome. Am J Gastroenterol 2000;95:596–604.
[100] Kaschula RO. Mixed juvenile, adenomatous and intermediate polyposis coli: report of a case. Dis Colon Rectum 1971;14:368–74.
[101] Sarles JC, Consentino B, Leandri R, et al. Mixed familial polyposis syndromes. Int J Colorectal Dis 1987;2:96–9.
[102] Whitelaw SC, Murday VA, Tomlinson IP, et al. Clinical and molecular features of the hereditary mixed polyposis syndrome. Gastroenterology 1997;112:327–34.
[103] Rozen P, Samuel Z, Brazowski E. A prospective study of the clinical, genetic, screening, and pathologic features of a family with hereditary mixed polyposis syndrome. Am J Gastroenterol 2003;98:2317–20.
[104] Cao X, Eu KW, Kumarasinghe MP, et al. Mapping of hereditary mixed polyposis syndrome (HMPS) to chromosome 10q23 by genomewide high-density single nucleotide polymorphism (SNP) scan and identification of BMPR1A loss of function. J Med Genet 2006;43:e13.
[105] Thomas HJW, Whitelaw SC, Cottrell SE, et al. Genetic mapping of the hereditary mixed polyposis syndrome to chromosome 6q. Am J Hum Genet 1996;58:770–6.
[106] Jeevaratnam P, Cottier DS, Browett PJ, et al. Familial giant hyperplastic polyposis predisposing to colorectal cancer: a new hereditary bowel cancer syndrome. J Pathol 1996;179:20–5.

[107] Tomlinson I, Rahman N, Frayling I, et al. Inherited susceptibility to colorectal adenomas and carcinomas: evidence for a new predisposition gene on 15q14-q22. Gastroenterology 1999;116:789–95.
[108] Park WS, Park JY, Oh RR, et al. A distinct tumor suppressor gene locus on chromosome 15q21.1 in sporadic form of colorectal cancer. Cancer Res 2000;60:70–3.
[109] Jaeger EE, Woodford-Richens KL, Lockett M, et al. An ancestral Ashkenazi haplotype at the HMPS/CRAC1 locus on 15q13-q14 is associated with hereditary mixed polyposis syndrome. Am J Hum Genet 2003;72:1261–7.
[110] Peng H, Cao X, Li HH, et al. [Haplotype and linkage analysis in Chinese hereditary mixed polyposis syndrome]. Zhonghua Wei Chang Wai Ke Za Zhi 2005;8:312–315 [in Chinese].
[111] Brazowski E, Misonzhnick-Bedny F, Rozen P. Cyclooxygenase-2 expression in the hereditary mixed polyposis syndrome. Dig Dis Sci 2004;49:1906–11.
[112] Riley HD, Smith WR. Macrocephaly, pseudopapilledema and multiple hemangiomata: a previously undescribed heredofamilial syndrome. Pediatrics 1960;26:293–300.
[113] Lloyd KM II, Dennis M. Cowden's disease. A possible new symptom complex with multiple system involvement. Ann Intern Med 1963;58:136–42.
[114] Bannayan GA. Lipomatosis, angiomatosis, and macrencephalia. A previously undescribed congenital syndrome. Arch Pathol 1971;92:1–5.
[115] Ruvalcaba RH, Myhre S, Smith DW. Sotos syndrome with intestinal polyposis and pigmentary changes of the genitalia. Clin Genet 1980;18:413–6.
[116] Arch EM, Goodman BK, Van Wesep RA, et al. Deletion of PTEN in a patient with Bannayan-Riley-Ruvalcaba syndrome suggests allelism with Cowden disease. Am J Med Genet 1997;71:489–93.
[117] Celebi JT, Tsou HC, Chen FF, et al. Phenotypic findings of Cowden syndrome and Bannayan-Zonana syndrome in a family associated with a single germline mutation in PTEN. J Med Genet 1999;36:360–4.
[118] Marsh DJ, Kum JB, Lunetta KL, et al. PTEN mutation spectrum and genotype-phenotype correlations in Bannayan-Riley-Ruvalcaba syndrome suggest a single entity with Cowden syndrome. Hum Mol Genet 1999;8:1461–72.
[119] Zigman AF, Lavine JE, Jones MC, et al. Localization of the Bannayan-Riley-Ruvalcaba syndrome gene to chromosome 10q23. Gastroenterology 1997;113:1433–7.
[120] Sogol PB, Sugawara M, Gordon HE, et al. Cowden's disease: familial goiter and skin hamartomas. A report of three cases. West J Med 1983;139:324–8.
[121] Carlson GJ, Nivatvongs S, Snover DC. Colorectal polyps in Cowden's disease (multiple hamartoma syndrome). Am J Surg Pathol 1984;8:763–70.
[122] Albrecht S, Haber RM, Goodman JC, et al. Cowden syndrome and Lhermitte-Duclos disease. Cancer 1992;70:869–76.
[123] Eng C, Murday V, Seal S, et al. Cowden syndrome and Lhermitte-Duclos disease in a family: a single genetic syndrome with pleiotropy? J Med Genet 1994;31:458–61.
[124] Nelen MR, Padberg GW, Peeters EA, et al. Localization of the gene for Cowden disease to chromosome 10q22–23. Nat Genet 1996;13:114–6.
[125] Eng C. Will the real Cowden syndrome please stand up: revised diagnostic criteria. J Med Genet 2000;37:828–30.
[126] Gorlin RJ, Cohen MM Jr, Condon LM, et al. Bannayan-Riley-Ruvalcaba syndrome. Am J Med Genet 1992;44:307–14.
[127] Brownstein MH, Mehregan AH, Bikowski JB, et al. The dermatopathology of Cowden's syndrome. Br J Dermatol 1979;100:667–73.
[128] Brownstein MH, Mehregan AH, Bilowski JB. Trichilemmomas in Cowden's disease. JAMA 1977;238:26.
[129] Walton BJ, Morain WD, Baughman RD, et al. Cowden's disease: a further indication for prophylactic mastectomy. Surgery 1986;99:82–6.
[130] Fackenthal JD, Marsh DJ, Richardson AL, et al. Male breast cancer in Cowden syndrome patients with germline PTEN mutations. J Med Genet 2001;38:159–64.

[131] Longy M, Coulon V, Duboue B, et al. Mutations of PTEN in patients with Bannayan-Riley-Ruvalcaba phenotype. J Med Genet 1998;35:886–9.
[132] Williard W, Borgen P, Bol R, et al. Cowden's disease. A case report with analyses at the molecular level. Cancer 1992;69:2969–74.
[133] Carlson HE, Burns TW, Davenport SL, et al. Cowden disease: gene marker studies and measurements of epidermal growth factor. Am J Hum Genet 1986;38:908–17.
[134] Hanssen AM, Werquin H, Suys E, et al. Cowden syndrome: report of a large family with macrocephaly and increased severity of signs in subsequent generations. Clin Genet 1993;44:281–6.
[135] Liaw D, Marsh DJ, Li J, et al. Germline mutations of the PTEN gene in Cowden disease, an inherited breast and thyroid cancer syndrome. Nat Genet 1997;16:64–7.
[136] Lynch ED, Ostermeyer EA, Lee MK, et al. Inherited mutations in PTEN that are associated with breast cancer, Cowden disease, and juvenile polyposis. Am J Hum Genet 1997; 61:1254–60.
[137] Nelen MR, van Staveren WC, Peeters EA, et al. Germline mutations in the PTEN/MMAC1 gene in patients with Cowden disease. Hum Mol Genet 1997;6:1383–7.
[138] Marsh DJ, Coulon V, Lunetta KL, et al. Mutation spectrum and genotype-phenotype analyses in Cowden disease and Bannayan-Zonana syndrome, two hamartoma syndromes with germline PTEN mutation. Hum Mol Genet 1998;7:507–15.
[139] Li J, Yen C, Liaw D, et al. PTEN, a putative protein tyrosine phosphatase gene mutated in human brain, breast, and prostate cancer. Science 1997;275:1943–7.
[140] Leslie NR, Downes CP. PTEN function: how normal cells control it and tumour cells lose it. Biochem J 2004;382:1–11.
[141] Sansal I, Sellers WR. The biology and clinical relevance of the PTEN tumor suppressor pathway. J Clin Oncol 2004;22:2954–63.
[142] Simpson L, Parsons R. PTEN: life as a tumor suppressor. Exp Cell Res 2001;264:29–41.
[143] Zhou XP, Waite KA, Pilarski R, et al. Germline PTEN promoter mutations and deletions in Cowden/Bannayan-Riley-Ruvalcaba syndrome result in aberrant PTEN protein and dysregulation of the phosphoinositol-3-kinase/Akt pathway. Am J Hum Genet 2003;73: 404–11.
[144] Marsh DJ, Dahia PL, Zheng Z, et al. Germline mutations in PTEN are present in Bannayan-Zonana syndrome. Nat Genet 1997;16:333–4.
[145] Sarquis MS, Agrawal S, Shen L, et al. Distinct expression profiles for PTEN transcript and its splice variants in Cowden syndrome and Bannayan-Riley-Ruvalcaba syndrome. Am J Hum Genet 2006;79:23–30.
[146] Higginbottom MC, Schultz P. The Bannayan syndrome: an autosomal dominant disorder consisting of macrocephaly, lipomas, hemangiomas, and risk for intracranial tumors. Pediatrics 1982;69:632–4.
[147] Cronkhite LW Jr, Canada WJ. Generalized gastrointestinal polyposis; an unusual syndrome of polyposis, pigmentation, alopecia and onychotrophia. N Engl J Med 1955;252: 1011–5.
[148] Jarnum S, Jensen H. Diffuse gastrointestinal polyposis with ectodermal changes. A case with severe malabsorption and enteric loss of plasma proteins and electrolytes. Gastroenterology 1966;50:107–18.
[149] Johnson JG, Gilbert E, Zimmermann B, et al. Gardner's syndrome, colon cancer, and sarcoma. J Surg Oncol 1972;4:354–62.
[150] Burke AP, Sobin LH. The pathology of Cronkhite-Canada polyps. A comparison to juvenile polyposis. Am J Surg Pathol 1989;13:940–6.
[151] Egawa T, Kubota T, Otani Y, et al. Surgically treated Cronkhite-Canada syndrome associated with gastric cancer. Gastric Cancer 2000;3:156–60.
[152] Murata I, Yoshikawa I, Endo M, et al. Cronkhite-Canada syndrome: report of two cases. J Gastroenterol 2000;35:706–11.

[153] Goto A. Cronkhite-Canada syndrome: epidemiological study of 110 cases reported in Japan. Nippon Geka Hokan 1995;64:3–14.
[154] Daniel ES, Ludwig SL, Lewin KJ, et al. The Cronkhite-Canada syndrome. An analysis of clinical and pathologic features and therapy in 55 patients. Medicine (Baltimore) 1982;61:293–309.
[155] Takeuchi Y, Yoshikawa M, Tsukamoto N, et al. Cronkhite-Canada syndrome with colon cancer, portal thrombosis, high titer of antinuclear antibodies, and membranous glomerulonephritis. J Gastroenterol 2003;38:791–5.
[156] Yashiro M, Kobayashi H, Kubo N, et al. Cronkhite-Canada syndrome containing colon cancer and serrated adenoma lesions. Digestion 2004;69:57–62.

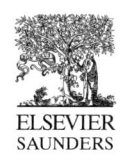

Hereditary Colorectal Cancer Syndromes: Familial Adenomatous Polyposis and Lynch Syndrome

Wigdan Al-Sukhni, MD[a,b,]*,
Melyssa Aronson, MSc, (C) CGC[c],
Steven Gallinger, MD, MSc[a,b]

[a]*Division of General Surgery, Department of Surgery, University of Toronto, 1225-600 University Avenue, Toronto, Ontario, Canada M5G 1X5*
[b]*Samuel Lunenfeld Research Institute, 1225-600 University Avenue, Toronto, Ontario, Canada M5G 1X5*
[c]*Dr. Zane Cohen Digestive Disease Clinical Research Centre, 60 Murray Street, 3rd floor, Toronto, Ontario, Canada M5T 3L9*

Familial adenomatous polyposis

Familial adenomatous polyposis (FAP) is an autosomal dominant disease with an estimated lifetime risk of 1 in 8000 to 15,000 births [1]. The earliest known description of multiple colorectal polyps is found in a German medical journal in 1721, and the first histologically confirmed adenomatous polyposis case was published in Russia by Sklifasowski in 1881 [2]. About 100 years later, the discovery that FAP is caused by mutations in the *APC* gene subsequently led to recognizing the role of *APC* in most sporadic colorectal carcinomas (CRC), contributing to the development of the Vogelstein adenoma-carcinoma molecular sequence for CRC [3].

The first polyposis registry was established in 1924 at St. Mark's hospital in the United Kingdom, by Dukes and Lockhart-Mummery [2]. Since then, many such registries have been developed worldwide. Adopting a multidisciplinary approach to managing FAP has allowed earlier diagnosis and intervention and improvements in prognosis and quality of life [2].

---

* Corresponding author. Division of General Surgery, Department of Surgery, University of Toronto, 1225-600 University Avenue, Toronto, Ontario, Canada M5G 1X5. (W. Al-Sukhni).
 E-mail address: wigdan.al.sukhni@utoronto.ca (W. Al-Sukhni).

Clinical features

FAP is characterized by the presence of more than 100 colorectal polyps, typically developing in puberty. The polyps are adenomatous and usually less than 1 cm in size. They may be pedunculated or sessile, with tubular, villous, or tubulovillous histology. Severe cases are associated with carpeting of the colon. FAP accounts for less than 1% of all colorectal cancer cases, and the risk for developing cancer is nearly 100% (usually left-sided) by the fourth or fifth decade if prophylactic colectomy is not performed [4].

A milder form of the disease, called attenuated adenomatous polyposis coli (AAPC), is also recognized, wherein subjects develop fewer than 100 colonic adenomas, which tend to be smaller and flatter than FAP polyps, predominantly in the right side of the colon [4]. CRC occurs later in AAPC, with a mean age at diagnosis of 50 to 52 years [5].

The upper gastrointestinal tract is also affected in FAP (Fig. 1A). At least 60% of patients develop duodenal polyps [6], and cumulative lifetime prevalence is as high as 90% to 98% [4,7]. Most of these adenomas occur on the ampulla or in the periampullary region (Fig. 1B). Duodenal polyposis is usually staged according to the Spigelman criteria (Table 1), based on the number, size, histology, and degree of dysplasia in polyps. Spigelman and colleagues reported a rate of 11% stage IV polyposis in patients who had FAP prospectively studied at St. Mark's Hospital [8]; more recently, Saurin and colleagues [9] reported a 43% cumulative risk for developing stage IV duodenal polyposis by age 60 and 50% by age 70. Of note, adenomatous changes have also been identified in macroscopically normal duodenal mucosa of patients who have FAP [8]. Based on Sellner's study of small bowel adenomas and carcinomas, it is recognized that the adenoma-to-carcinoma sequence of colorectal neoplasia also applies to upper gastrointestinal (GI) polyps [10]. The cumulative lifetime risk for duodenal cancer in patients who have FAP has been reported as 1% to 10% [6,11,12]. A prospective study of 99 patients who had FAP reported the risk for duodenal cancer as 36% for Spigelman stage IV, 2% for stages III and II, and 0% for stage I polyposis [11]; a retrospective review of patients by the Swedish Polyposis Registry described a 21% risk for duodenal cancer in patients who had stage IV polyposis [12]. Prospective endoscopic studies have demonstrated progression in stage of polyposis over time [13], and the incidence and severity of periampullary neoplasia has been found to segregate in FAP families [14].

Gastric polyps also occur in FAP, with rates as high as 81% to 84% [15]. Most are fundic gland polyps; histologic features include cystic dilatation and irregular budding of the fundic gland. Up to 25% show foveolar epithelial dysplasia, but cancer is rare [16]. Gastric adenomas are also found, limited to the antrum and occurring in smaller numbers and at lesser frequency than fundic gland polyps [6]. Some have suggested an etiologic link between

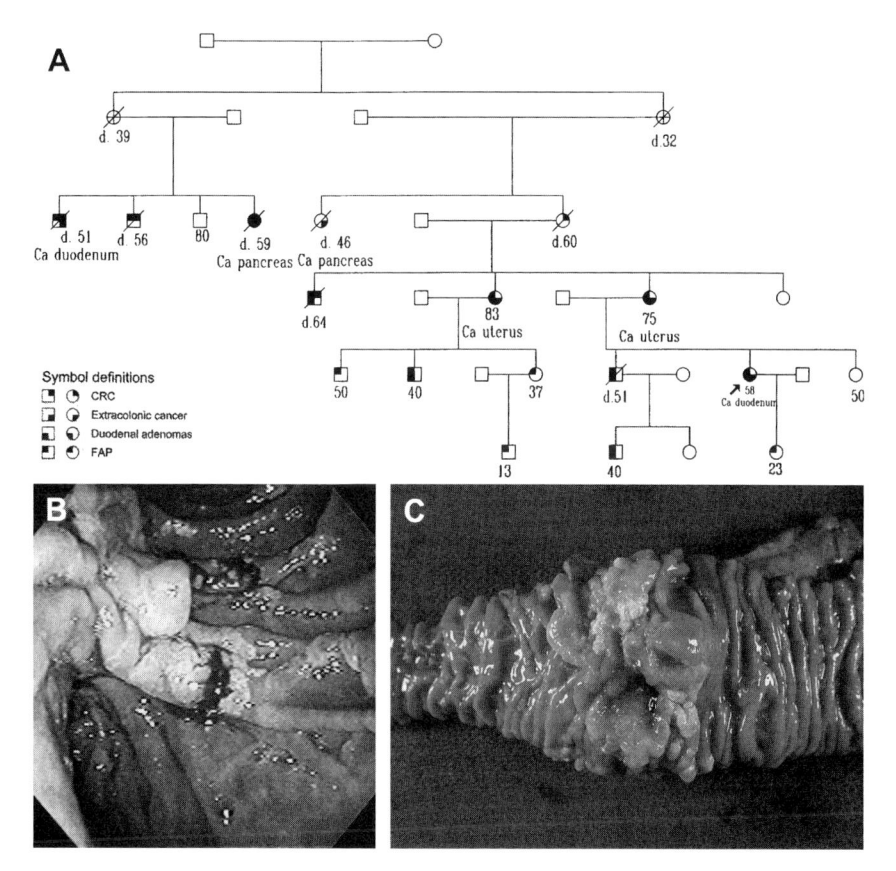

Fig. 1. (*A*) FAP pedigree demonstrating segregation of duodenal polyposis. Arrow points to patient represented in *B* and *C*. One other relative is known to have died of duodenal cancer; two other relatives whose cause of death was stated as pancreatic cancer in autopsy reports may have had misdiagnosed duodenal cancer. (*B*) Endoscopic image of duodenal adenomatous polyp in patient who had FAP. (*C*) Despite surveillance and attempts at endoscopic control of duodenal polyps, patient developed duodenal adenocarcinoma requiring pancreaticoduodenectomy. Resected duodenal specimen shown with tumor.

duodenogastric bile reflux and gastric adenomas [17]. Unlike duodenal polyposis, there is no strong evidence linking gastric polyposis and gastric cancer in patients who have FAP, although some studies have reported rates of gastric cancer in East Asian populations that are greater than the expected risk for the general population [18]. The incidence of small bowel adenomas and small bowel cancer in FAP has been estimated at less than 10% and less than 1%, respectively [19].

Other than gastrointestinal polyposis, FAP is also associated with several extraintestinal manifestations. One cause of significant morbidity is desmoid tumors, fibrinous masses that are not malignant but are locally invasive. Although desmoids can arise from fibroblasts throughout the body,

Table 1
Spigelman classification of duodenal polyps

Points[a]	Polyp number	Polyp size (mm)	Histologic type	Dysplasia
1	1–4	1–4	Tubular	Mild
2	5–20	5–10	Tubulovillous	Moderate
3	>20	>10	Villous	Severe

[a] Stage 0, 0 points; stage I, 1–4 points; stage II, 5–6 points; stage III, 7–8 points; stage IV, 9–12 points.

Data from Spigelman AD, Williams CB, Talbot IC, et al. Upper gastrointestinal cancer in patients with familial adenomatous polyposis. Lancet 1989;2:783–5.

intra-abdominal desmoids are most frequent in FAP, often occurring in the small bowel mesentery [7]. The most common complication is obstruction of the small bowel or ureters, but other potential problems include occlusion of mesenteric blood vessels, thrombosis of larger veins, and compression of peripheral nerves [4]. Desmoids have been reported as a cause of death in up to 21% of patients who have FAP [20]. The cause of desmoid tumors has been attributed to surgical trauma, hormonal exposure, and mutations in specific regions of the *APC* gene. An analysis of 930 patients who had FAP from the polyposis registry at Mount Sinai Hospital in Toronto identified desmoid tumors in 14% of patients, with a significantly higher prevalence in females than males; in females who had an early colectomy compared with those who had a late colectomy; and in patients who had *APC* mutations at the 3′ end of the gene compared with mutations at the 5′ end, particularly mutations occurring 3′ to codon 1399 [21].

Other malignancies, including thyroid cancer, hepatoblastoma, and brain tumors have also been associated with FAP. Herraiz and colleagues [22] reported papillary thyroid carcinoma in 12% of 51 patients who had FAP; however, this is much higher than the 1% to 2% reported in other studies [23]. Hepatoblastoma has been reported in 0.4% to 0.6% of children from FAP families, significantly higher than the general population rate of 1/100,000 [24]. Medulloblastoma is the most common brain tumor in FAP, with a risk 92 times that of the general population [25]. Pancreatic lesions, including adenocarcinoma, intraductal papillary neoplasm, mucinous pancreatic tumors, and high-grade pancreatic intraepithelial neoplasia, have also been reported in association with FAP [26–29].

Turcot syndrome can refer to the association of either FAP (when the underlying mutation is in the *APC* gene) or Lynch syndrome with brain tumors (mutation in mismatch repair [MMR] genes). (See Lynch Syndrome section). Gardner syndrome is an older term referring to the association of multiple colonic adenomatous polyps, osteomas of skull and mandible, multiple epidermal cysts, supernumerary and impacted teeth, fibromatosis, and congenital hypertrophy of the retinal pigment epithelium (CHRPE). It is in fact a phenotypic subtype of FAP, because the underlying genetic basis is still the *APC* gene [4].

Genetics and diagnosis

Using genetic linkage and positional cloning techniques, truncating mutations in the *APC* gene on chromosome 5q were shown to be the cause of most cases of FAP in 1991. Subsequently, somatic mutations of the *APC* gene were demonstrated to be important early events in 60% to 80% of sporadic colorectal cancer and adenomas [30]. *APC* is a large gene, with 15 exons, and genotype/phenotype correlations have been demonstrated. Profuse polyposis (>1000) has been correlated with mutations in the middle of the gene (codons 1250–1464). Two hotspots, codon 1061 and 1309 mutations, account for 11% and 13% of all germline mutations, respectively. The codon 1309 mutation is associated with younger onset of disease [31]. Attenuated FAP is seen with mutations at the 3' and 5' ends of the gene and in the alternatively spliced region of exon 9 [32]. Extracolonic manifestations have been associated with specific genotypes, including desmoids (3' end, downstream of codon 1400) and CHRPE (codons 311–1444) [33,34]. Nieuwenhuis and Vasen [35] recently reviewed the literature on genotype–phenotype correlations in FAP and noted that the site of mutation does not always accurately predict a phenotype, however, presumably because of additional factors, such as modifier genes.

Most mutations in the *APC* gene lead to protein truncation, and the protein-truncation assay was originally used to detect truncated protein products using RNA and DNA from peripheral blood lymphocytes. Other mutation detection techniques include conformation-sensitive gel electrophoresis, denaturing high performance liquid chromatography (dHPLC), single-stranded conformational polymorphism, denaturing gradient gel electrophoresis, and sequencing of the coding region. Successful detection of *APC* mutations in patients who have classic FAP is approximately 80% to 90% but less than 10% for patients who have AAPC [36]. Multiplex ligation-dependent probe amplification (MLPA) and Southern blot can be used to detect large insertions or deletions that account for 15% of patients who have classic FAP [37].

Unlike common truncating *APC* mutations in FAP, a nontruncating missense mutation caused by a single nucleotide substitution in the gene I1307K occurs in approximately 6% of the Ashkenazi Jewish population and may double the risk for colorectal polyps and cancer in heterozygous carriers. Rather than causing significant impairment of the *APC* protein, this variant predisposes to increased rate of somatic mutation of the gene in carriers. The lifetime risk for developing cancer is only 10% to 15% in carriers, and the age at diagnosis is not significantly younger than the general population [1].

Another gene in which mutations predispose to increased risk for somatic *APC* mutations is the *MYH* gene. In 2002, Al-Tassan and colleagues [38] described a British family in which siblings presented with colorectal polyposis or cancer but were negative for germline *APC* mutations. Their tumor

DNA, however, had inactivating mutations of the *APC* gene, which were characterized by G→T transversions. Such a mutation usually occurs because of formation of the oxidative metabolism byproduct 8-oxoguanine, and it is normally repaired by the base-excision repair gene *MYH*. Al-Tassan and colleagues identified germline biallelic *MYH* mutations in these patients, thus providing the first evidence linking heritable defects in base-excision repair to tumorigenesis. Subsequently, other studies have confirmed the association between germline *MYH* mutations and increased risk for CRC [39,40]. Population-based studies have reported biallelic germline *MYH* mutations in 0.7% to 3% of unselected patients who had CRC [41], and in approximately one third of individuals who had an attenuated polyposis phenotype who tested negative for *APC* mutations [42]. Despite a clearly elevated risk for CRC among carriers of biallelic mutations, possibly approaching 100% lifetime risk, the risk for polyposis and cancer in monoallelic carriers remains unclear [43]. Although some studies did not find a significantly increased risk for cancer in monoallelic mutation carriers [44,45], indicating a recessive mode of inheritance, others have suggested a codominant effect for *MYH* mutations in which monoallelic mutations predispose to a risk higher than the general population but lower than biallelic mutations. One kin-cohort study that assessed risk for cancer in first-degree relatives of *MYH* mutation carriers found a 3-fold increased risk for CRC in relatives of monoallelic carriers and 50-fold increased risk in relatives of biallelic carriers [46]. It has been suggested that lack of significant association in previous reports may be because of underpowered studies. At this time, testing for *MYH* mutations is recommended for patients presenting with clinical features of FAP but who test negative for germline *APC* mutations, and in patients who have a recessive pattern of CRC inheritance especially if the affected case has many synchronous or metachronous adenomatous polyps; colonoscopy is recommended for biallelic mutation carriers starting at age 25 to 30 every 2 years [39]. Although two pathogenic mutations, Y165C and G382D, are most common in whites of North European descent, 82 other germline mutations have been identified in different populations [47]. It is recommended that genetic testing include sequencing of the entire *MYH* gene, especially in apparently heterozygous Y165C and G382D carriers, because two thirds of patients who had mutations in one clinic-based study [42] and one third of mutation carriers in another series were found to have an "uncommon" variant [45]. Some reports have identified cases of upper GI polyposis in *MYH* mutation carriers, so upper GI surveillance is also warranted [45].

FAP is an autosomal dominant disease with affected parents having a 50% chance of passing the *APC* mutation to their children. Approximately 10% to 25% of patients who have FAP present with an apparent de novo mutation [48,49]. In most de novo cases, the mutation arises during embryogenesis with no risk for inheritance to siblings. In 11% to 20% of apparent de novo mutations, however, parents have somatic mosaicism of their *APC* mutation identified in somatic tissue cells but not in peripheral lymphocytes [48]. Despite having a mutation that is expected to cause classic FAP, they may present with a less severe phenotype because of the mosaicism. There have also been reports on gonadal mosaicism, wherein the parent is unaffected but his or her germline cells (eggs or sperm) carry the mutation. In these families, the siblings would have a risk for inheriting the *APC* mutation [50]. Patients who have apparent de novo mutations should therefore be investigated for nonpaternity, and other transmission mechanisms to assess risk to siblings.

Screening/surveillance

The American Gastroenterological Association recommends annual flexible sigmoidoscopy starting at age 10 to 12 years for all individuals who have an *APC* mutation and for families that have a clinical diagnosis of FAP but with no identified *APC* mutation. On identification of colonic or rectal adenomas, surgery should be discussed. Individuals who test negative for the known *APC* mutation in their family do not need colorectal cancer screening beyond general population guidelines. Members of families in which a known *APC* mutation has been identified, but who have not undergone genetic testing, should also start sigmoidoscopic screening at age 10 to 12 years, which should proceed annually until age 25, after which it may be performed every 2 years until age 35, then every 3 years until age 50, then using general population guidelines if there is no evidence of polyposis [4,51].

For AAPC, the guidelines are slightly modified to account for the later age of onset: an initial colonoscopy is recommended at age 15, and if no polyps are found, subsequent annual colonoscopies may be performed from age 20 onward in individuals who have a known *APC* mutation, or every 2 years if no specific mutation is identified. If polyps are identified at baseline colonoscopy, annual colonoscopy and polypectomy or colectomy is recommended [4].

The risk for duodenal polyposis and carcinoma is high in FAP. It is currently recommended that patients who have FAP undergo initial upper endoscopy around age 20 years, with good visualization of the periampullary region using a side-viewing scope [52]. Mild duodenal polyposis (stage I or II) may be followed at 3- to 5-year intervals, whereas patients who have more advanced polyposis (stage III or IV) should be scoped at 6- to 12-month intervals and considered for endoscopic ultrasound evaluation and chemoprevention or surgical intervention [53]. Biopsies of polyps should be taken to determine the Spigelman stage, and some advocate random biopsies if no polyps are visualized to rule out microadenomas [53].

Although upper endoscopy is currently the main tool for duodenal/periampullary cancer screening, it is not 100% effective in detecting adenomas or altering the progression from advanced polyposis to carcinoma [4]. Moreover, it is inadequate in assessing the small bowel beyond the ligament of

Treitz. The role of video capsule endoscopy (VCE) in screening patients who have FAP has been investigated in several studies, but remains controversial. Although some have found VCE helpful in identifying distal small bowel polyps [54], others have found capsule endoscopy to underestimate the number of small bowel polyps and to be unreliable in detecting large polyps [55].

Some recommend thyroid ultrasound screening in patients who have CHRPE or *APC* mutations at the 5′ end of exon 15 because of the association of these findings with elevated risk for thyroid cancer [56], although most agree that simple thyroid palpation should suffice in most patients who have FAP. No standard guidelines exist regarding hepatoblastoma screening, but some recommend use of α-fetoprotein levels and liver ultrasound imaging to screen children in FAP families [24].

Surgery—colon and rectum

The need for prophylactic surgery for the prevention of colorectal cancer in patients who have FAP is undisputed. Certain controversies exist with respect to the type of surgery, however. Three main surgical options include: total proctocolectomy with permanent ileostomy (TPC + ileostomy); subtotal colectomy with ileo-rectal anastomosis (IRA); and proctocolectomy with ileal pouch–anal anastomosis (IPAA). Although TPC + ileostomy provides the lowest risk for gastrointestinal cancer and lowest risk for complications [57], it is rarely the first choice for patients who have FAP because of the disadvantages associated with a permanent ileostomy. It may be appropriate for patients who have poor preoperative sphincter function, who have a rectal cancer invading the sphincter or levator complex, or in whom a proctocolectomy is necessary but an IPAA is technically prohibitive (eg, because of shortening of small bowel mesentery by desmoid disease).

The choice between IRA and IPAA should take into consideration disease, patient, and operative factors. The main argument for IPAA is based on the risk for developing cancer in the remaining rectal stump after IRA. Estimates of this risk have varied widely, between 3% and 32% depending on the postoperative follow-up period [58,59]. Some experts have argued these estimates may be falsely elevated because of biases in studies conducted before the establishment of IPAA as a surgical technique [57,60]. A study by Church and colleagues [61] supports this hypothesis; it compared patients who had FAP undergoing surgery before and after 1983, when ileal pouches became an option, and found the rate of rectal cancer to be lower in patients treated in the pouch era (0% after 1983 versus 12.9% before 1983). Moreover, analysis of rectal cancer rates by age groups suggests that the risk for developing cancer after IRA is related to chronologic age rather than the postoperative follow-up period [60]. It is clear, though, that the risk for rectal cancer is proportional to the degree of polyposis, and most experts agree that the presence of more than 1000 colonic adenomas or more than 20 rectal adenomas, rectal adenoma greater than 3 cm in size, or rectal adenoma with severe dysplasia mandates proctocolectomy [62]. In addition to endoscopic findings, genetic information may be helpful in identifying patients at increased risk for rectal cancer. Patients carrying an *APC* mutation at codon 1309 are at elevated risk for developing carpeting polyposis of the rectum requiring secondary proctectomy after IRA, whereas mutations at the 5' end of the *APC* gene are associated with a lower number of polyps before and after IRA [63].

Although the risk for cancer is considerably reduced with proctocolectomy, it is not eliminated by IPAA. Polyps have been reported in the ileal pouch and at the anal transition zone, and a few cases of cancer developing in those locations after IPAA have also been reported [64]. Postoperative endoscopic surveillance is therefore necessary for patients who have FAP whether undergoing IRA (every 6 months) or IPAA (every 2–5 years, depending on findings and symptoms).

IPAA is technically a more complex procedure than IRA, and most surgeons perform IPAA as a two-stage procedure, with a temporary diverting loop ileostomy to allow healing of the anastomosis. As discussed by Kartheuser and colleagues [64], several controversies exist with respect to the technical performance of IPAA, including: the role of transanal mucosectomy with handsewn anastomosis versus double-stapled anastomosis, role of mesenteric lengthening, use of close rectal dissection to preserve pelvic nerves, omission of diverting ileostomy, and the role of laparoscopy. A major point of contention is the type of anastomosis, with some experts preferring the stapled approach because it is relatively easier to perform and has better functional outcome, whereas others insist on mucosectomy because of the theoretic risk for cancer in retained mucosa. A recent meta-analysis found mucosectomy was significantly associated with worse functional outcome, but not reaching statistical significance in its control of cuff polyposis [65]. Dissection of the rectum in the perimuscular plane, rather than the traditional total mesorectal excision approach, protects pelvic autonomic nerves and subsequent sexual function. It is more tedious in males who have a narrow pelvis and in obese patients, and is not appropriate for patients who have severe rectal dysplasia or cancer. Laparoscopic technique for prophylactic surgery is clearly attractive because most newly diagnosed patients who have FAP are young and asymptomatic before surgery. Recent reports support the use of laparoscopic IPAA as a safe alternative for patients who have FAP [64,66].

Surgery—duodenum

Ampullary or periampullary adenomatous polyps greater than 1 cm in size, or those that have high-grade dysplasia, ulceration, or villous changes, should be excised [60]. Options for endoscopic removal include mucosal resection, snare polypectomy, thermal ablation, and argon plasma coagulation [67]. Although endoscopic removal may be attractive as a less-invasive option than surgery, a downside is the relatively high recurrence rate, as high as 50% to 100%, and the risk for missing foci of carcinoma in incompletely resected polyps [53,68]. Moreover, endoscopic management is not free of complications, including hemorrhage (at a higher rate than colonic polypectomy) and pancreatitis (as high as 10%) [53]. Although it may be an option for management of patients who have early-stage polyposis, or in the case of individuals not fit for surgery, endoscopic management is not an ideal treatment for patients who have FAP with advanced-stage duodenal or ampullary polyps.

As with endoscopic excision, local surgical resection is less morbid but is associated with a high recurrence rate [13,67,69]. Pancreaticoduodenectomy is most likely to eliminate the risk for ampullary/periampullary neoplasia (Fig. 1C), but carries the greatest risk for perioperative morbidity and potentially long-term complications [53,70]. A slightly less morbid surgical option may be pancreas-preserving duodenectomy, in which the duodenum is dissected away from the head of the pancreas and the ampulla is anastomosed to the jejunum. Several reports have been published describing this technique, with various modifications [71]. Duodenal mucosa left behind remains a potential focus for development of cancer [53].

Surgery—desmoid

Surgical resection of desmoid tumors is controversial. For the most part, resection of abdominal wall or extremity tumors is safe, although associated with high recurrence rates [72]. Some have advocated the use of radiotherapy to complement surgery and reduce risk for recurrence, but it is unclear if this is indeed effective; also uncertain is the significance of resection margins to recurrence rate [72]. A high proportion of desmoids in FAP tend to be intra-abdominal, which are best left alone unless surgery is unavoidable, such as in the situation of a rapidly expanding tumor that is causing ureteral or bowel obstruction [73,74]. A study of patients from the St. Mark's registry found a 36% perioperative mortality rate associated with resection of mesenteric desmoid tumors, and 71% recurrence rate in survivors, with nearly half requiring parenteral nutrition because of significant loss of small bowel [75]. A more recent 10-year review of surgical treatment of desmoids in FAP reported no perioperative mortality and only 1 of 20 patients undergoing surgery required parenteral nutrition, however [73]. It is likely that better surgical experience with desmoid tumors has improved morbidity and mortality of the procedure, but the high recurrence rate (more than 80% in some reports) remains a significant problem.

Nonsurgical management

Because most patients who have FAP are young and generally asymptomatic before undergoing prophylactic surgery, there has been interest in the use of chemopreventive agents to delay or avoid surgery. Various drugs, including acetylsalicylic acid (ASA, aspirin), nonsteroidal anti-inflammatory drugs (NSAIDS), 5-aminosalicylates, statins, COX-2 inhibitors, ursodeoxycholic acid, and vitamins and micronutrients have been studied [76,77]. Several animal-model studies and clinical trials demonstrated the usefulness of NSAIDS in reducing the number of adenomatous polyps in FAP, with the most promising drug class being COX-2 inhibitors [78–80]. Animal models demonstrated that COX-2 is significantly overexpressed in large bowel neoplastic lesions [81]. COX-2 inhibitors are associated with fewer GI complications than their nonselective NSAID counterparts. The discovery of increased cardiovascular events in patients taking either Celecoxib or Vioxx in two large randomized trials caused controversy in their use, however, and Vioxx has been withdrawn from clinical use [82].

The role of ASA in chemoprevention in FAP was investigated by the Concerted Action for Polyp Preventions (CAPP1) trial, which randomized 227 subjects who had FAP to 600 mg ASA or 30 g indigestible starch versus placebo daily. Polyp number was not significantly affected by either treatment [83].

Nonsurgical therapy is preferred for intra-abdominal desmoid disease. First-line options include NSAIDS and antiestrogen agents; up to 50% of tumors regress with these noncytotoxic drugs [74]. If those fail, interferon-alpha or cytotoxic chemotherapy, including combinations of methotrexate, vinblastine, doxorubicin, and dacarbazine, are used primarily in cases of rapidly growing or life-threatening tumors. Other nonpharmacologic options for desmoids that have been tried include radiofrequency ablation and chemical ablation with acetic acid [74].

Lynch syndrome (hereditary nonpolyposis colon cancer)

In 1913, American pathologist Aldred Warthin published the pedigree of a family that had a high frequency of multiple-site cancers occurring at young ages. Subsequently, Lynch and colleagues identified other similar families, and the clinical entity in those patients came to be known as Lynch syndrome [84]. For many years, the terms "Lynch syndrome" and "hereditary nonpolyposis colon cancer" (HNPCC) have been applied interchangeably and inconsistently to describe various heritable CRC cases. The term "nonpolyposis" in HNPCC is somewhat misleading, because patients who have this syndrome do develop adenomatous polyps that seem to undergo accelerated carcinogenesis. Moreover, although predisposition to CRC is high, it may not be the primary malignancy affecting a patient who has Lynch syndrome. Most experts today therefore believe that Lynch syndrome is the better name, and it is appropriately defined as "a hereditary predisposition to malignancy that is explained by a germline mutation in a DNA mismatch repair gene" [85].

Lynch syndrome is an autosomal dominant condition with incomplete penetrance. As the most common cause of heritable CRC, it is estimated to account for about 2% of all CRC cases [86]. It is characterized by the development of colorectal or several extracolonic cancers at an earlier age than the general population; unlike FAP, the presence of multiple polyps is not a significant feature of Lynch syndrome [87]. Associated extracolonic tumors include endometrial, ovarian, stomach, small bowel, hepatobiliary, pancreatic, upper uroepithelial tract, and brain [84]. Turcot syndrome, a variant of FAP consisting of colorectal and brain cancers, can also be a variant of Lynch syndrome. The type of brain tumor in Lynch tends to be glioblastoma, whereas it is usually medulloblastoma in FAP [88]. Another variant of Lynch syndrome is Muir-Torre syndrome, characterized by cutaneous lesions (sebaceous adenomas, epitheliomas, carcinomas, or keratoacanthomas) and multiple visceral malignancies [52]. Certain cardinal clinical features have been described for Lynch syndrome (Box 1).

Some patients formerly classified as Lynch families meet the Amsterdam diagnostic criteria (see Genetics and Diagnosis section) but lack the defining genetic mutations and have microsatellite stable tumors. Although the risk for CRC in these subjects is higher than the general population, it is lower than in mutation-carrier Lynch patients, and they are also at much lower risk for extracolonic cancers. It has therefore been proposed that these patients be grouped separately as "familial colorectal cancer type X" [89].

Box 1. Cardinal features of Lynch syndrome

Earlier average age of CRC onset than in general population
Proximal colon involvement
Excess synchronous and metachronous CRCs
Autosomal dominant inheritance
Increased risk for malignancy at certain extracolonic sites, especially endometrial carcinoma, but also ovary, stomach, small bowel, hepatobiliary tract, pancreas, upper uroepithelial tract, and brain
CRC tumors tend to be poorly differentiated, have excess mucoid and signet-cell features, Crohn-like reaction, and excess tumor-infiltrating lymphocytes. Microsatellite instability common to most CRC tumors
Improved prognosis of CRC compared with sporadic cases of CRC
Accelerated carcinogenesis and interval CRC
Identification of germline mismatch repair mutation segregating with syndrome-affected individuals in family

---

Adapted from Merg A, Lynch HT, Lynch JF, et al. Hereditary colorectal cancer—Part II. Curr Probl Surg 2005;42(5):267–334; with permission.

Associated cancer risks

The following are estimated lifetime risks for various cancers in Lynch syndrome: CRC 24% to 75%, endometrial 27% to 71%, ovarian 3% to 13%, gastric 2% to 13%, urinary tract 1% to 12%, small bowel 4% to 7%, brain 1% to 4%, and hepatobiliary 2% [90]. It has been argued, however, that CRC risk in particular has been overestimated in studies that use patients selected by familial criteria without correcting for bias [91]. Cancer penetrance in Lynch syndrome depends on several factors, including gender and type of mutations in MMR genes. Pathologic features of CRC in Lynch syndrome include solid growth pattern, mucin production, poor differentiation, and lymphoid infiltration of tumor [84]. Endometrial and ovarian cancers in patients who have Lynch syndrome are diagnosed on average 10 years earlier than in the general population, but stage-matched survival does not seem to differ significantly relative to sporadic cases [92]. Similarly to CRC tumors, Lynch-associated endometrial tumors are characterized by poor differentiation and tumor-invading lymphocytes [93]; in contrast, ovarian cancer in Lynch syndrome tends to be moderately or well differentiated [94]. As in the case of FAP, gastric cancer is not common but has been observed more frequently in families from Far East populations [87]. The lifetime risk for developing small bowel cancer in patients who have Lynch syndrome was estimated to be 4.2% in a recent retrospective study, with a median age at diagnosis of 52 years [95]. Uroepithelial tumors tend to be transitional cell carcinoma when they occurred in patients who have Lynch syndrome, with a mean age at diagnosis of 58 years [87].

Genetics and diagnosis

Lynch syndrome is caused by germline MMR gene mutations, primarily *MLH1*, *MSH2*, *MSH6*, and *PMS2*, which recognize and correct errors that occur during DNA replication. *MSH2* and *MLH1* are the primary proteins in this process, joining with the others to form complexes. *MSH2* and *MLH1* are mutated in 80% to 90% of patients who have Lynch syndrome, and because they can use alternative proteins for binding, germline mutations in *MSH6* and *PMS2* tend to result in a less severe phenotype [96].

The interaction of these proteins is also demonstrated through immunohistochemistry testing (IHC), which stains normal and tumor tissue for the MLH1, MSH2, MSH6, and PMS2 proteins (Fig. 2). Most patients who have MMR germline mutations exhibit the IHC results noted in Table 2; however, false-positive and false-negative results do occur. This test is used as a preliminary tool, often in conjunction with microsatellite instability testing, to determine who may benefit from germline testing.

Mutations in MMR genes leading to a loss of DNA mismatch repair during replication result in insertion or deletion of repeats in microsatellites, polymorphic stretches of DNA consisting of up to a dozen repeats of four to six nucleotide sequences. A panel of microsatellites (both

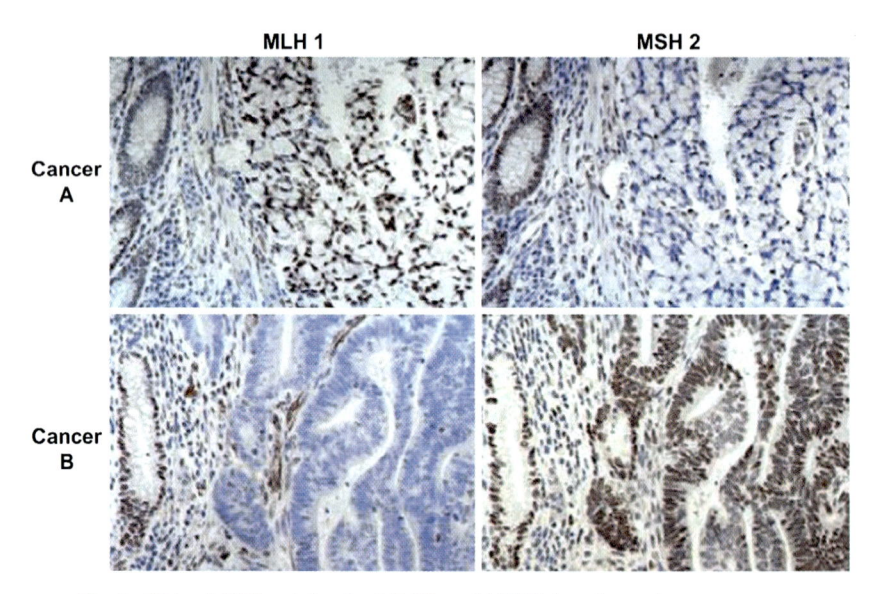

Fig. 2. Slide of IHC staining for MLH1 and MSH2 in colorectal cancer tumors.

mononucleotides and dinucleotides) is examined for expansion and contraction, known as microsatellite instability (MSI), comparing a colorectal tumor DNA to normal DNA. MSI can be categorized further into MSI-high (>30%–40% of markers are unstable), MSI-low (<30%–40% of markers are unstable), or microsatellite stable (none of the markers demonstrates instability) [97]. More than 90% of patients who have Lynch syndrome exhibit high microsatellite instability in their tumors [98].

Of note, approximately 15% of sporadic colorectal cancers also demonstrate microsatellite instability because of somatic methylation of both promoter regions of the *MLH1* gene early in tumorigenesis [99]. In those cases, MSI and IHC tumor results mimic those of a patient who has a germline *MLH1* mutation; however, these patients tend to be older at diagnosis without a strong family history of CRC.

There have been reports of heritable epimutations (germline hemiallelic methylation) of both *MLH1* and *MSH2* [100], despite that the process of embryogenesis causes epigenetic reprogramming. The inheritance of

Table 2
Immunohistochemistry testing results based on germline mutation

Germline mutation in:	Protein (− absent, + present)			
	MLH1	MSH2	MSH6	PMS2
MLH1	−	+	+	−
MSH2	+	−	−	+
MSH6	+	+	−	+
PMS2	+	+	+	−

MMR epimutations has been challenged, however [101]. It has also been shown that MMR mutation carriers can exhibit methylation of the *MLH1* promoter region, and its presence should not exclude a diagnosis of Lynch syndrome [102].

Mutations in the *BRAF* gene, a cytoplasmic serine/threonine kinase oncogene, are strongly correlated with *MLH1* methylation in patients who have sporadic MSI-H/MLH1-deficient tumors. A *BRAF* V600E mutation was seen in 31% to 83% of sporadic MSI-H CRC cases and has not yet been identified in patients who have known MMR mutations [103]. *BRAF* testing can be incorporated into an algorithm for genetic testing for Lynch syndrome to determine which patients who have MLH1-deficient tumors warrant germline testing.

Several different criteria have been developed to identify Lynch syndrome families. The Amsterdam I criteria (Box 2), developed in 1989, were primarily designed to assist in discovery of the genes that cause the syndrome. These criteria only address risk for CRC, however, and the Amsterdam II criteria were described in 1999 to include the risk for extracolonic tumors associated with Lynch syndrome (see Box 2). With the recognition of the genetic basis of Lynch syndrome due to germline mutations in MMR genes, the Bethesda guidelines were developed to identify patients presenting with CRC who should undergo genetic testing for tumor microsatellite instability (see Box 2). These guidelines include family history and age at diagnosis, but also include pathologic characteristics suggestive of a microsatellite-unstable tumor. The Bethesda criteria aim to improve sensitivity of detecting patients eligible for genetic testing while excluding sporadic MSI-positive tumors, based on age criteria. Various additional criteria have been developed to improve sensitivity and specificity of detecting patients who have Lynch syndrome [104,105].

Once identified, a cost-effective approach using *MSI*, *IHC*, and *BRAF* testing followed by germline analysis can be used to confirm a diagnosis of Lynch syndrome. Germline testing involves analyzing DNA from peripheral blood lymphocytes using dHPLC, sequencing and conversion testing to detect missense, nonsense, splice site, and frameshift mutations, in combination with MLPA to identify large deletions in an MMR gene. IHC is used to guide which MMR gene should be analyzed. Fig. 3 outlines an algorithm that can be used to test patients at risk for Lynch syndrome.

Lynch syndrome is most often transmitted in an autosomal dominant fashion, with one affected parent having a 50% chance of passing a mutated gene to the offspring. Most patients who have Lynch syndrome have a family history of cancer, but there is variable penetrance and cancer risks differ with the specific MMR gene affected in the family [106]. Lynch syndrome rarely arises as a new mutation (unlike FAP), although there have been reports of de novo *MLH1* and *MSH2* mutations [107]. Genotype–phenotype correlation with MMR mutations is poorly understood, but familial clustering of specific cancers, such as gastric and urologic cancer, has been reported

Box 2. Amsterdam I and Amsterdam II criteria and Bethesda guidelines

Amsterdam I criteria
At least three relatives who have histologically verified colorectal cancer:
1. One is a first-degree relative of the other two
2. At least two successive generations affected
3. At least one of the relatives who has colorectal cancer diagnosed at less than 50 years of age
4. Familial adenomatous polyposis has been excluded

Amsterdam II criteria
At least three relatives who have an HNPCC-associated cancer (colorectal cancer, endometrial, stomach, ovary, ureter/renal pelvis, brain, small bowel, hepatobiliary tract, or skin [sebaceous tumors]):
1. One is a first-degree relative of the other two
2. At least two successive generations affected
3. At least one of the HNPCC-associated cancers should be diagnosed at less than 50 years of age
4. Familial adenomatous polyposis has been excluded in any colorectal cancer cases

Tumors should be verified whenever possible.

Bethesda guidelines for testing of colorectal tumors for microsatellite instability
1. Individuals who have cancer in families that meet the Amsterdam criteria
2. Individuals who have two HNPCC-related cancers, including synchronous and metachronous colorectal cancers or associated extracolonic cancers[a]
3. Individuals who have colorectal cancer and a first-degree relative who has colorectal cancer or HNPCC-related extracolonic cancer or a colorectal adenoma; one of the cancers diagnosed at age less than 45 years and the adenoma diagnosed at age less than 40 years
4. Individuals who have colorectal cancer or endometrial cancer diagnosed at age less than 45 years
5. Individuals who have right-sided colorectal cancer with an undifferentiated pattern (solid/cribriform) on histopathology diagnosed at age less than 45 years[b]

6. Individuals who have signet-ring cell–type colorectal cancer diagnosed at age less than 45 years[c]
7. Individuals who have adenomas diagnosed at age less than 40 years

[a] Endometrial, ovarian, gastric, hepatobiliary, or small bowel cancer or transitional cell carcinoma of the renal pelvis or ureter.
[b] Solid/cribriform defined as poorly differentiated or undifferentiated carcinoma composed of irregular, solid sheets of large eosinophilic cells and containing small gland-like spaces.
[c] Composed of more than 50% signet ring cells.
Reproduced from Merg A, Lynch HT, Lynch JF, et al. Hereditary colorectal cancer—Part II. Curr Probl Surg 2005;42(5):267–334; with permission.

[106]. Homozygous and compound heterozygous mutations of *MLH1*, *MSH2*, *MSH6*, and *PMS2* have been reported, often in consanguineous families, with affected children exhibiting features of neurofibromatosis type 1 and high risk for childhood hematologic, brain, and gastrointestinal cancers [108].

Cancer surveillance

As with FAP, cancer screening plays a crucial role in the management of Lynch syndrome. Several studies have examined the role of colonoscopic surveillance in this population, although only two have been prospective studies [109,110]. All studies reported detection of colorectal polyps and cancers at an earlier stage in patients undergoing regular colonoscopy, and two studies also demonstrated a decrease in CRC-related mortality [90]. A prospective study by Jarvinen and colleagues [109] demonstrated a 63% decrease in CRC risk in patients having colonoscopy at 3-year intervals; the same group also reported recently a high cumulative risk for developing adenomatous polyps by age 60 in mutation carriers (68% men; 48% women), and a cumulative risk for CRC found by surveillance at intervals of 2 to 3 years of 35% in men and 22% in women by age 60 [110]. Given this risk for cancer development at 3-year intervals, most advocate 1- to 2-year surveillance, starting at age 20 to 25 years [90]. For patients identified as familial colorectal cancer type X, no clear evidence exists but surveillance is generally recommended at 3- to 5-year intervals, starting at age 45 to 50 or 10 years younger than the earliest diagnosed cases of CRC in the family, whichever comes first [51].

The evidence for gynecologic malignancy surveillance (endometrial and ovarian) in women from Lynch families is controversial [111]. Two studies suggested that a protocol of regular gynecologic examination, transvaginal ultrasound, and endometrial aspiration biopsy starting at age 30 to 35 may help in detecting premalignant and early cancerous endometrial or ovarian lesions. No study has demonstrated a reduction in mortality, however, and

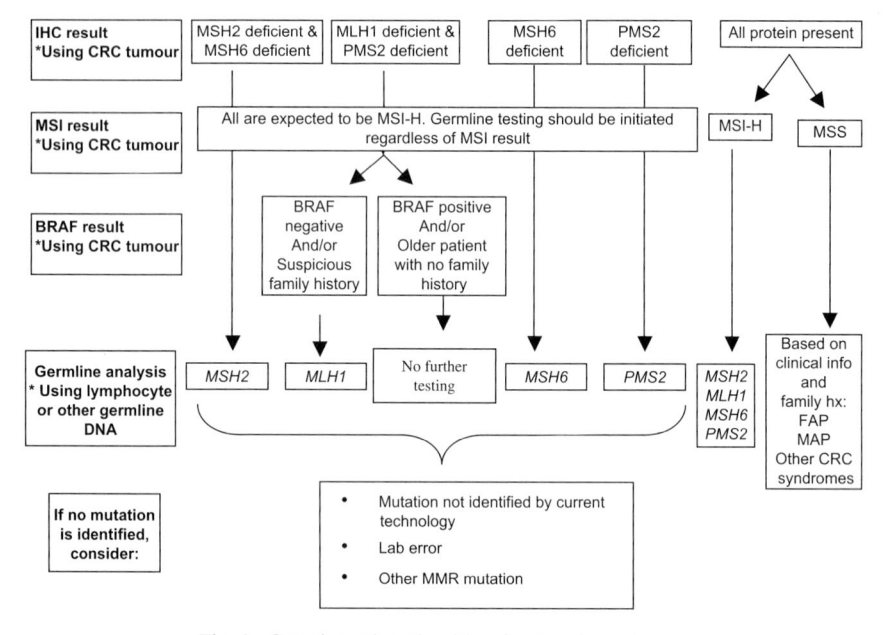

Fig. 3. Genetic testing algorithm for Lynch syndrome.

there is a high rate of false-positive results. Screening for the general population has not been adopted because of relatively low rates of cancer and generally good prognosis even in symptomatic patients, so no comparative evidence exists for the efficacy of these screening modalities. A recent decision-analysis study comparing female patients who had Lynch syndrome undergoing annual gynecologic examination versus annual ultrasound and biopsy screening versus total abdominal hysterectomy and bilateral salpingo-oophorectomy (TAHBSO) estimated an increased survival in the screening arm compared with the examination-only group, but acknowledged that such advantage may partly be because of a high false-positive rate that leads to surgery in the screening group [112] (see Surgical Management section).

Similarly, the evidence for screening for other extracolonic cancers in Lynch syndrome is limited. European and North American expert groups recommend the following: OGD screening at 1- to 2-year intervals starting at age 30 to 35 for gastric cancer in patients whose families show clustering of this malignancy, or for patients from populations with high incidence of gastric cancer; and urinalysis and urine cytology every 1 to 2 years starting at age 30 to 35 if urinary tract cancer occurs in the family [90,113].

Surgical management

In patients diagnosed with a colorectal tumor (invasive cancer or large polyp), the extent of resection in patients who have Lynch syndrome has been debated. Although no controlled studies have been performed, most experts advocate subtotal colectomy with ileorectal anastomosis. A decision analysis that compared subtotal to segmental resection for primary CRC in patients who had Lynch syndrome identified an improved life expectancy of 2.3 years in young patients (<47 years) undergoing subtotal colectomy. This analysis was limited by not adjusting for quality-of-life years, but the authors suggested that subtotal resection may improve quality of life for patients who have Lynch syndrome by reducing the need for subsequent colonoscopy and decreasing concern about development of secondary tumors [114].

The second surgical decision facing patients who have Lynch syndrome is the role of prophylactic surgery. Prophylactic surgery obviates the need for surveillance by colonoscopy (although proctoscopy/sigmoidoscopy would remain necessary). Because colorectal cancer penetrance in Lynch syndrome is variable and is likely significantly lower than the often-quoted 70% to 80% [91], and with recent reports suggesting a possible decreased risk in older patients [115], prophylactic colectomy is not generally advisable. Of course, more prospectively designed population studies are needed to adequately estimate penetrance and age-related risk for cancer in patients who have Lynch syndrome.

Prophylactic surgery also applies to gynecologic malignancy. The best evidence on this issue comes from a retrospective study of 315 women carrying MMR mutations, of whom 61 underwent prophylactic surgery. No endometrial or ovarian cancer developed at 10-year follow-up in the surgical group, compared with a 33% endometrial cancer and 5.5% ovarian cancer rate in the nonsurgical group [116]. Another recent study conducted a decision-analysis model that estimated the need to perform 6 and 28 prophylactic surgeries to reduce one case of endometrial and ovarian cancers, respectively [112]. Some experts recommend that TAHBSO be offered to female patients who have Lynch syndrome who would be undergoing laparotomy for CRC resection [113].

Nonsurgical management

There is obvious interest in identifying chemopreventive agents for CRC in Lynch syndrome. A double-blinded randomized controlled trial, the CAPP2 study, was undertaken to investigate the effect of 600 mg ASA and 30 g "resistant" starch on colorectal neoplasia in MMR mutation carriers. Although not published as yet, a recent presentation by CAPP2 investigators suggested that no significant chemopreventive effect was found for either treatment [117].

Oral contraceptives have been demonstrated to decrease the risk for endometrial and ovarian cancer in the general population, and but there are no data to guide recommendations on use of this medication as chemoprevention in patients who have Lynch syndrome [113].

Several studies have identified a differential effect of common chemotherapeutic agents for Stage II and III CRC depending on tumor microsatellite stability. A competent MMR system seems to be important to the cytotoxic effect of 5-fluoruracil (5-FU)–based treatments; in vitro studies demonstrated slower growth of MMR-proficient cells compared with MMR-deficient cells when exposed to pharmacologic doses of 5-FU [118]. Using data and biospecimens from three prospective randomized controlled chemotherapy trials, patients who had MSI-high tumors showed no benefit from 5-FU–based adjuvant chemotherapy, whereas chemotherapy did have a benefit for patients who had MSI-low or microsatellite-stable tumors [119]. Several other studies have confirmed these findings, including a study that specifically assessed patients from Lynch families [120]. A recent study of 40 young patients who had metastatic CRC, of whom 9 patients had MSI-high tumors, showed no significant survival difference between microsatellite stable and unstable tumors in response to two FOLFOX regimens (5-FU + oxaliplatin), but did note that MSI-high tumors seemed more sensitive to the higher-dose regimen [121].

To date, there is insufficient definitive evidence to avoid conventional adjuvant or palliative chemotherapy in the usually young patient who has Lynch syndrome, but other chemotherapeutic options for MSI-high CRCs are being investigated. In vitro studies have shown that MMR deficiency enhances apoptosis and sensitivity of CRC tumor cells to the topoisomerase inhibitor irinotecan (CPT-11) [122]. A retrospective study of patients who have metastatic CRC showed that MSI-positive patients had a better response to irinotecan therapy than microsatellite-stable patients [123], whereas another study found a significantly greater response to neoadjuvant irinotecan-based chemoradiotherapy for MSI-high rectal cancer compared with microsatellite-stable tumors [124].

Summary

FAP and Lynch syndrome represent the major forms of hereditary CRC, both inherited in an autosomal dominant manner. Understanding the genetic basis of these conditions has progressed rapidly, facilitating improved sensitivity and specificity in identifying at-risk individuals. Management of these patients includes close surveillance of the organs at risk, with implementation of surgical intervention when appropriate.

In FAP, prophylactic colectomy is generally indicated for all mutation carriers, usually at the end of the second to third decade. FAP also increases risk for duodenal polyposis and cancer, so careful upper GI surveillance is essential and aggressive surgical intervention may be necessary in stage IV duodenal polyposis. The role of prophylactic surgery in Lynch syndrome is less clear, but a subtotal colectomy is favored over a segmental resection when CRC is identified.

There is significant interest in identifying chemopreventive agents for FAP and Lynch syndrome, but the evidence remains inconclusive.

Acknowledgment

We thank Terri Berk for her input and access to FAP pedigree and endoscopy images.

References

[1] Gryfe R. Clinical implications of our advancing knowledge of colorectal cancer genetics: inherited syndromes, prognosis, prevention, screening and therapeutics. Surg Clin North Am 2006;86(4):787–817.
[2] Bulow S, Berk T, Neale K. The history of familial adenomatous polyposis. Fam Cancer 2006;5(3):213–20.
[3] Senda T, Iizuka-Kogo A, Onouchi T, et al. Adenomatous polyposis coli plays multiple roles in the intestinal and colorectal epithelia. Med Mol Morphol 2007;40(2):68–81.
[4] Merg A, Lynch H, Lynch J, et al. Hereditary colon cancer—Part I. Curr Probl Surg 2005; 42(4):195–256.
[5] Brensinger JD, Laken SJ, Luce MC, et al. Variable phenotype of familial adenomatous polyposis in pedigrees with 3' mutation in the *APC* gene. Gut 1998;43:548–52.
[6] Kashiwagi H, Spigelman AD. Gastroduodenal lesions in familial adenomatous polyposis. Surg Today 2000;30(8):675–82.
[7] Galiatsatos P, Foulkes WD. Familial adenomatous polyposis. Am J Gastroenterol 2006; 101(2):385–98.
[8] Spigelman AD, Williams CB, Talbot IC, et al. Upper gastrointestinal cancer in patients with familial adenomatous polyposis. Lancet 1989;2:783–5.
[9] Saurin JC, Guknecht C, Napoleon B, et al. Surveillance of duodenal adenomas in familial adenomatous polyposis reveals high cumulative risk of advanced disease. J Clin Oncol 2004;22(3):493–8.
[10] Sellner F. Investigations on the significance of the adenoma-carcinoma sequence in the small bowel. Cancer 1990;66(4):702–15.
[11] Groves CJ, Saunders BP, Spigelman AD, et al. Duodenal cancer in patients with familial adenomatous polyposis (FAP): results of a 10 year prospective study. Gut 2002;50(5). 636–41.
[12] Bjork J, Akerbrant H, Iselius L, et al. Periampullary adenomas and adenocarcinomas in familial adenomatous polyposis: cumulative risks and *APC* gene mutations. Gastroenterology 2001;121(5):1127–35.
[13] Heiskanen I, Kellokumpu I, Jarvinen H. Management of duodenal adenomas in 98 patients with familial adenomatous polyposis. Endoscopy 1999;31(6):412–6.
[14] Sanabria JR, Croxford R, Berk TC, et al. Familial segregation in the occurrence and severity of periampullary neoplasms in familial adenomatous polyposis. Am J Surg 1996;171(1): 136–40.
[15] Church JM, McGannon E, Hull-Boiner S, et al. Gastroduodenal polyps in patients with familial adenomatous polyposis. Dis Colon Rectum 1992;35(12):1170–3.
[16] Burt RW. Gastric fundic gland polyps. Gastroenterology 2003;125(5):1462–9.
[17] Mabrut JY, Romagnoli R, Collard JM, et al. Familial adenomatous polyposis predisposes to pathologic exposure of the stomach to bilirubin. Surgery 2006;140(5):818–23.
[18] Iwama T, Mishima Y, Utsunomiya J. The impact of familial adenomatous polyposis on the tumorigenesis and mortality at the several organs. Its rational treatment. Ann Surg 1993; 217(2):101–8.

[19] Kadmon M, Tandara A, Herfarth C. Duodenal adenomatosis in familial adenomatous polyposis coli. A review of the literature and results from the Heidelberg Polyposis Register. Int J Colorectal Dis 2001;16:63–75.
[20] Jones IT, Jagelman DG, Fazio VW, et al. Desmoid tumors in familial polyposis coli. Ann Surg 1986;204(1):94–7.
[21] Durno C, Mongo N, Bapat B, et al. Does early colectomy increase desmoid risk in familial adenomatous polyposis? Clin Gastroenterol Hepatol 2007;5(10):1190–4.
[22] Herraiz M, Barbesino G, Faquin W, et al. Prevalence of thyroid cancer in familial adenomatous polyposis syndrome and the role of screening ultrasound examinations. Clin Gastroenterol Hepatol 2007;5(3):367–73.
[23] Truta B, Allen BA, Conrad PG, et al. Genotype and phenotype of patients with both familial adenomatous polyposis and thyroid carcinoma. Fam Cancer 2003;2(2):95–9.
[24] Aretz S, Koch A, Uhlhaas S, et al. Should children at risk for familial adenomatous polyposis be screened for hepatoblastoma and children with apparently sporadic hepatoblastoma be screened for *APC* germline mutations? Pediatr Blood Cancer 2006;47(6):811–8.
[25] Hamilton SR, Liu B, Parsons RE, et al. The molecular basis of Turcot's syndrome. N Engl J Med 1995;332(13):839–47.
[26] Gupta C, Mazzara PF. High-grade pancreatic intraepithelial neoplasia in a patient with familial adenomatous polyposis. Arch Pathol Lab Med 2005;129(11):1398–400.
[27] Chetty R, Salahshor S, Bapat B, et al. Intraductal papillary mucinous neoplasm of the pancreas in a patient with attenuated familial adenomatous polyposis. J Clin Pathol 2005;58(1): 97–101.
[28] Maire F, Hammel P, Terris B, et al. Intraductal papillary and mucinous pancreatic tumour: a new extracolonic tumour in familial adenomatous polyposis. Gut 2002;51(3):446–9.
[29] DiMagno EP. Pancreatic cancer: clinical presentation, pitfalls and early clues. Ann Oncol 1999;10(S4):140–2.
[30] Narayan S, Roy D. Role of *APC* and DNA mismatch repair genes in the development of colorectal cancers. Mol Cancer 2003;2:41–55.
[31] Caspari R, Friedl W, Mandl M, et al. Familial adenomatous polyposis: mutation at codon 1309 and early onset of colon cancer. Lancet 1994;343(8898):629–32.
[32] Soravia C, Berk T, Madlensky L, et al. Genotype-phenotype correlations in attenuated adenomatous polyposis coli. Am J Hum Genet 1998;62:1290–301.
[33] Couture J, Mitri A, Legace R, et al. A germline mutation at the extreme 3' end of the *APC* gene results in a severe desmoid phenotype and is associated with overexpression of beta-catenin in the desmoid tumour. Clin Genet 2000;57(3):205–12.
[34] Caspari R, Olschwang S, Friedl W, et al. Familial adenomatous polyposis: desmoid tumors and lack of ophthalmic lesions (CHRPE) associated with *APC* mutations beyond codon 1444. Hum Mol Genet 1995;4:337–40.
[35] Nieuwenhuis MH, Vasen HF. Correlations between mutation site in APC and phenotype of familial adenomatous polyposis (FAP): a review of the literature. Crit Rev Oncol Hematol 2007;61:153–61.
[36] Friedl W, Caspari R, Sengteller M, et al. Can *APC* mutation analysis contribute to therapeutic decisions in familial adenomatous polyposis? Experience from 680 FAP families. Gut 2001;48:515–21.
[37] Michils G, Tejpar S, Thoelen R, et al. Large deletions of the *APC* gene in 15% of mutation-negative patients with classical polyposis (FAP): a Belgian study. Hum Mutat 2005;25: 125–34.
[38] Al-Tassan N, Chmiel NH, Maynard J, et al. Inherited variants of *MYH* associated with somatic G:C→T:A mutations in colorectal tumors. Nat Genet 2002;30:227–32.
[39] Chow E, Thirlwell C, Macrae F, et al. Colorectal cancer and inherited mutations in base-excision repair. Lancet Oncol 2004;5(10):600–6.
[40] Farrington SM, Tenesa A, Barnetson R, et al. Germline susceptibility to colorectal cancer due to base-excision repair gene defects. Am J Hum Genet 2005;77:112–9.

[41] Russell AM, Zhang J, Luz J, et al. Prevalence of *MYH* germline mutations in Swiss *APC* mutation-negative polyposis patients. Int J Cancer 2006;118(8):1937–40.
[42] Croitoru ME, Cleary SP, Monga N, et al. Germline *MYH* mutations in a clinic-based series of Canadian multiple colorectal adenoma patients. J Surg Oncol 2007;95(6):499–506.
[43] David S, O'Shea Y, Kunda S. Base-excision repair of oxidative DNA damage. Nature 2007; 447(7147):941–50.
[44] Balaguer F, Castellvi-Bel S, Castells A, et al. Identification of *MYH* mutation carriers in colorectal cancer: a multicenter, case-control, population-based study. Clin Gastroenterol Hepatol 2007;5(3):379–87.
[45] Bouguen G, Manfredi S, Blayau M, et al. Colorectal adenomatous polyposis associated with *MYH* mutations: genotype & phenotype characteristics. Dis Colon Rectum 2007; 50(10):1612–7.
[46] Jenkins MA, Croitoru ME, Monga N, et al. Risk of colorectal cancer in monoallelic and biallelic carriers of *MYH* mutations: a population-based case-family study. Cancer Epidemiol Biomarkers Prev 2006;15(2):312–4.
[47] Cheadle JP, Sampson JR. MUTYH-associated polyposis—from defect in base excision repair to clinical genetic testing. DNA Repair (Amst) 2007;6(3):274–9.
[48] Aretz S, Stienen D, Friedrichs N, et al. Somatic *APC* mosaicism: a frequent cause of FAP. Hum Mutat 2007;28(10):985–92.
[49] Bisgaard ML, Fenger K, Bulow S, et al. Familial adenomatous polyposis (FAP): frequency, penetrance, and mutation rate. Hum Mutat 1994;3:121–5.
[50] Schwab A, Tuohy TM, Condie M, et al. Gonadal mosaicism and familial adenomatous polyposis. Fam Cancer 2008;7:173–7.
[51] Winawer S, Fletcher R, Rex D, et al. Colorectal cancer screening and surveillance: clinical guidelines and rationale-update based on new evidence. Gastroenterology 2003;124(2): 544–60.
[52] Johnson JC, DiSario JA, Grady WM. Surveillance and treatment of periampullary and duodenal adenomas in familial adenomatous polyposis. Curr Treat Options Gastroenterol 2004;7(2):79–89.
[53] Gallagher MC, Phillips RK, Bulow S. Surveillance and management of upper gastrointestinal disease in familial adenomatous polyposis. Fam Cancer 2006;5(3):263–73.
[54] Burke CA, Santisi J, Church J, et al. The utility of capsule endoscopy small bowel surveillance in patients with polyposis. Am J Gastroenterol 2005;100(7):1498–502.
[55] Wong RF, Tuteja AK, Haslem DS, et al. Video capsule endoscopy compared with standard endoscopy for the evaluation of small-bowel polyps in persons with familial adenomatous polyposis (with video). Gastrointest Endosc 2006;64(4):530–7.
[56] Cetta F, Montalto G, Gori M, et al. Germline mutations of the *APC* gene in patients with familial adenomatous polyposis-associated thyroid carcinoma: results from a European cooperative study. J Clin Endocrinol Metab 2000;85(1):286–92.
[57] Church J. In which patients do I perform IRA, and why? Fam Cancer 2006;5:237–40.
[58] De Cosse JJ, Bülow S, Neale K, et al. Rectal cancer risk in patients treated for familial adenomatous polyposis. The Leeds Castle Polyposis Group. Br J Surg 1992;79(12):1372–5.
[59] Bulow C, Vasen H, Jarvinen H, et al. Ileorectal anastomosis is appropriate for a subset of patients with familial adenomatous polyposis. Gastroenterology 2000;119(6):1454–60.
[60] Guillem JG, Wood WC, Moley JF, et al. ASCO/SSO review of current role of risk-reducing surgery in common hereditary cancer syndromes. Ann Surg Oncol 2006;13(10): 1296–321.
[61] Church J, Burke C, McGannon E, et al. Risk of rectal cancer in patients after colectomy and ileorectal anastomosis for familial adenomatous polyposis: a function of available surgical options. Dis Colon Rectum 2003;46(9):1175–81.
[62] Church J, Simmang C. Standards Task Force; American Society of Colon and Rectal Surgeons; Collaborative Group of the Americas on Inherited Colorectal Cancer and the Standards Committee of The American Society of Colon and Rectal Surgeons. Practice

parameters for the treatment of patients with dominantly inherited colorectal cancer (familial adenomatous polyposis and hereditary nonpolyposis colorectal cancer). Dis Colon Rectum 2003;46:1001–12.

[63] Valanzano R, Ficari F, Curia MC, et al. Balance between endoscopic and genetic information in the choice of ileorectal anastomosis for familial adenomatous polyposis. J Surg Oncol 2007;95(1):28–33.

[64] Kartheuser A, Stangherlin P, Brandt D, et al. Restorative proctocolectomy and ileal pouch-anal anastomosis for familial adenomatous polyposis revisited. Fam Cancer 2006;5(3):241–60.

[65] Chambers WM, McC Mortensen NJ. Should ileal pouch-anal anastomosis include mucosectomy? Colorectal Dis 2007;9(5):384–92.

[66] Zhang H, Hu S, Zhang G, et al. Laparoscopic versus open proctocolectomy with ileal pouch-anal anastomosis. Minim Invasive Ther Allied Technol 2007;16(3):187–91.

[67] Alarcon FJ, Burke CA, Church JM, et al. Familial adenomatous polyposis. Efficacy of endoscopic and surgical treatment for advanced duodenal adenomas. Dis Colon Rectum 1999;42:1533–6.

[68] Brosens LA, Keller JJ, Offerhaus GJ, et al. Prevention and management of duodenal polyps in familial adenomatous polyposis. Gut 2005;54(7):1034–43.

[69] Dixon E, Vollmer CM, Sahajpal A, et al. Transduodenal resection of peri-ampullary lesions. World J Surg 2005;29(5):649–52.

[70] Gallagher M, Shankar A, Groves C, et al. Pylorus-preserving pancreaticoduodenectomy for advanced duodenal disease in familial adenomatous polyposis. Br J Surg 2004;91(9): 1157–64.

[71] Imamura M, Komoto I, Doi R, et al. New pancreas-preserving total duodenectomy technique. World J Surg 2005;29(2):203–7.

[72] Lev D, Kotilingam D, Wei C, et al. Optimizing treatment of desmoid tumors. J Clin Oncol 2007;25(13):1785–91.

[73] Latchford AR, Sturt NJ, Neale K, et al. A 10-year review of surgery for desmoid disease associated with familial adenomatous polyposis. Br J Surg 2006;93(10):1258–64.

[74] Sakorafas GH, Nissotakis C, Peros G. Abdominal desmoid tumors. Surg Oncol 2007;16(2): 131–42.

[75] Clark SK, Neale KF, Landgrebe JC, et al. Desmoid tumours complicating familial adenomatous polyposis. Br J Surg 1999;86:1185–9.

[76] Khor TO, Cheung WK, Prawan A, et al. Chemoprevention of familial adenomatous polyposis in Apc(Min/+) mice by phenethyl isothiocyanate (PEITC). Mol Carcinog 2007;47(5): 321–5.

[77] Shen G, Khor TO, Hu R, et al. Chemoprevention of familial adenomatous polyposis by natural dietary compounds sulforaphane and dibenzoylmethane alone and in combination in ApcMin/+ mouse. Cancer Res 2007;67(20):9937–44.

[78] Steinbach G, Lynch PM, Phillips RK, et al. The effect of celecoxib, a cyclooxygenase-2 inhibitor, in familial adenomatous polyposis. N Engl J Med 2000;342:1946–52.

[79] Phillips RK, Wallace MH, Lynch PM, et al. A randomised, double blind, placebo controlled study of celecoxib, a selective cyclooxygenase 2 inhibitor, on duodenal polyposis in familial adenomatous polyposis. Gut 2002;50(6):857–60.

[80] Higuchi T, Iwama T, Yoshinaga K, et al. A randomized, double-blind, placebo-controlled trial of the effects of rofecoxib, a selective cyclooxygenase-2 inhibitor, on rectal polyps in familial adenomatous polyposis patients. Clin Cancer Res 2003;9(13):4756–60.

[81] Spychalski M, Dizki L, Dizki A. Chemoprevention of colorectal cancer – a new target needed? Colorectal Dis 2007;9(5):397–401.

[82] Bresalier RS, Sandler RS, Quan H, et al, Adenomatous Polyp Prevention on Vioxx (APPROVe) Trial Investigators. Cardiovascular events associated with rofecoxib in a colorectal adenoma chemoprevention trial. N Engl J Med 2005;352:1092–102.

[83] Burn J. Invited commentary. Fam Cancer 2006;5:295–6.

[84] Merg A, Lynch HT, Lynch JF, et al. Hereditary colorectal cancer-part II. Curr Probl Surg 2005;42(5):267–333.
[85] Jass JR. Hereditary non-polyposis colorectal cancer: the rise and fall of a confusing term. World J Gastroenterol 2006;12(31):4943–50.
[86] Lynch HT, Boland CR, Gong G, et al. Phenotypic and genotypic heterogeneity in the Lynch syndrome: diagnostic, surveillance and management implications. Eur J Hum Genet 2006;14(4):390–402.
[87] Vasen H. Review article: the Lynch syndrome (hereditary nonpolyposis colorectal cancer). Aliment Pharmacol Ther 2007;26(S2):113–26.
[88] Paraf F, Jothy S, Van Meir EG. Brain tumor-polyposis syndrome: two genetic diseases? J Clin Oncol 1997;15(7):2744–58.
[89] Lindor NM, Rabe K, Petersen GM, et al. Lower cancer incidence in Amsterdam-I criteria families without mismatch repair deficiency: familial colorectal cancer type X. JAMA 2005; 293(16):1979–85.
[90] Vasen HF, Moslein G, Alonso A, et al. Guidelines for the clinical management of Lynch syndrome (hereditary non-polyposis cancer). J Med Genet 2007;44(6):353–62.
[91] Alarcon F, Lasset C, Carayol J, et al. Estimating cancer risk in HNPCC by the GRL method. Eur J Hum Genet 2007;15:831–6.
[92] Vasen HF, Watson P, Mecklin JP, et al. The epidemiology of endometrial cancer in hereditary nonpolyposis colorectal cancer. Anticancer Res 1994;14(4B):1675–8.
[93] van den BM, van den HM, Jongejan E, et al. More differences between HNPCC-related and sporadic carcinomas from the endometrium as compared to the colon. Am J Surg Pathol 2004;28:706–11.
[94] Watson P, Butzow R, Lynch HT, et al. The clinical features of ovarian cancer in hereditary nonpolyposis colorectal cancer. Gynecol Oncol 2001;82(2):223–8.
[95] ten Kate GL, Kleibeuker JH, Nagengast FM, et al. Is surveillance of the small bowel indicated for Lynch syndrome families? Gut 2007;56(9):1198–201.
[96] Boland CR, Koi M, Chang DK, et al. The biochemical basis of microsatellite instability and abnormal immunohistochemistry and clinical behaviour in Lynch Syndrome: from bench to bedside. Fam Cancer 2007;7(1):41–52.
[97] Boland CR, Thibodeau SN, Hamilton SR, et al. A national cancer institute workshop on microsatellite instability for cancer detection and familial predisposition: development of international criteria for the determination of microsatellite instability in colorectal cancer. Cancer Res 1998;58:5248–57.
[98] Hampel H, Frankel WL, Martin E, et al. Screening for Lynch syndrome. N Engl J Med 2005;66(15):7810–7.
[99] Burgart LJ. Testing for defective DNA mismatch repair in colorectal carcinoma: a practical guide. Arch Pathol Lab Med 2005;129(11):1385–9.
[100] Hitchins MP, Wong JJ, Suthers G, et al. Inheritance of a cancer-associated MLH1 germline epimutation. N Engl J Med 2007;356(7):697–705.
[101] Jass JR. Hereditary and DNA methylation in colorectal cancer. Gut 2007;56(1):154–5.
[102] Rahner N, Friedrichs N, Steinke V, et al. Coexisting somatic promoter hypermethylation and pathogenic *MLH1* germline mutation in Lynch syndrome. J Pathol 2008;214: 10–6.
[103] Loughrey MB, Waring PM, Tan A, et al. Incorporation of somatic *BRAF* mutation testing into an algorithm for the investigation of hereditary non-polyposis colorectal cancer. Fam Cancer 2007;6(3):301–10.
[104] Barnetson RA, Tenesa A, Farrington SM, et al. Identification and survival of carriers of mutations in DNA mismatch-repair genes in colon cancer. N Engl J Med 2006;354(26): 2751–63.
[105] Chen S, Wang W, Lee S, et al. Prediction of germline mutations and cancer risk in the Lynch syndrome. JAMA 2006;296(12):1479–87.

[106] Geary J, Sasieni P, Houlston R, et al. Gene-related cancer spectrum in familial with hereditary non-polyposis colorectal cancer (HNPCC). Fam Cancer 2008;7:163–72.
[107] Smith L, Tesoriero A, Mead L, et al. Large genomic alterations in hMSH2 and hMLH1 in early-onset colorectal cancer; identification of a large complex de novo hMLH1 alteration. Clin Genet 2006;70:250–2.
[108] Gallinger S, Aronson M, Shayan K, et al. Gastrointestinal cancers and neurofibromatosis type 1 features in children with a germline homozygous MLH1 mutation. Gastroenterology 2004;126(2):576–85.
[109] Jarvinen HJ, Aarnio M, Mustonen H, et al. Controlled 15-year trial on screening for colorectal cancer in families with hereditary nonpolyposis colorectal cancer. Gastroenterology 2000;118:829–34.
[110] Mecklin JP, Aarnio M, Laara E, et al. Development of colorectal tumors in colonoscopic surveillance in Lynch syndrome. Gastroenterology 2007;133(4):1093–8.
[111] Renkonen-Sinisalo L, Butzow R, Leminen A, et al. Surveillance for endometrial cancer in hereditary nonpolyposis colorectal cancer syndrome. Int J Cancer 2007;120:821–4.
[112] Chen L, Yang K, Little S, et al. Gynecologic cancer prevention in Lynch syndrome/hereditary nonpolyposis colorectal cancer families. Obstet Gynecol 2007;110(1):18–25.
[113] Lindor NM, Petersen GM, Hadley DW, et al. Recommendations for the care of individuals with an inherited predisposition to Lynch syndrome: a systematic review. JAMA 2006; 296(12):1507–17.
[114] de Vos tot Nederveen Cappel WH, Buskens E, van Duijvendijk P, et al. Decision analysis in the surgical treatment of colorectal cancer due to a mismatch repair gene defect. Gut 2003; 52:1752–5.
[115] Jenkins MA, Baglietto L, Dowty JG, et al. Cancer risks for mismatch repair gene mutation carriers: a population-based early onset case-family study. Clin Gastroenterol Hepatol 2006;4(4):489–98.
[116] Schmeler KM, Lynch HT, Chen LM, et al. Prophylactic surgery to reduce the risk of gynecologic cancers in the Lynch syndrome. N Engl J Med 2006;354(3):261–9.
[117] Burn J. Chemoprevention in hereditary colorectal cancer: where are we headed? In: 11th Annual Meeting of the Collaborative Group of the Americas on Inherited Colorectal Cancer. La Jolla: October 21-22, 2007.
[118] Carethers JM, Chauhan DP, Fink D, et al. Mismatch repair proficiency and in vitro response to 5-fluorouracil. Gastroenterology 1999;117:123–31.
[119] Ribic CM, Sargent DJ, Moore MJ, et al. Tumor microsatellite instability status as a predictor of benefit from fluorouracil-based adjuvant chemotherapy for colon cancer. N Engl J Med 2003;349:247–57.
[120] de Vos tot Nederveen Cappel WH, Meulenbeld HJ, Kleibeuker JH, et al. Survival after adjuvant 5-FU treatment for Stage III colon cancer in hereditary nonpolyposis colorectal cancer. Int J Cancer 2004;109:468–71.
[121] Des Guetz G, Mariani P, Cucherousset J, et al. Microsatellite instability and sensitivity to FOLFOX treatment in metastatic colorectal cancer. Anticancer Res 2007;27(4C):2715–9.
[122] Magrini R, Bhonde MR, Hanski ML, et al. Cellular effects of CPT-11 on colon carcinoma cells: dependence on p53 and hMLH1 status. Int J Cancer 2002;101:23–31.
[123] Fallik D, Borrini F, Boige V, et al. Microsatellite instability is a predictive factor of the tumor response to irinotecan in patients with advanced colorectal cancer. Cancer Res 2003;63:5738–44.
[124] Charara M, Edmonston TB, Burkholder S, et al. Microsatellite status and cell cycle associated markers in rectal cancer patients undergoing combined regimen of 5-FU and CPT-11 chemotherapy and radiotherapy. Anticancer Res 2004;24(5B):3161–7.

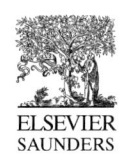

Management of Women Who Have a Genetic Predisposition for Breast Cancer

Ismail Jatoi, MD, PhD[a],*, William F. Anderson, MD, MPH[b]

[a]Breast Care Center, National Naval Medical Center, Uniformed Services University, 8901 Wisconsin Avenue, Bethesda, MD 20889, USA
[b]Biostatistics Branch, Division of Cancer Epidemiology and Genetics, National Cancer Institute, National Institutes of Health, Department of Health and Human Services, Bethesda, MD 20852, USA

Breast cancer is a major public health problem, affecting 12.3% or one in eight of all women in the United States (123/1000 women) during their lifetime [1]. The three most important risk factors for breast cancer, in decreasing order of importance, are gender, aging, and family history [2]. Although many women have no immediate family members who have had breast cancer, some clearly do. Since the nineteenth century, there have been numerous reports of families suffering from multiple cases of breast cancer. In 1866, Paul Broca, a French surgeon, published the first such description, reporting that 10 of 24 women through five successive generations of his wife's family had died of breast cancer [3].

Approximately 5% to 10% of all breast cancers in the United States occur in women who have a genetic predisposition, and most of these are attributable to mutations in the breast cancer susceptibility gene 1 (*BRCA1*) and breast cancer susceptibility gene 2 (*BRCA2*) [4,5]. Other genes also are associated with breast cancer, including *p53*, *PTEN*, *STK11/LKB1*, *CDH 1*, *ATM*, and *CHEK 2* [6]. The lifetime risk of breast cancer

---

The views or opinions expressed in this article are those of the authors and should not be construed as representing the official views of the Departments of the Army, Navy, or Defense.

This research was supported in part by the Intramural Research Program of the National Institutes of Health/National Cancer Institute.

*Corresponding author.

E-mail address: ismail.jatoi@us.army.mil (I. Jatoi).

(penetrance) varies considerably among women who carry these mutations. The high-penetrance mutations (eg, *BRCA1, BRCA2, p53, PTEN, STK11/ LKB1, CDH1*) are associated with a high lifetime risk of breast cancer (40%–85%), whereas the low-to-moderate penetrance mutations (eg, *ATM, CHEK 2*) are associated with a lower risk [6]. These mutations are associated with an increased risk for other cancers and diseases as well as breast cancer. Thus, these mutations are linked with a diverse spectrum of syndromes that includes the hereditary breast and ovarian cancer syndrome (*BRCA1* and *BRCA2*), Li-Fraumeni syndrome (*p53*), Cowden's disease (*PTEN*), Peutz-Jeghers syndrome (*STK11/LKB1*), hereditary diffuse gastric carcinoma syndrome (*CDH 1*), ataxia-telangiectasia (*ATM*), and a Li-Fraumeni syndrome variant (*CHEK 2*) [6,7]. Many of these syndromes are discussed in other articles in this issue. This article focuses on the hereditary breast and ovarian cancer syndromes, which are responsible for more than half of the known cases of hereditary breast cancer. Much of the discussion focuses on the management of breast cancer risk, but *BRCA* mutation carriers also are at increased risk for ovarian cancer [8]. Therefore, issues pertinent to the management of ovarian cancer risk in *BRCA* mutation carriers are discussed briefly. Finally, issues relevant to breast cancer treatment in mutation carriers are discussed.

Hereditary breast and ovarian cancer syndrome

BRCA1 and *BRCA2* are tumor-suppressor genes, identified in chromosomes 17 and 13, respectively, coding for proteins intimately involved in cellular growth and differentiation [9,10]. In the United States approximately 1 woman in 250 carries a mutation in these genes, predisposing these women to an increased risk for breast and ovarian cancer [11]. The *BRCA1* and *BRCA2* gene mutations are transmitted in an autosomal dominant manner and therefore may originate from either the maternal or paternal side [12]. Each offspring of a *BRCA1* or *BRCA2* mutation carrier has a 50% chance of inheriting that mutation, and a carefully documented family history is essential for the initial assessment of any woman concerned about a hereditary predisposition to breast cancer. If a woman has multiple close relatives (mother, sisters, daughters, grandmothers, aunts) who have had breast and ovarian cancer diagnosed at an early age (before age 50 years), close relatives who have had bilateral breast cancer, close male relatives (father, brothers, uncles, grandfathers, sons) who have had breast cancer, and/or if the woman is of Ashkenazi Jewish ancestry, a hereditary predisposition to breast cancer might be suspected [13]. Even in women who have one or more of these risk factors, however, the likelihood of a *BRCA1* or *BRCA2* mutation is quite low [14].

The *BRCA1* and *BRCA2* genes were cloned in 1994 and 1995, respectively, and genetic testing for breast cancer susceptibility was adopted widely soon afterwards [15,16]. Numerous mutations now have been identified in each of these genes, and different mutations within the same gene are associated with different risks for breast and ovarian cancer [12]. Among women who have *BRCA1* and *BRCA2* mutations, the lifetime risk of breast cancer is 36% to 85%, and the lifetime risk of ovarian cancer is 16% to 60% [17,18]. These risk estimates, however, were derived from large families with many affected members. Although family members share mutations in the *BRCA* genes, they share other genes as well and often live in a similar environment. Thus, these risk estimates partly reflect the impact of other genetic or environmental factors and may not indicate the risk of breast and ovarian cancer among mutation carriers in the general population. Also, risk estimates often were derived from families outside the United States. Chen and colleagues [19] recently have estimated that, in the United States population, the cumulative breast cancer risk by age 70 years for *BRCA1* and *BRCA2* mutation carriers is 46% and 43%, respectively, and the cumulative risk for ovarian cancer is 39% and 22% [19]. These estimates point out that many women who have *BRCA* mutations never develop breast or ovarian cancer.

Alterations in the *BRCA1* or *BRCA2* genes are more common in certain ethnic and geographic populations (eg, Ashkenazi Jewish, Norwegian, Dutch, Icelandic), and specific mutations (founder mutations) often are clustered in particular ethnic groups [20]. For example, alterations in the *BRCA1* or *BRCA2* gene occur in approximately 2.5% of individuals of Ashkenazi Jewish decent, and three specific mutations (two in the *BRCA1* gene and one in the *BRCA2* gene) are ubiquitous in these individuals [21]. The three founder mutations frequently observed in persons of Ashkenazi Jewish heritage are 185delAG (*BRCA1*), 5383insC (*BRCA1*), and 617delT (*BRCA2*). The risk of breast cancer is similar in carriers of the two founder *BRCA1* gene mutations (approximately 65%) but is lower in carriers of the founder *BRCA2* mutation (43%) [22]. Individuals of Ashkenazi Jewish heritage should be tested for all three founder mutations, because two or more may coexist in the same family.

Clearly, women who have BRCA mutations have a markedly increased risk of developing breast and ovarian cancer at an early age. Men who have *BRCA1* or *BRCA2* mutations (particularly *BRCA2*) also are at increased risk for breast cancer, although that risk is considerably lower than it is in women. Recently, it was estimated that the cumulative risk, by age 70 years, of breast cancer is about 1.2% for male *BRCA1* mutation carriers and about 6.8% for male *BRCA2* mutation carriers [23]. Carriers of the *BRCA1* and *BRCA2* mutations also are at increased risk for other cancers, notably cancers of the prostate and pancreas [24]. Women who have a strong family history for breast cancer may consider genetic testing, particularly if they wish to pursue strategies to lower their risk.

Genetic testing

Many organizations, including the US Preventive Services Task Force (USPTF) and the American Society of Clinical Oncology, recommend against genetic testing in women who have a low risk for the *BRCA* mutation [25,26]. In low-risk individuals, the potential risks of genetic testing outweigh the benefits. For instance, in a woman without a family history of breast cancer, how might one interpret an alteration in the *BRCA* gene that never has been strongly linked to cancer? Such an alteration might be less pathogenic than other mutations or even phenotypically silent. Thus, indiscriminate genetic testing may produce needless anxiety and lead to unnecessary prophylactic surgery or other treatments. Women might be labeled falsely as having a genetic predisposition to breast cancer, with adverse ethical, legal, financial, and social consequences.

Over the years, a number of empiric models were developed to estimate a woman's risk of developing breast cancer (eg, the Gail, Claus, Tyrer-Cuzick, and BRCAPRO models) [6]. There now are models that specifically estimate the likelihood for deleterious *BRCA* mutations (eg, the Myriad Genetic Laboratories, Couch, BRCAPRO, and Tyrer models) [6,13]. These models incorporate information about personal or family history of breast and ovarian cancer as well as Ashkenazi Jewish background [27]. If a woman has a 10% or greater probability of carrying a *BRCA1* or *BRCA2* gene mutation, genetic testing should be considered [28]. Informed consent should be obtained before genetic testing, and the potential risks and benefits should be discussed in detail. Women should understand that the *BRCA* test is "predictive" rather than "diagnostic" [29]. Diagnostic tests confirm the diagnosis of a particular condition (eg, an extra chromosome 21 in an infant confirms the diagnosis of Down's syndrome), whereas predictive tests reveal the likelihood of developing a particular disease (in this case, breast cancer) but do not confirm that an individual will develop the disease.

The first person tested for the *BRCA* mutation should be a family member most likely to test positive, generally an individual who has developed breast cancer at a young age or an individual who has ovarian cancer [27]. If a mutation is found in that family member, other members of the family should be tested for the same mutation. In a family in which a *BRCA1* or *BRCA2* mutation has been identified, individuals who do not carry the mutation are not at increased risk for breast or ovarian cancer. At worst, their risk is similar to that of the overall population, but it might be even less, because risk estimates of the overall population include women who carry the *BRCA1* and *BRCA2* mutations.

If a *BRCA* mutation is not found in a family member who has breast or ovarian cancer, the test is not informative and does not provide useful information to other family members. In such instances, the cluster of breast cancer cases within a family might be attributable to mutations other than those in the *BRCA1* or *BRCA2* genes or to environmental or lifestyle factors. If no family members who have cancer are alive or available for testing, the options for testing should be weighed and considered on an individual basis.

Management options for mutation carriers

To reduce cancer-related mortality, women who have *BRCA1* or *BRCA2* mutations may wish to consider screening, chemoprevention, or prophylactic surgery (Fig. 1). The impact of these interventions on cancer-related mortality is not understood fully, however, because no randomized, prospective trials have addressed their impact specifically in mutation carriers. The results of clinical trials indicate that breast cancer screening is beneficial in the overall population and that chemoprevention is useful in high-risk populations. Additionally, the results of retrospective and nonrandomized prospective studies indicate that these risk-reducing strategies benefit mutation carriers.

Screening

There always has been a widespread belief that the early detection of cancer is beneficial. For individuals at high risk for developing cancer, intensive cancer screening often is recommended, even if proper evidence to support such a recommendation is lacking. For example, it long was assumed that screening with sputum cytology and/or chest radiographs would reduce lung cancer mortality among smokers. Eventually, the results of four randomized, controlled trials proved this assumption wrong [30]. This example

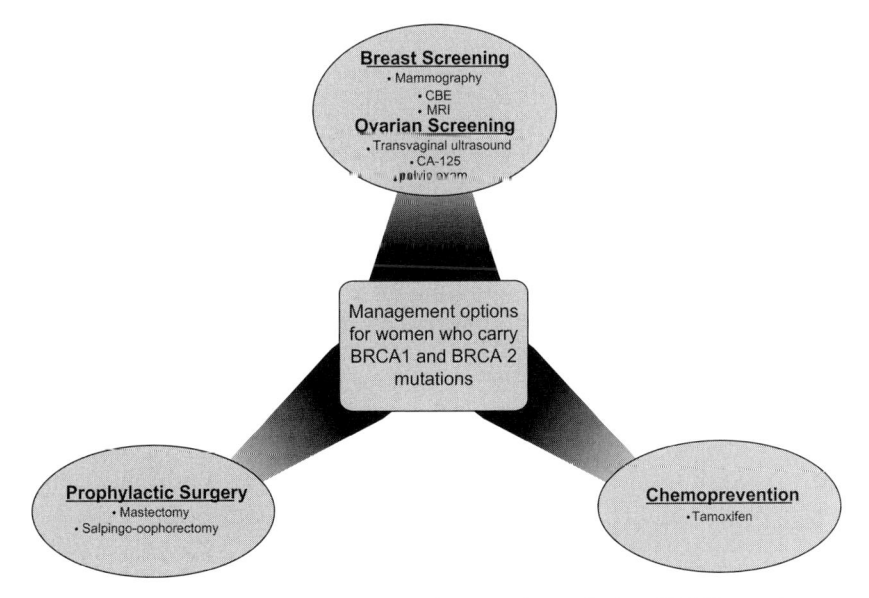

Fig. 1. Management options for women who carry the *BRCA1* or *BRCA2* mutations.

illustrates why the impact of screening on cancer-related mortality should be ascertained through large, randomized, prospective trials whenever feasible. Such trials, however, probably are not feasible in women who have a genetic predisposition for breast cancer, so screening recommendations in these women often are based on the results of randomized, controlled trials undertaken in the general population. Although other types of studies (eg, retrospective and case-control control) have been used to assess the efficacy of screening, those studies have limitations, particularly in lead time, length, and selection biases [30,31].

"Survival" refers to the interval of time from diagnosis of cancer to death, and "lead-time bias" refers to the interval between the diagnosis of cancer by screening and usual clinical detection [30,31]. As a result of "lead-time bias," one might conclude that screening improves survival, when in fact it simply extends the period of time over which the cancer is observed. The only way to exclude the effect of lead-time bias is to test the efficacy of screening in a randomized, controlled trial, with mortality as the end point. Thus, even though screening may result in the early detection of cancer, early detection alone never should justify its use. It is necessary to conduct randomized, controlled trials to prove that a particular screening modality reduces mortality.

In addition to "lead-time bias," retrospective studies are subject to length bias and selection biases [30,31]. "Length bias" refers to the fact that slower-growing cancers exist in the preclinical phase for a longer period of time and therefore are more likely to be detected by screening. In contrast, faster-growing tumors exist for a shorter period of time in the preclinical phase and are more likely to be detected clinically in the intervals between screening sessions. Retrospective comparisons of screen-detected and clinically detected cancers might reveal that screen-detected cancers have better outcomes, but this finding could reflect, in part, the more indolent biology of the screen-detected cancers. Thus, length bias reflects the differences in tumor biology between the screen-detected and clinically detected cancers. There also are differences in the characteristics of women who volunteer for screening and those who do not; these differences result in selection bias. Women who volunteer for cancer screening generally are more health conscious (eg, eat nutritional foods, exercise regularly) than those who decline screening. As a result, women who volunteer for screening may have better outcomes after a cancer diagnosis, and these outcomes might be attributable in part to their lifestyle.

The only way to exclude lead-time, length, and selection biases is to conduct randomized, prospective trials with mortality as the end point. For breast cancer, five screening modalities commonly are considered: mammography, ultrasound, MRI, clinical breast examination (CBE), and breast self-examination (BSE) (screening CBE differs from screening BSE in that it requires the use of trained personnel) [30–32]. Nine randomized, prospective trials have assessed the impact of mammography screening (with or without

CBE) on breast cancer mortality in the general population: the Health Insurance Plan (HIP) of New York, Malmo, Two-County, Stockholm, Gothenburg, Edinburgh, Canadian National Breast Screening Study I (CNBSS I), Canadian National Breast Screening Study II (CNBSS II), and Age Trials [30,31,33]. Currently, a trial is underway in India to assess the impact of screening CBE alone in the general population [31]. Additionally, two trials, conducted in St. Petersburg, Russia, and in Shanghai, China, have assessed the impact of screening BSE on breast cancer mortality in the general population [34,35]. To date, no randomized, prospective trials have assessed the impact of ultrasound or MRI screening on breast cancer mortality. At least six nonrandomized prospective studies have shown that in high-risk patients MRI is more sensitive than mammography [36], but no randomized, prospective trials have assessed the impact of any of these screening modalities specifically in mutation carriers.

Several overviews (meta-analyses) of the mammography screening trials have been published [37,38]. These meta-analyses indicate that, in the general population, the impact of screening differs in younger and older women. For women who are over the age of 50 years at the start of these trials, a significant 20% to 25% reduction in breast cancer mortality is attributable to screening, evident after 7 to 9 years of follow-up. In contrast, for women below age 50 years at the start of these trials, the benefit of mammography screening emerges gradually, with a significant reduction in mortality (about 18%) appearing after 12 or more years of follow-up. These meta-analyses did not include the results of the Age trial, the most recent randomized clinical trial to examine the efficacy of screening mammography in women aged 40 to 49 years [33]. This trial showed that breast cancer deaths in the screened group were decreased, but that decrease did not reach statistical significance (relative risk, 0.83; 95% confidence interval [CI], 0.66–1.04).

Although mammography screening seems to be efficacious in the general population, its impact on mutation carriers is not known. Some investigators have suggested that, because the *BRCA1* and *BRCA2* genes code for proteins involved in DNA repair, low-dose radiation from mammography might be particularly detrimental in mutation carriers, potentially increasing their risk for breast cancer [39]. Additional data are needed to determine if this concern is valid, but recent studies seem to indicate that it is not [40,41].

To date, no randomized, controlled trials have compared CBE screening alone with no screening, although four of the nine mammography screening trials (HIP, Edinburgh, CNBSS I, CNBSS II) also included CBE as a screening modality [31]. The results of these four trials suggest that screening CBE can detect cancers effectively, and Barton and colleagues [42] estimate that screening CBE has a sensitivity of approximately 54% and a specificity of about 94%. Additionally, two randomized, controlled trials have examined the effect of screening BSE alone on breast cancer mortality in the general population [34,35]. The first of these trials conducted by the World Health Organization recruited women between the years 1985 and 1989 in

St. Petersburg, Russia. The other was initiated between the years 1989 and 1991 in Shanghai, China. In the control and study arms of these trials, breast cancer detection and mortality rates were nearly identical, but the number of breast biopsies performed was nearly twofold higher in the screened group. Thus, false-positive results are common with BSE screening and may lead to unnecessary biopsies.

At least six prospective, nonrandomized studies have evaluated annual MRI screening (in conjunction with mammography) in women at increased risk for developing breast cancer (Fig. 2) [36]. These studies were conducted in the United States, the Netherlands, Canada, the United Kingdom, Germany, and Italy, and participants either were documented *BRCA1* or *BRCA2* mutation carriers or had a very strong family history of breast cancer. In some of these studies, ultrasound and/or CBE also were used as screening modalities. The sensitivity of MRI ranged from 77% to 100%, whereas the sensitivity of mammography or ultrasound was only 16% to 40%. There are, however, no data from randomized prospective trials to indicate whether the improved detection rates associated with MRI screening translate to a reduction in breast cancer mortality. Although MRI is more sensitive than mammography, its specificity is lower. Kriege and colleagues [43] found that the specificity of MRI was 88%, compared with 95% for mammography. The lower specificity of MRI leads to higher recall and false-positive rates. The danger of false-positive screening results is unnecessary biopsies.

As mentioned earlier, evidence concerning the efficacy of breast cancer screening is derived from trials undertaken in the general population. To date, no randomized clinical trials have been designed to assess the benefit

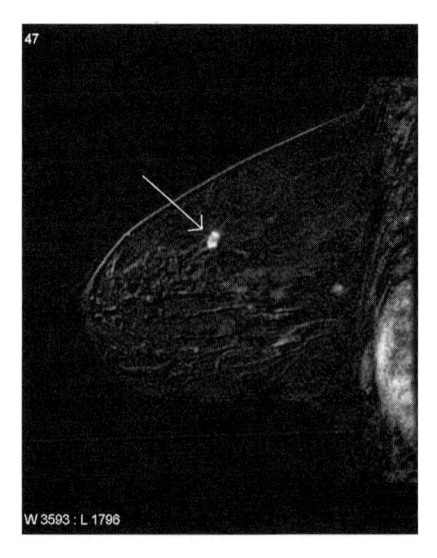

Fig. 2. Breast cancer (*arrow*) detected on screening MRI.

of these screening modalities in mutation carriers. Nonetheless, several organizations have published screening guidelines for women who have a hereditary predisposition for breast cancer. The National Comprehensive Cancer Network recommends monthly BSE starting at age 18 years, CBE every 6 months starting at age 25 years, annual mammography starting at age 25 years, and annual breast MRI starting at age 25 years [6]. The American Cancer Society recommends annual BSE and annual breast MRI [44], beginning at age 30 years and continuing for as long as a woman is in good health. The USPTF, however, maintains that there is insufficient evidence at the present time to recommend for or against breast cancer screening in mutation carriers [26]. Given the uncertainty surrounding the efficacy of breast cancer screening among mutation carriers, it seems prudent to discuss its potential for benefit and harm with each patient.

BRCA mutation carriers also are at considerable risk for developing ovarian cancer. As yet, no data from randomized clinical trials (either in the general population or in high-risk women) indicate whether ovarian cancer screening reduces cancer-related mortality. Furthermore, there are no reliable methods for detecting ovarian cancer early. Nonetheless, a number of screening tests have been investigated for potential use, particularly the serum marker CA-125 and transvaginal ultrasound [45]. CA-125 is a protein produced by more than 90% of advanced epithelial ovarian cancers. Transvaginal ultrasound is the most promising imaging method for the early detection of ovarian cancer. Combining transvaginal ultrasound and CA-125 results in a higher sensitivity for ovarian cancer detection than either method alone but increases false-positive rates. Although *BRCA* mutation carriers generally have been urged to undergo screening with transvaginal ultrasound and CA-125, a recent study suggests that this screening may not detect tumors at a sufficiently early stage to influence prognosis [46].

Prophylactic surgery

To reduce cancer risk, *BRCA1* and *BRCA2* mutation carriers may wish to consider prophylactic surgery. These patients are at increased risk both for breast and ovarian tumors and for tumors arising from the fallopian tubes [47]. Thus, *BRCA* mutation carriers should consider prophylactic mastectomy and prophylactic salpingo-oophorectomy (rather than oophorectomy alone). Patients concerned about the potential impact of prophylactic mastectomy on body image may elect to undergo salpingo-oophorectomy alone because it is a "hidden" procedure and may reduce the risk of both ovarian and breast cancer risk. These patients generally opt for continued surveillance of the breasts. Alternatively, nulliparous women may consider prophylactic mastectomy initially and delay salpingo-oophorectomy until after childbearing. Again, no randomized, prospective trials have assessed the impact of these procedures, although the results of several retrospective studies indicate that they dramatically reduce cancer risk. Patients should be made aware that these procedures do not eliminate cancer risk entirely.

Hartmann and colleagues [48] conducted a retrospective analysis of women who had a family history of breast cancer and who underwent prophylactic mastectomy at the Mayo Clinic between 1960 and 1993. To estimate the number of breast cancers expected in the absence of prophylactic mastectomy, the authors applied the Gail model for women at moderate risk. For women at high risk, the authors compared those who underwent prophylactic mastectomy with their sisters who did not. In this study, prophylactic mastectomy reduced the incidence of breast cancer by 90%, and other studies have shown similar results [49–51].

Three procedures are used commonly for prophylactic mastectomy: total, skin-sparing, and subcutaneous (nipple-sparing) mastectomy (Table 1) [47]. Total mastectomy involves removal of the breast tissue, nipple, areola, and much of the skin overlying the breast. In contrast, skin-sparing mastectomy involves removal of the breast tissue, nipple, and areola, but preserves skin overlying the breast. Skin-sparing mastectomy facilitates breast reconstruction and results in a better cosmetic outcome than total mastectomy [52]. The reduction in breast cancer risk seems to be similar for total mastectomy and skin-sparing mastectomy. Subcutaneous mastectomy, which involves removal of the breast tissue but leaves the nipple and areola intact, seems to be less effective [47].

Breast reconstruction usually is undertaken at the time of prophylactic mastectomy. Reconstruction is feasible with either prostheses alone or autogenous tissue (with or without prostheses) [53]. If a patient opts for prosthesis alone, the prosthesis generally is placed below the pectoralis major muscle at the time of mastectomy. Alternatively, an expander can be placed and inflated gradually over a period of several weeks by injecting solution through a port. This process creates a ptosis, and the injectable port and expander subsequently are removed and replaced with a permanent prosthesis. In some instances, the expander is left in place as the permanent prosthesis. If the patient chooses reconstruction with autogenous tissue, then either a latissimus dorsi flap or the transverse rectus abdominis muscle (TRAM) flap might be considered [54]. The latissimus dorsi flap does not provide sufficient tissue bulk, and a prosthesis usually is placed beneath the flap. The

Table 1
Types of prophylactic mastectomy

Procedure	Description of procedure	Recommendation
Skin-sparing mastectomy	Removal of breast, nipple, areola	Preferred
Total mastectomy	Removal of breast, nipple, areola, and skin overlying breast	Acceptable
Subcutaneous mastectomy	Removal of breast; preserves nipple and areola	Not recommended

TRAM flap provides considerable tissue bulk, and a prosthesis usually is not required. Although it might result in an aesthetically more appealing outcome, the TRAM procedure is technically more challenging and carries a greater risk of complications.

Among *BRCA* mutation carriers, the risk of ovarian cancer is considerably less than that of breast cancer. There are, however, no reliable means of detecting ovarian cancer early, and it is more lethal than breast cancer. Thus, mutation carriers often are urged to undergo bilateral salpingo-oophorectomy after completion of childbearing. Kauff and colleagues [55] and Rebbeck and colleagues [28] reported that prophylactic surgery (either salpingo-oophorectomy or oophorectomy) reduces the risk of ovarian cancer by about 90% in mutation carriers. Additionally, premenopausal oophorectomy in mutation carriers was associated with about a 50% reduction in breast cancer risk [28,55]. After removal of the ovaries, *BRCA* mutation carriers still are at small risk for developing papillary serous carcinoma of the peritoneum, so continued surveillance is warranted.

Chemoprevention

Tamoxifen is a selective estrogen-receptor modulator widely used in the treatment of estrogen receptor–positive breast cancers [56]. More than 20 years ago, Cuzick and Baum [57] reviewed the results of women who received tamoxifen following surgery for breast cancer and found that it reduced the risk of contralateral breast cancer. This observation led to the hypothesis that tamoxifen could prevent breast cancer, and four randomized, prospective trials were initiated to test this hypothesis. These trials were the Royal Marsden trial [58], the National Surgical Adjuvant Breast and Bowel Project (NSABP) P-1 trial [59], the Italian trial [60], and the International Breast Intervention Study-1 trial [61], all of which assigned women randomly to receive either tamoxifen (20 mg daily) or placebo for at least 5 years. An overview of these trials showed that the administration of tamoxifen reduced the risk of invasive breast cancer by about 38% (95% CI, 28%–46%; $P < .0001$) [62]. Tamoxifen now is approved as a chemopreventive agent for women at high risk for breast cancer.

No randomized, prospective trial has tested the impact of tamoxifen specifically in *BRCA* mutation carriers, although each of the four trials mentioned earlier undoubtedly included women who had *BRCA* mutations. A subgroup analysis of the NSABP P-1 trial failed to show a significant benefit of tamoxifen in preventing breast cancers in *BRCA* mutation carriers, but such a benefit could not be excluded completely [63]. A case-control study, however, did find that tamoxifen was effective in preventing breast cancer in *BRCA* mutation carriers. In that study, Narod and colleagues [64] compared *BRCA* mutation carriers who had bilateral breast cancer with those who had unilateral disease. Women were interviewed or given a self-administered questionnaire to ascertain whether they had been treated with tamoxifen after surgery for their first breast cancer. In these mutation carriers the multivariate odds ratio for contralateral breast cancer associated with tamoxifen use was 0.50 (95% CI, 0.28–0.89). Tamoxifen was associated with a lower risk of contralateral breast cancer in *BRCA1* mutation carriers (odds ratio, 0.38; 95% CI, 0.19–0.74) than in *BRCA2* mutation carriers (odds ratio, 0.63; 95% CI, 0.20–1.50), even though *BRCA1* mutation carriers are more likely to develop estrogen receptor–negative tumors (83% of the breast cancers developing in *BRCA1* mutation carriers and 14% of those in *BRCA2* mutation carriers are estrogen receptor–negative).

The differential response rates among *BRCA* mutation carriers in the NSABP P-1 trial [59] and in the case-control study of Narod and colleagues [64] might be related to the timing of chemoprevention. Sixty percent of the P-1 participants were 50 years old or older, whereas nearly 90% of the case-control participants were younger than 50 years. Given that premenopausal oophorectomy is effective in preventing *BRCA1* tumors [65], tamoxifen also possibly should be administered before menopause.

Tamoxifen increases the risk of endometrial cancer and thromboembolism by twofold or more [66]. Raloxifene is a selective estrogen modulator that seems to have a better safety profile (lower risk of uterine cancer and thromboembolism) than tamoxifen [67]. A large, randomized, prospective trial compared the impact of tamoxifen and raloxifene in lowering the risk of breast cancer in postmenopausal women and found that the two were equally efficacious [67]. Much less is known about the potential impact of raloxifene in reducing breast cancer risk in *BRCA* mutation carriers, however.

Thus, women who carry the BRCA mutations have three major options to consider, with significant trade-offs. Screening is the most commonly used option but frequently is associated with false-positive results that produce needless anxiety. Additionally, cancers missed on screening (false-negative results) might affect outcome adversely. Although prophylactic surgery may reduce the risk of breast and ovarian cancer by 90%, mastectomy may affect a woman's perception of her body image, and oophorectomy prevents childbearing. Even though chemoprevention may reduce the risk of breast cancer by as much as 50%, it increases the risk of endometrial cancer and venous thromboembolism by more than twofold. Clinicians should discuss the potential risks and benefits of these options with *BRCA* mutation carriers. Finally, the timing of intervention may be important, but this issue is not well defined and could differ for *BRCA1* and *BRCA2* carriers [68]. Ultimately, the best choice is the one made by a fully informed patient.

Breast cancer treatment

If a *BRCA* mutation carrier develops breast cancer, options for local therapy should be weighed carefully. Radiotherapy can be administered safely after breast-conserving surgery in *BRCA* mutation carriers, although these patients are at increased risk for developing second primary cancers (particularly contralateral breast cancers) [69]. Pierce and colleagues [70] followed 160 mutation carriers and 445 matched controls diagnosed with breast cancer following breast-conserving surgery. Mutation carriers who had not undergone oophorectomy had an increased risk of ipsilateral breast tumor recurrence; those who had undergone oophorectomy did not. Many women who have *BRCA* mutations opt for bilateral mastectomy, however. A recent study of women who had *BRCA1* or *BRCA2* mutations who had been diagnosed with unilateral breast cancer found that bilateral mastectomy was accepted more widely in North America than in Europe [71]. In the United States, nearly half of all *BRCA* mutation carriers opted for bilateral mastectomy. At the time of mastectomy, a sentinel biopsy generally should be performed in the axilla on the side affected by breast cancer. If the sentinel node contains metastatic disease, a complete axillary dissection is indicated. Patients who have significant involvement of the axillary lymph nodes (generally with four or more lymph nodes containing metastatic disease) should consider postmastectomy radiotherapy [72].

For *BRCA* mutation carriers who are diagnosed with breast cancer, the choice of systemic therapy is determined by standard prognostic and predictive factors [69]. There are no treatments specifically tailored for patients who have *BRCA* mutations. Decisions concerning systemic therapy are based both on nodal status and tumor size and, more importantly, on estrogen receptor status and *HER-2* status of the tumor. Thus, *BRCA* mutation carriers who are diagnosed with breast cancer should receive the same systemic treatments as patients who have sporadic breast cancer, based on standard prognostic and predictive factors.

Summary

Genetic testing now makes it possible to identify women who have a greatly increased risk for developing breast cancer. Not all women who have a family history of breast cancer are appropriate candidates for genetic testing, however. Women must be informed about the potential risks and benefits of genetic testing, and those who are found to carry mutations in the *BRCA1* or *BRCA2* genes should be advised of all management options. Three strategies commonly are employed to manage *BRCA* mutation carriers: screening, prophylactic surgery, and chemoprevention. No randomized prospective trials have addressed the impact of these interventions in mutation carriers, however, and their potential risks and benefits should be discussed with each patient. Ultimately, many patients may elect more than one option (eg, screening initially and then prophylactic surgery after completing childbearing). Thus, physicians who manage patients who have *BRCA* mutations should be prepared to follow these patients over a span of many years.

References

[1] Jemal A, Siegel R, Ward E, et al. Cancer statistics, 2008. CA Cancer J Clin 2008;58(2):71–96.
[2] Hankinson SE, Colditz GA, Willett WC. Towards an integrated model for breast cancer etiology: the lifelong interplay of genes, lifestyle, and hormones. Breast Cancer Res 2004; 6(5):213–8.
[3] van de Vijver MJ. The pathology of familial breast cancer: the pre-BRCA1/BRCA2 era: historical perspectives. Breast Cancer Res 1999;1(1):27–30.
[4] Anderson K, et al. Cost-effectiveness of preventive strategies for women with a BRCA1 or a BRCA2 mutation. Ann Intern Med 2006;144(6):397–406.
[5] Thull DL, Vogel VG. Recognition and management of hereditary breast cancer syndromes. Oncologist 2004;9(1):13–24.
[6] Robson M, Offit K. Clinical practice. Management of an inherited predisposition to breast cancer. N Engl J Med 2007;357(2):154–62.
[7] Emery J, Lucassen A, Murphy M. Common hereditary cancers and implications for primary care. Lancet 2001;358(9275):56–63.
[8] Rubinstein WS. Surgical management of BRCA1 and BRCA2 carriers: bitter choices slightly sweetened. J Clin Oncol 2005;23(31):7772–4.
[9] Wooster R, Neuhausen SL, Mangion J, et al. Localization of a breast cancer susceptibility gene, BRCA2, to chromosome 13q12-13. Science 1994;265(5181):2088–90.
[10] Hall JM, Lee MK, Newman B. Linkage of early-onset familial breast cancer to chromosome 17q21. Science 1990;250(4988):1684–9.
[11] Narod SA, Foulkes WD. BRCA1 and BRCA2: 1994 and beyond. Nat Rev Cancer 2004;4(9): 665–76.
[12] Iau PT, Macmillan RD, Blamey RW. Germ line mutations associated with breast cancer susceptibility. Eur J Cancer 2001;37(3):300–21.
[13] U.S. Protective Services Task Force. Genetic risk assessment and BRCA mutation testing for breast and ovarian cancer susceptibility: recommendation statement. Ann Intern Med 2005;143(5):355–61.
[14] Frank TS, Deffenbaugh AM, Reid JE, et al. Clinical characteristics of individuals with germ-line mutations in BRCA1 and BRCA2: analysis of 10,000 individuals. J Clin Oncol 2002; 20(6):1480–90.
[15] Miki Y, Swensen J, Shattuck-Eidens D, et al. A strong candidate for the breast and ovarian cancer susceptibility gene BRCA1. Science 1994;266(5182):66–71.
[16] Wooster R, Bignell G, Lancaster J, et al. Identification of the breast cancer susceptibility gene BRCA2. Nature 1995;378(6559):789–92.
[17] Chen S, Parmigiani G. Meta-analysis of BRCA1 and BRCA2 penetrance. J Clin Oncol 2007; 25(11):1329–33.
[18] Levy-Lahad E, Friedman E. Cancer risks among BRCA1 and BRCA2 mutation carriers. Br J Cancer 2007;96(1):11–5.
[19] Chen S, Iversen ES, Friebel T, et al. Characterization of BRCA1 and BRCA2 mutations in a large United States sample. J Clin Oncol 2006;24(6):863–71.
[20] Ferla R, Calo Y, Cascio S, et al. Founder mutations in BRCA1 and BRCA2 genes. Ann Oncol 2007;18(Suppl 6):vi93–8.
[21] Narod SA, Offit K. Prevention and management of hereditary breast cancer. J Clin Oncol 2005;23(8):1656–63.
[22] Antoniou AC, Pharoah PD, Narod S, et al. Breast and ovarian cancer risks to carriers of the BRCA1 5382insC and 185delAG and BRCA2 6174delT mutations: a combined analysis of 22 population based studies. J Med Genet 2005;42(7):602–3.
[23] Tai YC, Domchek S, Parmigiani G, et al. Breast cancer risk among male BRCA1 and BRCA2 mutation carriers. J Natl Cancer Inst 2007;99(23):1811–4.
[24] Garber JE, Offit K. Hereditary cancer predisposition syndromes. J Clin Oncol 2005;23(2): 276–92.

[25] American Society of Clinical Oncology. Policy statement update: genetic testing for cancer susceptibility. J Clin Oncol 2003;21(12):2397–406.
[26] Nelson HD, Huffman LH, Fu R, et al. Genetic risk assessment and BRCA mutation testing for breast and ovarian cancer susceptibility: systematic evidence review for the U.S. Preventive Services Task Force. Ann Intern Med 2005;143(5):362–79.
[27] Berliner JL, Fay AM. Risk assessment and genetic counseling for hereditary breast and ovarian cancer: recommendations of the National Society of Genetic Counselors. J Genet Couns 2007;16(3):241–60.
[28] Rebbeck TR, Lynch HT, Neuhausen SL, et al. Prophylactic oophorectomy in carriers of BRCA1 or BRCA2 mutations. N Engl J Med 2002;346(21):1616–22.
[29] Taylor MR. Genetic testing for inherited breast and ovarian cancer syndromes: important concepts for the primary care physician. Postgrad Med J 2001;77(903):11–5.
[30] Jatoi I, Anderson WF. Cancer screening. Curr Probl Surg 2005;42(9):620–82.
[31] Jatoi I. Breast cancer screening. Am J Surg 1999;177(6):518–24.
[32] Jatoi I. Screening clinical breast examination. Surg Clin North Am 2003;83(4):789–801.
[33] Moss SM, Cuckle H, Evans A, et al. Effect of mammographic screening from age 40 years on breast cancer mortality at 10 years' follow-up: a randomised controlled trial. Lancet 2006; 368(9552):2053–60.
[34] Semiglazov VF, Moisenko VM, Manikhas AG, et al. Interim results of a prospective randomized study of self-examination for early detection of breast cancer (Russia/St.Petersburg/WHO)). Vopr Onkol 1999;45(3):265–71 [in Russian].
[35] Thomas DB, Gao DL, Ray RM, et al. Randomized trial of breast self-examination in Shanghai: final results. J Natl Cancer Inst 2002;94(19):1445–57.
[36] Liberman L. Breast cancer screening with MRI—what are the data for patients at high risk? N Engl J Med 2004;351(5):497–500.
[37] Hendrick RE, Smith RA, Rutledge JH 3rd, et al. Benefit of screening mammography in women aged 40–49: a new meta-analysis of randomized controlled trials. J Natl Cancer Inst Monogr 1997;22:87–92.
[38] Kerlikowske K, Grady D, Rubin SM, et al. Efficacy of screening mammography. A meta-analysis. JAMA 1995;273(2):149–54.
[39] Vaidya JS, Baum M. Benefits and risks of screening mammography in women with BRCA1 and BRCA2 mutations. JAMA 1997;278(4):290.
[40] Narod SA, Lubinski J, Ghadirian P, et al. Screening mammography and risk of breast cancer in BRCA1 and BRCA2 mutation carriers: a case-control study. Lancet Oncol 2006;7(5): 402–6.
[41] Goldfrank D, Chuai S, Bernstein JL, et al. Effect of mammography on breast cancer risk in women with mutations in BRCA1 or BRCA2. Cancer Epidemiol Biomarkers Prev 2006; 15(11):2311–3.
[42] Barton MB, Harris R, Fletcher SW. The rational clinical examination. Does this patient have breast cancer? The screening clinical breast examination: should it be done? How? JAMA 1999;282(13):1270–80.
[43] Kriege M, Brekelmans CT, Boetes C, et al. Efficacy of MRI and mammography for breast-cancer screening in women with a familial or genetic predisposition. N Engl J Med 2004; 351(5):427–37.
[44] Saslow D, Boetes C, Burke W, et al. American Cancer Society guidelines for breast screening with MRI as an adjunct to mammography. CA Cancer J Clin 2007;57(2):75–89.
[45] Anderiesz C, Quinn MA. Screening for ovarian cancer. Med J Aust 2003;178(12):655–6.
[46] Stirling D, Evans DG, Pichert G, et al. Screening for familial ovarian cancer: failure of current protocols to detect ovarian cancer at an early stage according to the international Federation of gynecology and obstetrics system. J Clin Oncol 2005;23(24): 5588–96.
[47] Guillem JG, Wood WC, Moley JF, et al. ASCO/SSO review of current role of risk-reducing surgery in common hereditary cancer syndromes. J Clin Oncol 2006;24(28):4642–60.

[48] Hartmann LC, Schaid DJ, Woods JE, et al. Efficacy of bilateral prophylactic mastectomy in women with a family history of breast cancer. N Engl J Med 1999;340(2):77–84.
[49] Meijers-Heijboer H, van Geel B, van Putten WL, et al. Breast cancer after prophylactic bilateral mastectomy in women with a BRCA1 or BRCA2 mutation. N Engl J Med 2001; 345(3):159–64.
[50] Rebbeck TR, Friebel T, Lynch HT, et al. Bilateral prophylactic mastectomy reduces breast cancer risk in BRCA1 and BRCA2 mutation carriers: the PROSE Study Group. J Clin Oncol 2004;22(6):1055–62.
[51] Hartmann LC, Sellars TA, Schaid DJ, et al. Efficacy of bilateral prophylactic mastectomy in BRCA1 and BRCA2 gene mutation carriers. J Natl Cancer Inst 2001;93(21):1633–7.
[52] Ueda S, Tamaki Y, Yano K, et al. Cosmetic outcome and patient satisfaction after skin-sparing mastectomy for breast cancer with immediate reconstruction of the breast. Surgery 2008;143(3):414–25.
[53] Carlson GW. Breast reconstruction. Surgical options and patient selection. Cancer 1994; 74(Suppl 1):436–9.
[54] Bostwick J III, Carlson GW. Reconstruction of the breast. Surg Oncol Clin N Am 1997;6(1): 71–89.
[55] Kauff ND, Satagopan JM, Robson ME, et al. Risk-reducing salpingo-oophorectomy in women with a BRCA1 or BRCA2 mutation. N Engl J Med 2002;346(21):1609–15.
[56] Baum M, Brinkley DM, Dossett JA, et al. Improved survival among patients treated with adjuvant tamoxifen after mastectomy for early breast cancer. Lancet 1983;2(8347):450.
[57] Cuzick J, Baum M. Tamoxifen and contralateral breast cancer. Lancet 1985;2(8449):282.
[58] Powles TJ, Jones AL, Ashley JE, et al. The Royal Marsden Hospital pilot tamoxifen chemoprevention trial. Breast Cancer Res Treat 1994;31(1):73–82.
[59] Fisher B, Jones AL, Ashley JE, et al. Tamoxifen for prevention of breast cancer: report of the National Surgical Adjuvant Breast and Bowel Project P-1 Study. J Natl Cancer Inst 1998; 90(18):1371–88.
[60] Veronesi U, Maisonneuve P, Sacchini V, et al. Tamoxifen for breast cancer among hysterectomised women. Lancet 2002;359(9312):1122–4.
[61] Cuzick J, Forbes J, Edwards R, et al. First results from the International Breast Cancer Intervention Study (IBIS-I): a randomised prevention trial. Lancet 2002;360(9336):817–24.
[62] Cuzick J, Powles T, Veronesi U, et al. Overview of the main outcomes in breast-cancer prevention trials. Lancet 2003;361(9354):296–300.
[63] King MC, Wieand S, Hale K, et al. Tamoxifen and breast cancer incidence among women with inherited mutations in BRCA1 and BRCA2: National Surgical Adjuvant Breast and Bowel Project (NSABP-P1) Breast Cancer Prevention Trial. JAMA 2001;286(18):2251–6.
[64] Narod SA, Brunet JS, Ghadirian P, et al. Tamoxifen and risk of contralateral breast cancer in BRCA1 and BRCA2 mutation carriers: a case-control study. Hereditary Breast Cancer Clinical Study Group. Lancet 2000;356(9245):1876–81.
[65] Rebbeck TR, Levin AM, Eisen A, et al. Breast cancer risk after bilateral prophylactic oophorectomy in BRCA1 mutation carriers. J Natl Cancer Inst 1999;91(17):1475–9.
[66] Fisher B, Constantino JP, Wickerhan DL, et al. Tamoxifen for the prevention of breast cancer: current status of the National Surgical Adjuvant Breast and Bowel Project P-1 study. J Natl Cancer Inst 2005;97(22):1652–62.
[67] Vogel VG, Constantino JP, Wickerhan DL, et al. Effects of tamoxifen vs raloxifene on the risk of developing invasive breast cancer and other disease outcomes: the NSABP Study of Tamoxifen and Raloxifene (STAR) P-2 trial. JAMA 2006;295(23):2727–41.
[68] Anderson WF, Brawley OW, Chang S. Oophorectomy in carriers of BRCA mutations. N Engl J Med 2002;347:1037–40.
[69] Domchek SM, Armstrong K, Weber BL. Clinical management of BRCA1 and BRCA2 mutation carriers. Nat Clin Pract Oncol 2006;3(1):2–3.

[70] Pierce LJ, Strawderman M, Narod SA, et al. Effect of radiotherapy after breast-conserving treatment in women with breast cancer and germline BRCA1/2 mutations. J Clin Oncol 2000;18(19):3360–9.
[71] Metcalfe KA, Lubinski J, Ghadirian P, et al. Predictors of contralateral prophylactic mastectomy in women with a BRCA1 or BRCA2 mutation: the Hereditary Breast Cancer Clinical Study Group. J Clin Oncol 2008;26(7):1093–7.
[72] Recht A, Edge SB, Solin LJ, et al. Postmastectomy radiotherapy: clinical practice guidelines of the American Society of Clinical Oncology. J Clin Oncol 2001;19(5):1539–69.

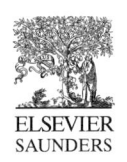

Multiple Endocrine Neoplasia Syndromes

Glenda G. Callender, MD,
Thereasa A. Rich, MS, CGC, Nancy D. Perrier, MD*

Department of Surgical Oncology, The University of Texas M. D. Anderson Cancer Center, 1400 Holcombe Boulevard, Unit 444, Houston, TX, USA

The multiple endocrine neoplasia (MEN) syndromes are rare autosomal-dominant conditions that predispose affected individuals to benign and malignant tumors of the pituitary, thyroid, parathyroids, adrenals, endocrine pancreas, paraganglia, or nonendocrine organs. The classic MEN syndromes include MEN type 1 (MEN1) and MEN type 2 (MEN2). However, several other hereditary conditions should also be considered in the category of MEN: von Hippel-Lindau syndrome (VHL), the familial paraganglioma syndromes, Cowden syndrome, Carney complex, and hyperparathyroidism jaw-tumor syndrome. In addition, there are other familial endocrine neoplasia syndromes with an unknown genetic basis that might also fall into the category of MEN.

The MEN syndromes differ from other hereditary cancer syndromes in that most tumor growth occurs in hormone-secreting glands. This feature has two primary consequences of clinical importance. First, the excess hormone production often results in well-defined hormonal syndromes with characteristic symptoms and medical sequelae. Second, the excess hormone production serves as a sensitive tumor marker that is useful for making a diagnosis, determining response to therapy, and screening asymptomatic patients.

This article reviews the clinical features, diagnosis, and surgical management of the various MEN syndromes and genetic risk assessment for patients presenting with one or more endocrine neoplasms. Table 1 provides an overview of all of the hereditary syndromes discussed in this chapter.

---

* Corresponding author.
  E-mail address: nperrier@mdanderson.org (N.D. Perrier).

Table 1
Overview of endocrine neoplasia syndromes

Syndrome	Mutated gene	Manifestations
MEN1	*MEN1*	Primary hyperparathyroidism (usually four-gland hyperplasia), anterior pituitary adenomas, tumors of endocrine pancreas and duodenum, foregut carcinoids
MEN subtype 2A	*RET* proto-oncogene	Medullary thyroid cancer, pheochromocytoma, primary hyperparathyroidism (usually single adenoma), cutaneous lichen amyloidosis, Hirschsprung disease
MEN subtype 2B	*RET* proto-oncogene	Medullary thyroid cancer, pheochromocytoma, marfanoid body habitus, facial features resulting from mucosal neuromas, ganglioneruomatosis of the gastrointestinal tract
Familial medullary thyroid cancer	*RET* proto-oncogene	Medullary thyroid cancer in at least four family members, with documented absence of other endocrinopathies
Hyperparathyroidism-jaw tumor syndrome	*HRPT2*	Primary hyperparathyroidism (usually single adenoma), ossifying fibromas of maxilla or mandible, renal cysts and hamartomas, 15% risk of parathyroid carcinoma
Familial isolated hyperparathyroidism	*MEN1, HRPT2, CASR*, other	Nonsyndromic primary hyperparathyroidism
Familial hypocalciuric hypercalcemia	*CASR*	Benign hypercalcemia; medical management only
VHL	*VHL*	Pheochromocytoma, retinal and central nervous system hemangioblastoma, renal cysts and clear cell carcinoma, pancreatic cysts and islet cell tumors, endolymphatic sac tumors, papillary cystadenomas of the epididymis and broad ligament
Familial pheochromocytoma/ paraganglioma syndrome	*SDHB, SDHC, SDHD*	Multiple paragangliomas and pheochromocytoma
Neurofibromatosis type I	*NF1*	Pheochromocytoma, characteristic physical features (eg, café-au-lait spots, neurofibromas, axillary and inguinal freckling)

Table 1
(continued)

Syndrome	Mutated gene	Manifestations
Cowden syndrome	PTEN	Nonmedullary thyroid cancer (usually follicular rather than papillary); benign and malignant tumors of skin, oral mucosa, breast, and uterus
Familial adenomatous polyposis	APC	Hundreds of adenomatous colon polyps, colon cancer, cribriform morular variant of papillary thyroid cancer
Carney complex	PRKAR1A	Endocrine tumors (including thyroid, pituitary, primary pigmented nodular adrenocortical disease), characteristic skin pigmentation, myxomas, melanotic schwannomas
Familial nonmedullary thyroid cancer	Unknown	Nonsyndromic nonmedullary thyroid cancer

Multiple endocrine neoplasia type 1

Overview

MEN1 is characterized by tumors in the parathyroid glands, anterior pituitary, endocrine pancreas, and duodenum (see Table 1). However, a wide range of other tumors can occur in MEN1, including foregut carcinoids, adrenocortical adenomas, thyroid nodules, and such nonendocrine tumors as meningiomas, ependymomas, and leiomyomas. Lipomas, facial angiofibromas, and collagenomas are also common and can be useful in visually identifying the MEN1 syndrome in patients with otherwise equivocal features.

MEN1 is an autosomal-dominant condition that occurs as a result of inactivating mutations of the MEN1 gene (*MEN1*), located on chromosome 11q13. *MEN1* has 10 exons (the first exon is noncoding) and produces a 610-amino-acid protein called menin. Although the function of menin is still not fully understood, menin has roles in DNA replication and repair, transcription, and chromatin modification and generally behaves as a tumor suppressor [1]. No genotype-phenotype correlations have been found for MEN1.

The prevalence of MEN1 is estimated to be 1 in 20,000 to 40,000 individuals, with approximately 10% of patients being the first affected person in their family (ie, the index patient) [2,3]. MEN1 is highly variable in terms of the number of organ systems involved and age at onset of tumors and symptoms, both within and between families. Most individuals with MEN1 are diagnosed with their first tumors in late adolescence or early adulthood. However, there are reports of tumor development in children as young as 5 years and diagnosis that is delayed until late in life [4]. The penetrance is estimated to be 80% by age 50 years, although biochemical screening detects tumors in 90% to 95% of patients by this age [5–7].

Risk assessment and surveillance

MEN1 should be considered in patients diagnosed with primary hyperparathyroidism under age 30 years, primary hyperparathyroidism resulting from multigland involvement, familial primary hyperparathyroidism, Zollinger-Ellison syndrome, multifocal pancreatic endocrine tumors, or two or more MEN1-related tumors. A clinical diagnosis of MEN1 is made in patients with tumors in two of the three most commonly affected endocrine organs (parathyroid, pituitary, and pancreatic/duodenal endocrine tumors) and in patients with one such tumor and a family history of MEN1. Of the tumors commonly seen in MEN1, pituitary adenomas are the least predictive for true MEN1 as approximately 10% of adults in the general population have a pituitary abnormality detected on MRI [8,9].

Genetic testing for MEN1 is available through several commercial laboratories and should be offered to patients in whom a diagnosis of MEN1 is being considered. The benefit of offering genetic testing is that a diagnosis of MEN1 at an early age allows patients to be monitored for the development of subsequent MEN1-related tumors. However, the sensitivity of genetic testing varies, depending on the combination of affected organs and whether the patient is an index or familial case, and mutations can be identified in only 75% to 90% of patients with a clinical diagnosis of MEN1. This is important because a negative test result cannot definitively rule out risk for further MEN1-related tumors. Follow-up screening recommendations in such cases are controversial and require careful consideration of the index of suspicion of MEN1 based on the patient's personal and family history.

Routine surveillance of presymptomatic patients and treated patients who are currently without evidence of disease involves a combination of annual biochemical testing for all tumor types and imaging studies (CT or MRI) every 1 to 3 years (Table 2) [10]. Pancreatic endocrine tumors in MEN1 patients may be nonfunctioning. Therefore, screening for these tumors with biochemical tests alone is inadequate. The goal of screening is to detect abnormalities at an early stage when tumors are most easily managed and the long-term effects of hormone hypersecretion can be avoided. The age at which screening should begin for each of the component tumors is controversial. Some advocate beginning screening as early as age 5 years. However, others advocate beginning screening in early adolescence owing to the rarity of life-threatening complications of MEN1 in young children [10]. Appropriate screening of presymptomatic MEN1 patients leads to earlier tumor detection by approximately 10 years [11].

Table 2
MEN1 screening guidelines

Tumor	Age to begin screening	Biochemical tests (annually)	Imaging (every 3 y)
Parathyroid	8 y	Serum calcium, parathyroid hormone	None
Gastrinoma	20 y	Serum gastrin	None
Insulinoma	5 y	Fasting serum glucose, insulin	None
Other enteropancreatic	20 y	Chromogranin A, glucagon, proinsulin	Octreotide scan, CT, or MRI
Anterior pituitary	5 y	Prolactin, insulinlike growth factor–1	Brain MRI
Foregut carcinoid	20 y	None	CT

Data from Brandi ML, Gagel RF, Angeli A, et al. Guidelines for diagnosis and therapy of MEN type 1 and type 2. J Clin Endocrinol Metab 2001; 86(12):5658–71.

Diagnosis and management of component tumors

Parathyroid tumors

Primary hyperparathyroidism resulting from benign four-gland hyperplasia is the most common presentation of parathyroid disease in MEN1 patients. Patients usually present in their early 20s and virtually all MEN1 patients are affected by parathyroid tumors by age 50 years [3]. If symptoms occur, they are similar to those of sporadic hyperparathyroidism: nephrolithiasis, decrease in bone mineral density leading to osteopenia or osteoporosis, fatigue, myopathy, peptic ulcer disease, and neurocognitive deficits, including depression and disordered sleep.

The diagnosis of hyperparathyroidism is confirmed by the presence of an elevated or high-normal serum calcium level in concordance with an inappropriately elevated serum parathyroid hormone level. A 24-hour urine collection documenting no evidence of hypocalciuria (urinary calcium excretion < 100 mg/24 h) should be performed to exclude the possibility of familial hypocalciuric hypercalcemia.

Parathyroidectomy is the cornerstone of the management of primary hyperparathyroidism in MEN1 patients. According to the 2007 National Comprehensive Cancer Network guidelines, there are two surgical options: (1) subtotal parathyroidectomy (leaving 50 mg of the most normal gland in situ), parathyroid cryopreservation, and transcervical thymectomy; or (2) total parathyroidectomy with parathyroid autotransplantation into the nondominant forearm, parathyroid cryopreservation, and transcervical thymectomy [12]. Controversy exists as to which operation should be performed at the outset. Initial subtotal parathyroidectomy is associated with a 30% to 40% rate of recurrent hyperparathyroidism, which often requires cervical reoperation [13,14]. However, initial total parathyroidectomy with autotransplantation results in permanent hypoparathyroidism in up to one third of patients because of autograft failure [14,15]. Our group has previously recommended subtotal parathyroidectomy and transcervical thymectomy with parathyroid cryopreservation but not autotransplantation at the first operation. Then, if hyperparathyroidism recurs, completion total parathyroidectomy, parathyroid autotransplantation into the nondominant forearm, and cryopreservation of the remaining parathyroid tissue are performed [16]. This approach balances the desire to avoid cervical reoperation for recurrent hyperparathyroidism with the morbidity of permanent hypoparathyroidism.

Transcervical thymectomy should always be performed during the first neck operation because MEN1 patients have an increased risk of supernumerary parathyroid glands, which are usually located ectopically, commonly in the thyrothymic ligament and in the thymus. In addition, MEN1 patients have an increased incidence of developing carcinoid tumors in the thymus.

It is important to identify MEN1 in patients presenting with apparently sporadic primary hyperparathyroidism. Unless MEN1 is recognized before the initial parathyroidectomy, the operative approach may not be appropriate. Thus, genetic testing should be offered to young patients, considered for patients presenting with suspected multigland primary hyperparathyroidism, and patients with a family history of hyperparathyroidism or any other MEN1-related disease.

Pituitary tumors

Between 20% and 60% of individuals with MEN1 develop adenomas of the anterior pituitary gland [2]. Pituitary adenomas are the initial manifestation of MEN1 in 10% to 20% of cases [17,18]. The typical age at which MEN1-related pituitary adenomas develop is in the second to fourth decade of life, with rare occurrences in children.

MEN1-related pituitary adenomas can secrete a number of different hormones. The most common functioning tumors produce prolactin, growth hormone, or corticotropin. Approximately 15% of tumors are nonfunctioning (no hormone production) [2].

MEN1-associated pituitary tumors are usually not malignant or multifocal. Most are macroadenomas (larger than 1 cm), and approximately one third are invasive and cause morbidity because of their mass effects (eg, headache, visual field defect, hypopituitarism, compression of adjacent structures, and mild hyperprolactinemia due to stalk compression) [18].

The preferred imaging modality for suspected pituitary tumors is MRI. The functional status is determined by biochemical evaluation of basal hormone levels (eg, prolactin, growth hormone, insulinlike growth factor-1, corticotropin).

Treatment of MEN1-related pituitary adenomas is the same as that of their sporadic counterparts and depends on tumor size and functional status. Treatment options include surgery (usually from a minimally invasive transsphenoidal approach), medication (for patients with prolactin– or growth-hormone–producing tumors), and radiation.

Prolactin-secreting tumors, or prolactinomas, are by far the most common functioning pituitary adenomas in MEN1. Women usually present with oligomenorrhea, amenorrhea, or galactorrhea, and men with sexual dysfunction or gynecomastia. Familial occurrences of prolactinoma are rare outside of MEN1. The diagnosis of prolactinoma is made by the presence of serum prolactin levels greater than 250 ng/mL and identification of an adenoma on MRI. When serum prolactin levels are elevated but less than 100 ng/mL, the pituitary adenomas are usually nonfunctioning, and the mild hyperprolactinemia is usually due to stalk compression.

Growth hormone–producing tumors, or somatotropinomas, are rare in MEN1 (less than 10% of functioning tumors) and result in gigantism if the tumor develops before puberty or acromegaly in adults. Acromegaly is characterized by enlargement of the hands, feet, and lower jaw; frontal bossing; and coarsening facial features. The diagnosis of growth hormone–producing tumors is established by the presence of elevated insulinlike growth factor-1. Plasma growth hormone levels may be normal or elevated.

Corticotropin-producing tumors are rare in MEN1 (accounting for less than 5% of functioning tumors) and cause cortisol overproduction, resulting in Cushing syndrome. The diagnosis of pituitary-dependent Cushing syndrome is made in the presence of excess cortisol production (best shown by a high 24-hour urinary level of free cortisol) and normal to elevated corticotropin in the presence of a pituitary abnormality on MRI. Though rare, Cushing syndrome is an important diagnosis to recognize because of the morbidities and cardiovascular complications associated with long-term cortisol excess.

Nonfunctioning pituitary tumors may present as symptoms related to their mass effect but are more typically detected incidentally or on routine screening in patients with MEN1.

Pancreatic and duodenal tumors

Approximately 75% of individuals with MEN1 develop neuroendocrine tumors of the pancreatic islet cells or duodenum, with a prevalence approaching 100% on autopsy series [19]. Pancreatic endocrine tumors are the most significant source of MEN1-specific morbidity and mortality, mainly because of their potential for malignant transformation but also from complications of hormone overproduction [20].

In contrast to sporadic pancreatic endocrine tumors, MEN1-associated pancreatic endocrine tumors develop earlier, are almost always multifocal, and occur throughout the pancreas. However, because total pancreatectomy to treat these tumors would result in insulin-dependent diabetes and pancreatic exocrine insufficiency, both of which are associated with considerable morbidity, the timing and extent of pancreatic resection for MEN1-related pancreatic endocrine tumors remain controversial.

Gastrinoma (Zollinger-Ellison syndrome) affects approximately 40% of patients with MEN1 and may present as abdominal pain, esophagitis, and peptic ulcer disease [10]. Patients with ulcers that are multiple, found in atypical locations, fail to respond to medical therapy, recur after adequate therapy, or are discovered in association with diarrhea or hyperparathyroidism should undergo evaluation for gastrinoma. The diagnosis is made by measuring a serum gastrin level drawn when the patient has discontinued proton-pump inhibitors for at least 2 weeks. The gastrin level is usually greater than 1000 pg/mL in a patient with gastrinoma. If the gastrin level is equivocal, a secretin stimulation test can be performed, with a resulting rise in the gastrin level of more than 200 pg/mL confirming the diagnosis.

Gastrinomas are often multiple in patients with MEN1 and can occur both within the gastrinoma triangle (the area between the confluence of the cystic and common bile duct, the junction of the second and third portions of the duodenum, and the junction of the neck and body of the pancreas) and in the body of the pancreas and the distal duodenum. Tumor localization is best performed by a combination of octreotide scan, CT, and endoscopic ultrasonography. At least 40% of gastrinomas have metastasized to the lymph nodes at the time of diagnosis; liver metastases are more unusual [21–23].

Gastrinoma management is controversial, and no consensus has been achieved regarding surgical management. Medical control of acid hypersecretion has been revolutionized by the introduction of proton-pump inhibitors. When MEN1 patients have hyperparathyroidism as well as gastrinoma, parathyroidectomy is a reasonable first approach because the procedure has been shown to reduce fasting gastrin levels and basal acid output as well as parathyroid hormone levels [24,25]. However, medical management and correction of the hypercalcemia do not address the malignant potential of gastrinomas, which is considerable. Some investigators have advocated an aggressive approach, which involves early surgical intervention for any MEN1 patient with biochemical or radiographic evidence of gastrinoma [26–29]. Other investigators recommend medical management until tumors reach 2.5 to 3 cm in diameter [30,31]. The rationale for the conservative approach is that the risk of distant metastasis is small for gastrinomas less than 2.5 to 3 cm and pancreatic resection carries a high incidence of morbidity [20,23,32]. A reasonable surgical approach includes distal pancreatectomy, enucleation of lesions in the pancreatic head and uncinate process that are palpable or visible with intraoperative ultrasonography, regional lymphadenectomy, and duodenotomy with local resection of any tumors found in the duodenum.

Insulinoma affects approximately 10% of MEN1 patients and classically presents as "Whipple's triad" of fasting or exercise-induced hypoglycemia, plasma glucose level less than 50 mg/dL, and reversal of symptoms with administration of glucose. The diagnosis is confirmed with a monitored 72-hour fast in which plasma glucose and insulin levels are measured every 4 to 6 hours. An inappropriately high insulin level in the presence of a low glucose level (insulin-to-glucose ratio greater than 0.4) is indicative of insulinoma.

Insulinomas may be multifocal and located throughout the pancreas. CT and endoscopic ultrasonography are the best tests for localization. Octreotide scanning is of limited value, as insulinomas express few somatostatin receptors. Unlike other pancreatic endocrine tumors, insulinomas are usually benign [33].

Insulinomas should be managed surgically. Although only a few small series have been reported in the literature, it seems that a rational surgical approach includes distal pancreatectomy with enucleation of any disease in the pancreatic head or uncinate process that is palpable or visible by intraoperative ultrasonography [34].

The other functioning pancreatic endocrine tumors affect less than 5% of patients with MEN1. Glucagonoma may present as the characteristic syndrome of diabetes, weight loss, anemia, and migratory necrolytic erythema. However, in MEN1 patients, glucagonomas are usually found on routine screening while they are still small and asymptomatic. A serum glucagon level greater than 1000 pg/mL confirms the diagnosis of glucagonoma, although a secretin stimulation test may be useful in equivocal situations. Glucagonomas are usually located in the pancreatic body and tail and are best localized with a combination of octreotide scan, CT, and endoscopic ultrasonography. When symptomatic, glucagonomas tend to be large and malignant [35].

Vasoactive intestinal peptide tumors (VIPomas) present as the syndrome of severe intermittent watery diarrhea, hypokalemia, and achlorhydria. Patients may also describe flushing. The diagnosis is made by fasting plasma vasoactive intestinal peptide (VIP) levels greater than 200 pg/mL. VIPomas are usually located in the body and tail of the pancreas and are localized with an octreotide scan, CT, and endoscopic ultrasonography. Their potential for malignancy is considerable [36].

Somatostatinoma presents as cholelithiasis, diabetes, and steatorrhea. The diagnosis is confirmed by a fasting somatostatin level of greater than 100 pg/mL. Somatostatinomas can be located in the pancreas or duodenum and are localized with an octreotide scan, CT, and endoscopic ultrasonography. These tumors have some potential to metastasize, although they are so rare that the incidence of metastatic disease is difficult to quantify [37].

Nonfunctioning pancreatic endocrine tumors represent up to 71% of surgically treated MEN1-associated pancreatic endocrine tumors [34]. Symptoms can arise as a result of local growth or metastatic disease. The diagnosis is made with CT, endoscopic ultrasonography, or MRI. These tumors are often malignant, metastasizing both to the lymph nodes and to the liver [37]. Pancreatic polypeptidoma is considered together with the nonfunctioning pancreatic endocrine tumors because oversecretion of pancreatic polypeptide does not produce a clinical syndrome.

Glucagonoma, somatostatinoma, VIPoma, and nonfunctioning pancreatic endocrine tumors are so unusual that it is difficult to support management guidelines with data. However, a logical approach includes optimal medical management of any resulting syndrome and imaging studies for tumor localization. If disease cannot be localized, it seems appropriate to observe these patients with serial imaging. When disease can be localized, a reasonable surgical approach is that described by Thompson: distal pancreatectomy to the level of the superior mesenteric vein, enucleation of any palpable or ultrasonographically visible lesions in the pancreatic head or uncinate process, and regional lymphadenectomy [27]. In patients with elevated gastrin levels, duodenotomy with local excision of any visible tumors should also be performed. Although this procedure leaves behind islet cell tissue in the head and uncinate process of the pancreas, it strikes a balance between a complete oncologic operation and the morbidity associated with the insulin-dependent diabetes and pancreatic exocrine insufficiency that result from total pancreatectomy.

Other manifestations of multiple endocrine neoplasia type 1

Over 40 different tumor types have been reported in patients with MEN1. Although these are not part of the diagnostic criteria for MEN1, their presence can help to support a diagnosis of MEN1.

Foregut (thymic, bronchial, or gastric) carcinoid tumors occur in 5% to 10% of patients with MEN1. Carcinoid tumors associated with MEN1 tend to be nonfunctioning and do not usually produce the "carcinoid syndrome." Carcinoids typically develop after age 50 years and are usually detected incidentally. The exception is thymic carcinoids, which tend to be aggressive and carry a poor prognosis [38]. Carcinoid tumors represent the second-leading MEN1-specific cause of death [20].

Approximately half of MEN1 patients develop adenomas, hyperplasia, or "fullness" of the adrenal cortex [39]. In most cases, the adrenal lesions are nonfunctioning, are not malignant, and are discovered incidentally. Rarely, pheochromocytoma, hyperaldosteronism, hypercortisolism, or adrenocortical carcinomas have been reported in MEN1, so biochemical evaluation is indicated when an adrenal lesion is identified on imaging. Management of MEN1-associated adrenal lesions is the same as management in sporadic cases.

Thyroid tumors, such as follicular adenomas, goiters, and, occasionally, nonmedullary thyroid carcinoma, are observed in at least 25% of MEN1 patients. However, this observation is likely a consequence of the increased frequency of neck imaging in MEN1 patients rather than an inherent increase in risk [40].

Benign facial angiofibromas (persistent acnelike papules composed of blood vessels and connective tissue) occur in 88% of MEN1 patients. Collagenomas (elastic nonpigmented or hypopigmented raised nodules) of the neck, upper limbs, and chest occur in 72% of MEN1 patients. Such angiofibromas and collagenomas can be useful in making a diagnosis of MEN1 in patients with otherwise equivocal features, particularly because these skin tumors are uncommon in the general population [41,42]. Subcutaneous or visceral lipomas occur in about one third of patients with MEN1, compared with about 6% of the general population. Uterine or esophageal leiomyomas, meningiomas, and spinal ependymomas also occur at a higher frequency in individuals with MEN1 than in the general population [43–46].

Multiple endocrine neoplasia type 2

Overview

The hallmark of MEN2 is a very high lifetime risk of developing medullary thyroid carcinoma (MTC)—more than 95% in untreated patients. Three clinical subtypes—MEN2A, MEN2B, and familial MTC (FMTC)—have been defined based on the risk of pheochromocytoma, hyperparathyroidism, and the presence or absence of characteristic physical features (see Table 1). The prevalence of MEN2 has been estimated at 1 in 35,000 individuals [2].

MEN2 occurs as a result of germline *activating* missense mutations of the RET (*RE*arranged during *T*ransfection) proto-oncogene. *RET*, a 21-exon proto-oncogene located on chromosome 10q11.2, encodes a receptor tyrosine kinase that functions as a signal transducer upon interaction with the glial-derived neurotrophic factor family of ligands. Binding of these ligands induces dimerization of RET receptors, autophosphorylation of intracellular tyrosine residues, and ultimately cell growth and survival mediated by the mitogen-activated protein kinase intracellular signaling cascade [47]. Mutations in *RET* associated with MEN2 cause ligand-independent activation of the downstream pathways and result in unregulated cell growth and survival. MEN2-associated mutations are almost always located in exons 10, 11, or 13 through 16, although mutations in exons 5 and 8 have been reported on rare occasions [48,49]. A definitive diagnosis of MEN2 in cases of apparently sporadic MTC and in patients with an equivocal family history usually depends on the identification of a germline *RET* mutation.

Strong genotype-phenotype correlations exist with respect to clinical subtype, age at onset, and aggressiveness of MTC in MEN2. These are used to determine the age at which prophylactic thyroidectomy should occur and whether screening for pheochromocytoma or hyperparathyroidism is necessary. The presence or absence of specific *RET* mutations can also impact management in patients presenting with apparently sporadic MTC. Therefore, genetic testing should be performed before surgical intervention in all patients diagnosed with MTC.

Multiple endocrine neoplasia subtype 2A

MEN2A is the most common subtype of MEN2 and is associated with MTC and the risk of developing pheochromocytoma (approximately 50% of patients) and primary hyperparathyroidism (20%–30% of patients) [50]. The typical age at onset of biochemical evidence of MTC in untreated patients with MEN2A is 15 to 20 years. However, MTC is frequent in children ages 10 years and younger [51–53]. Most patients with MEN2A have an affected parent. However, an apparently negative family history must be interpreted with caution as the diagnosis of MTC in family members may be delayed until late in life [54].

At least 95% of individuals with MEN2A have an identifiable *RET* mutation [55,56]. By far the most common mutation associated with MEN2A occurs at the cysteine residue at codon 634 in exon 11 (85% of MEN2A families). Mutations of cysteine residues at codons 609, 611, 618, and 620 in exon 10 account for the majority of the remainder of the MEN2A-associated mutations. However, mutations of codons 630, 666, 768, 790, 791, 804, and 891 have also been reported [51,57].

A small number of families with MEN2A have been reported to have pruritic cutaneous lichen amyloidosis or Hirschsprung disease. Cutaneous lichen amyloidosis is an itchy skin rash that develops on the upper portion of the back. Cutaneous lichen amyloidosis can be present before the onset of MTC, and identification of this skin lesion should prompt an evaluation for MEN2A. Cutaneous lichen amyloidosis has been associated only with mutations of codon 634. Hirschsprung disease is the congenital absence of the autonomic ganglia of various parts of the large intestine and results in colonic dilation, constipation, and obstruction, usually presenting in the neonatal period. Hirschsprung disease has been associated with exon 10 *RET* mutations [58].

Multiple endocrine neoplasia subtype 2B

MEN2B is the rarest subtype of MEN2 and is associated with MTC, a risk of pheochromocytoma (50% of patients), and a characteristic physical appearance that results from mucosal neuromas in the tongue, lips, and eyelids [59]. The characteristic facial features include enlarged lips, a "bumpy" tongue, and eversion of the eyelids (Fig. 1). Often patients have a thin and lanky (marfanoid) body habitus with increased joint mobility and decreased subcutaneous fat. Patients with MEN2B frequently have thickening of the corneal nerves or ganglioneuromatosis of the gastrointestinal tract, which can result in abdominal distention, megacolon, constipation, or diarrhea. The physical traits are usually evident in early childhood. The risk of hyperparathyroidism is not elevated in MEN2B.

Patients with MEN2B have the earliest onset and most aggressive type of MTC. Without prophylactic thyroidectomy at a young age (before 1 year of age), most patients with MEN2B develop metastatic MTC in childhood or adolescence [53]. Most MEN2B patients are index cases and thus do not have the benefit of early genetic screening and prophylactic thyroidectomy that would result from the identification of an affected parent. This means that the diagnosis often relies on recognition of the characteristic physical features associated with this rare subtype. Unfortunately, most

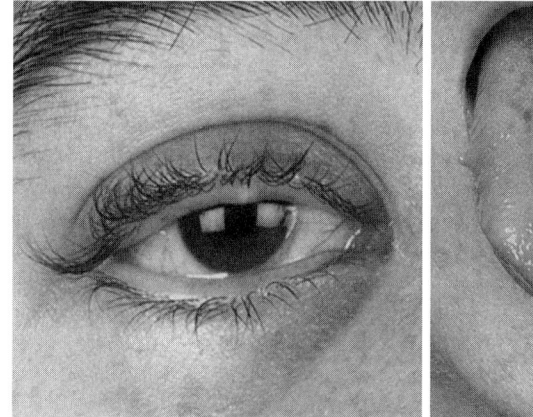

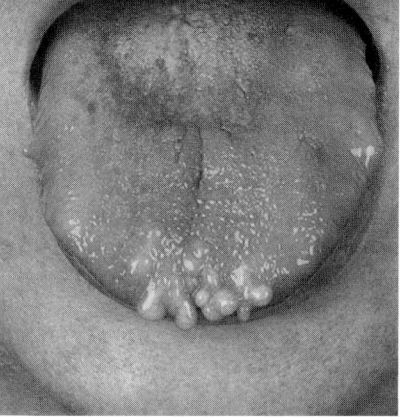

Fig. 1. MEN2B phenotype illustrating neuromas of the tongue and eyelid and eyelid eversion.

MEN2B patients experience a delay in diagnosis until palpable thyroid tumors are present, at which time MTC metastases are usually already present [60].

At least 98% of patients with MEN2B have an identifiable *RET* mutation. The mutation is almost invariably M918T. However, some individuals with MEN2B have been found to have the mutation A883F [61,62].

Familial medullary thyroid carcinoma

Patients with FMTC develop MTC but are not at increased risk for other tumors. The classification of FMTC is clinical and must be strict: Only families in which four or more cases of MTC exist with documented absence of pheochromocytoma and hyperparathyroidism should be considered to have FMTC [61]. Families with fewer than four affected members or young families without pheochromocytoma or hyperparathyroidism should be considered to have "unclassified MEN2" and screened as MEN2A patients until they meet criteria for MEN2A or FMTC. There is a broad overlap in the spectrum of *RET* mutations seen in FMTC and MEN2A, so genetic testing alone cannot always predict MEN2 subtype. In addition, mutations in codons once classified as associated with FMTC have since been found in families with MEN2A. Thus, the designation of FMTC must be used cautiously.

MTC in FMTC families tends to be the least aggressive MTC seen among all the MEN2 subtypes and tends to have the oldest age at onset, although age at onset varies considerably even among family members with the same mutation [63–65]. Certain mutations in exons 13 through 15 (except for codon 883 mutations) may be associated with reduced penetrance of MTC [63,66,67]. Mutations of codons 790, 791, or 804 may be associated with an increased risk of papillary thyroid carcinoma as well as of MTC [68].

Risk assessment and surveillance

MEN2 accounts for approximately 25% of all cases of MTC and approximately 7% of individuals presenting with apparently sporadic MTC [69]. *RET* genetic testing is considered the standard of care for newly identified MTC patients, regardless of age at diagnosis or family history. The identification of a mutation provides essential risk information for the patient's family members, and genotype-phenotype correlations can help estimate the patient's risk of developing additional endocrinopathies (eg, pheochromocytoma, primary hyperparathyroidism), provide prognostic information, and guide the surgical management of MTC.

Almost all MEN2 patients eventually develop MTC. Early detection is difficult, and the treatment options for locally advanced and metastatic disease are limited. Thus, given the acceptably low morbidity and mortality associated with thyroidectomy, it is recommended that patients at risk of inheriting a *RET* mutation undergo predictive genetic testing and that gene carriers undergo prophylactic surgical removal of the thyroid during childhood.

An international consensus conference of experts in MEN syndromes was held in 1999 to provide management guidelines for individuals with the most commonly observed *RET* codon mutations [10]. Mutations were classified into one of three levels, which are used to recommend the age at which prophylactic thyroidectomy should occur in affected patients. Level 1 mutations are associated with the least aggressive and latest onset of MTC. Some level 1 codons are also associated with reduced penetrance of MTC. Therefore, there was no consensus about at which age level 1 mutation carriers should undergo prophylactic thyroidectomy. Several panel members recommended age 5 or 10 years, whereas others felt that serial ultrasounds and calcitonin measurement could be used to delay thyroidectomy [66]. Level 2 mutations are associated with moderately aggressive MTC. Individuals with level 2 mutations should undergo prophylactic thyroidectomy by age 5 years. Codon 609 mutations were recently reclassified from level 1 to level 2 based on the diagnosis of MTC in a 5-year-old with a codon 609 mutation [70]. Level 3 mutations are associated with the most aggressive MTC and include the MEN2B-related mutations. Individuals with level 3 mutations should undergo prophylactic thyroidectomy by 6 months of age, with some experts advocating even earlier surgery. Table 3 is a summary of the most commonly observed *RET* codon mutations according to the level of risk for development of MTC as described above [10,70].

Diagnosis and management of component tumors

Medullary thyroid carcinoma

MTC is a rare cancer that develops from the calcitonin-producing cells of the thyroid (C-cells). MEN2-associated MTC typically occurs at a younger

Table 3
Genotype-phenotype correlations in MEN2

MEN2 subtype	RET codon mutations	Level of risk for development and aggressiveness of MTC	Age before which prophylactic thyroidectomy is recommended
MEN2A or FMTC	768, 790, 791, 804, 891	1 (lowest risk)	5–10 y
MEN2A or FMTC	609, 611, 618, 620, 630, 634	2 (intermediate risk)	5 y
MEN2B	883, 918, 922	3 (highest risk)	6 mo

Data from Brandi ML, Gagel RF, Angeli A, et al. Guidelines for diagnosis and therapy of MEN type 1 and type 2. J Clin Endocrinol Metab 2001; 86(12):5658–71; and Machens A, Ukkat J, Brauckhoff M, et al. Advances in the management of hereditary medullary thyroid cancer. J Intern Med 2005; 257(1):50–9.

age than sporadic MTC and is more often associated with C-cell hyperplasia (the precursor lesion of hereditary MTC) and multifocality or bilaterality [71]. Both C-cell hyperplasia and MTC cause an increased production of calcitonin from the C-cells, and serum measurements of calcitonin are used to monitor the presence and progression of MTC.

MTC usually presents as neck pain, a palpable neck mass, or diarrhea associated with significant hypercalcitoninemia. Approximately 50% of index patients with MEN2 have locally advanced or distant metastatic MTC by the time a thyroid mass is palpable. Diarrhea associated with hypercalcitoninemia is generally a poor prognostic indicator [72,73].

Total extracapsular thyroidectomy is indicated to manage MTC in the setting of MEN2, but the extent of neck dissection and the management of devascularized parathyroid glands differ depending upon the patient's MEN2 subtype and whether the intervention is prophylactic or therapeutic. An algorithm for management of these issues is found in Table 4 [74].

MTC associated with MEN2A and FMTC is generally less aggressive than MTC associated with MEN2B. Thus, prophylactic thyroidectomy need not include lymph node dissection in the setting of a low-risk patient with MEN2A or FMTC. Central (level VI) neck dissection should be considered based on variables such as specific *RET* mutation, age, serum calcitonin level, and preoperative cervical ultrasound findings. In the setting of MEN2B, however, central (level VI) neck dissection should be performed routinely with prophylactic thyroidectomy. In addition, strong consideration should be given to lateral (levels IIA, III, IV, and V) neck dissection, based on the estimated risk of MTC.

In patients with a malignant neuroendocrine thyroid nodule and no lymphadenopathy noted on cervical ultrasound, the extent of neck dissection that should accompany therapeutic thyroidectomy is generally determined based on the level of risk associated with their particular *RET* mutation. In MEN2A and FMTC patients with a level 1 (lowest risk)

Table 4
Operative management of MEN2-associated medullary thyroid carcinoma

Indication for surgery	Extent of neck dissection[a]	Management of devascularized parathyroid glands
Prophylactic thyroidectomy in MEN2A or FMTC	Central (level VI) neck dissection based on *RET* mutation, age, serum calcitonin level, and ultrasound	*RET* mutation consistent with MEN2A: cryopreserve/autograft in forearm *RET* mutation consistent with FMTC: autograft in neck (parathyroids normal)
Prophylactic thyroidectomy in MEN2B	Central (level VI) neck dissection routinely; lateral (levels IIA, III, IV, and V) neck dissection based on age, serum calcitonin level, and ultrasound	Autograft in neck (parathyroids normal)
Therapeutic thyroidectomy in MEN2A or FMTC[b]	Level 1 *RET* mutation: central (level VI) neck dissection routinely Level 2 *RET* mutation: central (level VI) neck dissection routinely; bilateral or ipsilateral lateral (levels IIA, III, IV, and V) neck dissection based on age, serum calcitonin level, and ultrasound	*RET* mutation consistent with MEN2A: cryopreserve/autograft in forearm *RET* mutation consistent with FMTC: autograft in neck (parathyroids normal)
Therapeutic thyroidectomy in MEN2B[b]	Central (level VI) neck dissection and bilateral lateral (levels IIA, III, IV, and V) neck dissection	Autograft in neck (parathyroids normal)
Therapeutic thyroidectomy in sporadic MTC[b]	Central (level VI) neck dissection and ipsilateral lateral (levels IIA, III, IV, and V) neck dissection	Autograft in neck (parathyroids normal)

[a] Any disease visible by ultrasound in the central or lateral neck requires a central (level VI) or lateral (levels IIA, III, IV, and V) neck dissection respectively.
[b] Patients with a malignant thyroid nodule and a normal ultrasound of the lateral neck.
Data from Kouvaraki M, Perrier N, Rich T, et al. The surgical treatment of MEN-1. In: Pollock R, Curley S, Ross M, et al, editors. Advanced therapy in surgical oncology, Hamilton (Canada): BC Decker Inc.; 2008. p. 449–64.

mutation, central (level VI) neck dissection should be performed routinely. In MEN2A and FMTC patients with a level 2 (intermediate risk) mutation, central (level VI) neck dissection should be performed routinely, and consideration should be given to ipsilateral or bilateral lateral (levels IIA, III, IV, and V) neck dissection, based on age and serum calcitonin level. In MEN2B patients (level 3, highest risk mutation), central (level VI), and bilateral lateral (levels IIA, III, IV, and V) neck dissection should be performed routinely.

The management of devascularized or removed parathyroid glands is fairly straightforward. If the patient's *RET* mutation is consistent with MEN2A, parathyroid glands should be cryopreserved or autografted in the forearm because these patients are at increased risk for the future development of hyperparathyroidism. Eliminating a reoperative neck procedure is ideal. If the patient's *RET* mutation is consistent with FMTC or MEN2B, devascularized parathyroid glands may be simply autografted in the neck, as patients with these MEN2 subtypes have normal parathyroid glands and are not at increased risk for future hyperparathyroidism.

Pheochromocytoma

Pheochromocytomas are rare catecholamine-secreting tumors of the adrenal medulla. MEN2-associated pheochromocytomas secrete adrenergic catecholamines and may be detected by routine biochemical screening of MEN2 patients or present as hypertension, palpitations, headache, tachycardia, or sweating. Diagnosis is confirmed by measuring 24-hour urinary levels of total metanephrines and catecholamines or plasma free metanephrines. A recent study demonstrated that plasma free metanephrines have high sensitivity and specificity for detecting pheochromocytoma and should be the test of choice in patients at high risk of pheochromocytoma, such as those with hereditary syndromes [75,76]. Imaging studies such as CT, MRI, metaiodobenzylguanidine scintiscan, or positron emission tomography are useful for localization.

Compared with sporadic pheochromocytoma, MEN2-associated pheochromocytoma is frequently bilateral and rarely malignant [77,78]. Consequently, bilateral adrenalectomy is often required, which will leave a patient dependent on replacement doses of corticosteroid drugs for life and at risk for acute adrenal insufficiency (Addisonian crisis), which can be life-threatening. A recent publication of the M.D. Anderson experience with cortex-sparing adrenalectomy in a series of hereditary pheochromocytomas found that cortex-sparing adrenalectomy led to corticosteroid independence in up to 65% of patients. Recurrent pheochromocytoma developed in only 10% of patients and metastatic disease was detected in none [79].

Based on the above findings, a reasonable approach to management of pheochromocytoma in MEN2 is as follows. A patient who presents with bilateral pheochromocytoma should undergo a unilateral cortex-sparing adrenalectomy and a total contralateral adrenalectomy. Pathologic confirmation of no medullary tissue at the margin should be considered to assure removal of the entire medulla. Preserving the cortex on only one side instead of both sides keeps the risk of recurrent pheochromocytoma low but still enables corticosteroid independence in many patients. A patient with unilateral pheochromocytoma and a normal contralateral adrenal gland should undergo unilateral total adrenalectomy. If such a patient should present later with a contralateral pheochromocytoma, a cortex-sparing adrenalectomy should be performed. A patient who has undergone a cortex-sparing adrenalectomy requires annual biochemical screening for recurrent pheochromocytoma.

In the event that a patient is diagnosed with pheochromocytoma and concurrent MTC or primary hyperparathyroidism, it is essential that the pheochromocytoma be surgically addressed first. In addition, because the consequences of operating on a patient with an undiagnosed pheochromocytoma can be devastating, MEN2 patients undergoing preoperative evaluation for thyroidectomy, parathyroidectomy, or any other surgical procedure must be screened for pheochromocytoma with measurement of plasma free metanephrines.

Parathyroid tumors

Hyperparathyroidism occurs in 20% to 30% of patients with MEN2A and can result from a single adenoma or from hyperplasia of all parathyroid glands. The clinical presentation and diagnosis are as described above for MEN1.

MEN2A patients invariably undergo prophylactic or therapeutic cervical operation for MTC at an early age and usually before hyperparathyroidism has developed. In these patients, enlarged parathyroid glands should be resected at the initial thyroid operation, even if the patient is eucalcemic. Normal glands, however, should be left in situ. If normal parathyroid glands are inadvertently removed or devascularized during thyroidectomy, they should be cryopreserved or autografted into the forearm, but not into the neck, as there remains a risk that hyperparathyroidism will develop in the future [74]. If parathyroid glands are autotransplanted into the neck, and the patient subsequently develops hyperparathyroidism, the need for reoperation amidst scar tissue increases the morbidity of the procedure. Most cases of hyperparathyroidism in MEN2A develop many years after thyroidectomy. Such cases should be managed as sporadic primary hyperparathyroidism would be managed [74].

Genetic risk assessment of patients with endocrine neoplasias

Overview

Two basic principles guide decisions about whether patients and their families could benefit from comprehensive genetic risk assessment. First, patients with more than one endocrine tumor or a family history of endocrine tumors should have a genetic risk assessment. Unlike common diseases and common cancers that may affect multiple family members by chance, endocrine tumors are rare, and it would be unusual to see more than one endocrine tumor in a single person or in multiple members of the same family by chance. Second, there are several red flag endocrine tumors that have a high likelihood of having an underlying genetic basis, even in the absence of a personal or family history suggestive of a particular syndrome. These red flag tumors include pheochromocytoma, paraganglioma, MTC, and parathyroid carcinoma.

Parathyroid disease

In the general population, primary hyperparathyroidism affects approximately 1 in 2000 individuals [80]. Women are diagnosed more than three times more frequently than men, with the peak incidence occurring between 50 and 60 years of age. Aside from a history of ionizing radiation, the only known risk factors for hyperparathyroidism are genetic susceptibilities, which include MEN1, MEN2A, and hyperparathyroidism-jaw tumor syndrome. A diagnosis of hyperparathyroidism, particularly in young patients (under age 30 years) and in patients with multigland disease, should prompt an assessment for features of syndromic disease and consideration of genetic testing.

MEN1 is the most common syndrome associated with hyperparathyroidism and may underlie 3% to 5% of cases of primary hyperparathyroidism. MEN1 is more prevalent in early-onset cases and in patients with multigland disease [81–83]. Genetic evaluation for MEN1 should be considered in patients with a family history of hyperparathyroidism, young onset of disease, multigland disease, or a family history of or symptoms suggestive of MEN1-associated endocrinopathies.

MEN2A accounts for a very small percentage of cases of hyperparathyroidism. Hyperparathyroidism is rarely the sentinel feature of MEN2A, so generally a diagnosis of MEN2A is considered only in hyperparathyroid patients who have a personal or family history or symptoms suggestive of MTC or pheochromocytoma.

Hyperparathyroidism-jaw tumor syndrome is an extremely rare autosomal-dominant condition associated with hyperparathyroidism (80% of patients), ossifying fibromas of the maxilla or mandible (one third of patients), kidney lesions, and risk of parathyroid carcinoma (15% of patients). Hyperparathyroidism typically presents in young adulthood and, unlike other forms of inherited hyperparathyroidism, is usually due to a single parathyroid adenoma (or carcinoma) that frequently has a cystic component. In most cases of hyperparathyroidism-jaw tumor syndrome, an inactivating germline mutation of the HRPT2 gene (*HRPT2*) on chromosome 1q25-31 can be identified. Clinical genetic testing for *HRPT2* mutations should be offered to all patients who have hyperparathyroidism and also jaw tumors or kidney lesions and to all patients with parathyroid carcinoma. In addition, it can be considered in patients with a family history of hyperparathyroidism, particularly if a patient has a cystic or atypical parathyroid adenoma.

Approximately 5% of cases of hyperparathyroidism are familial but are not associated with an endocrine neoplasia syndrome. These cases are termed familial isolated hyperparathyroidism. Some families with apparently isolated hyperparathyroidism have been found to harbor germline mutations in *MEN1* (10%–15%), *HRPT2* (5%–10%), or *CASR* (5%–10%) [84,85]. *CASR* mutations are typically associated with a condition called familial hypocalciuric hypercalcemia (previously referred to as benign familial hyperparathyroidism), in which the function of the extracellular calcium sensing receptors is reduced, resulting in mild to moderate hypercalcemia with inappropriately normal parathyroid hormone levels, relative hypocalciuria, and a renal calcium-to-creatinine clearance ratio of less than 0.01. In classic familial hypocalciuric hypercalcemia, the hypercalcemia is from benign causes, and parathyroidectomy is not indicated. At this time, it is unclear whether *MEN1*, *HRPT2*, and *CASR* mutations do in fact cause true isolated primary hyperparathyroidism or whether the families studied to date have incomplete or late-onset expression of the other aspects of a MEN syndrome. The majority of families with isolated hyperparathyroidism (75%–80%) do not have an identifiable mutation, although recent linkage studies suggest a new susceptibility locus on chromosome 2p13.3-14 [86].

Pheochromocytoma and paraganglioma

Pheochromocytomas and paragangliomas are histologically identical tumors. The former occur within the adrenal medulla and the latter in the sympathetic or parasympathetic paraganglia. The paraganglia are a system of neural crest-derived cells interspersed along major blood vessels and nerves from the base of the skull to the base of the pelvis; paraganglia respond to stress and changing levels of oxygen. The sympathetic paraganglia are located mainly in the chest, abdomen, and pelvis, whereas the parasympathetic paraganglia are located mostly in the head and neck, particularly near the carotid body or ganglion jugulare, vestibulare, or aortae.

Pheochromocytomas and sympathetic paragangliomas generally result in overproduction of catecholamines and cause the characteristic symptom triad of headache, palpitations, and sweating, as well as many other nonspecific symptoms. Tumor development within the parasympathetic paraganglia typically does not result in excessive catecholamine secretion, and tumors are usually asymptomatic until bulky enough to cause a visible or palpable neck mass, headaches, vocal cord disturbance, or cranial nerve deficit, such as tongue weakness, shoulder drop, hearing loss, tinnitus, or problems with balance. Parasympathetic paragangliomas of the head and neck region are also known as glomus tumors, chemodectomas, and nonchromaffin tumors. However, these terms are anatomically nonspecific. The preferred terminology is paraganglioma plus the associated anatomic position (eg, "carotid body paraganglioma").

Pheochromocytomas and paragangliomas should be considered red flag tumors, meaning that an unusually high proportion of individuals with these tumors have an underlying genetic condition. The majority of familial and syndromic cases of pheochromocytoma and paraganglioma can be attributed to VHL, MEN2A, MEN2B, a mutation in one of the familial pheochromocytoma/paraganglioma genes (*SDHB*, *SDHD*, and *SDHC*), or neurofibromatosis type 1. There are also familial cases in which no underlying genetic basis has been identified, suggesting the existence of additional susceptibility loci or limitations in current genetic testing techniques for the succinate dehydrogenase (SDH) genes.

Several retrospective studies have assessed the frequency of germline mutations in patients with apparently sporadic pheochromocytoma or paragangliomas (defined generally as patients without a suggestive family history and without any other clinical evidence of a particular syndrome) since the identification of *SDHD* and *SDHC* in 2000 and *SDHB* in 2001 [87–89]. Overall, the rate of detection of mutations in *SDHB*, *SDHD*, *RET*, and *VHL* in cases of apparently sporadic pheochromocytoma/paraganglioma has been estimated at approximately 25%. However, the mutation prevalence really ranges from less than 2% to nearly 70% if one takes into consideration age at diagnosis, adrenal or extra-adrenal tumor location, focality, biochemical phenotype, and presence of malignancy [90]. It is important to take these factors into consideration in providing risk information and genetic counseling for patients. Because of the multiple genes known to cause pheochromocytoma and paraganglioma, it is burdensome and expensive to evaluate each patient for all of the known genes. Fortunately, even for apparently sporadic tumors, each gene has distinguishing clinical features, so most cases can be narrowed down to one or two possible genes. Knowledge of which gene (if any) is involved enables counseling of the patient about the risk of various tumor types, risk of malignancy, and inheritance pattern. In addition, identifying a genetic basis allows for accurate risk assessment of a patient's family members.

Multiple endocrine neoplasia subtype 2A

Approximately 4% to 5% of cases of apparently sporadic pheochromocytoma occurring before age 50 years are due to mutations of *RET* and are thus associated with MEN2A [90]. MEN2A-associated pheochromocytomas almost always secrete epinephrine and may or may not secrete norepinephrines [91]. In addition, malignancy and extra-adrenal location are extremely rare in MEN2A. Therefore, all young patients presenting with apparently sporadic adrenergic pheochromocytoma should be offered testing for *RET* mutations, whereas patients with entirely noradrenergic, extra-adrenal, or malignant tumors are unlikely to benefit from *RET* testing.

Von Hippel-Lindau syndrome

VHL accounts for approximately 11% of apparently sporadic pheochromocytomas [90]. Pheochromocytomas in VHL are characterized by particularly young age at onset (often in childhood), frequent bilaterality or multifocality, possibility of extra-adrenal abdominal location and malignancy, and noradrenergic biochemical phenotype [91–93]. In addition to pheochromocytoma, VHL is characterized by hemangioblastomas in the retina and central nervous system, renal cysts and clear cell renal cell carcinoma, pancreatic cysts and islet cell tumors, endolymphatic sac tumors, and papillary cystadenomas of the epididymis and broad ligament.

In patients presenting with pheochromocytoma, VHL should be the first consideration if the patients are particularly young at diagnosis (VHL accounts for nearly half of pheochromocytomas presenting before age 20 years) and in patients whose tumors have a noradrenergic phenotype [90]. The clinician can also look for other features of VHL in a patient, such as renal or pancreatic cysts, and ask about a family history of VHL-associated diseases. Some patients with VHL are at risk only for pheochromocytoma and not for the other features of VHL. Thus, the absence of extra-adrenal VHL features, even in an older patient, cannot by itself rule out VHL.

The underlying genetic defect is within the VHL gene (*VHL*), a three-exon tumor suppressor gene located on chromosome 3p25. Genetic testing is clinically available for VHL, and by using a combination of sequencing and large deletion testing, the detection rate is thought to be 100%. Genetic testing is the most effective method to diagnose or rule out VHL in patients with suspected VHL and in patients presenting with apparently sporadic VHL-related disease [94].

Familial paraganglioma syndromes

The familial paraganglioma syndromes are characterized by susceptibility to multiple head and neck, thoracic and abdominal paragangliomas and pheochromocytoma. Three genes encoding subunits of the mitochondrial complex II (SDH complex)—*SDHB*, *SDHC*, and *SDHD*—have recently been found to be the underlying genetic cause of most familial cases of paragangliomas and of 8% to 50% of apparently sporadic paragangliomas [95,96].

The typical age at tumor development in patients with the familial paraganglioma syndromes is in the late 20s to early 30s. However, a wide range of ages at onset have been reported, and penetrance is incomplete [97]. The risk of various tumor types and of malignancy varies, as does the inheritance pattern, depending on the gene involved.

SDHB and *SDHD* are the most common genes underlying familial forms of paraganglioma. In *SDHB* mutation carriers, paragangliomas develop most often in the abdomen, frequently in the head and neck, and less commonly in the chest and adrenal gland. Paragangliomas in *SDHD* mutation carriers tend to develop most often in the head and neck. However, abdominal and thoracic paragangliomas and adrenal pheochromocytoma are also observed at a lower frequency [97,98]. *SDHC* mutations are rare and have been identified in only a handful of families, most of which presented with benign tumors of the head and neck [99].

SDHB-related paragangliomas have a high rate of malignancy, approaching 100% in some studies; whereas the risk of malignancy in *SDHD*-related paragangliomas is low, likely less than 2% [97,100]. As for other neuroendocrine tumors, malignancy cannot reliably be predicted based on tumor histology alone and is generally identified only by the presence of metastatic disease. Therefore, the presence of an SDH gene mutation provides important information regarding risk of malignancy.

The inheritance pattern is also different for the three SDH genes. *SDHB* and *SDHC* are inherited in an autosomal-dominant manner, whereas *SDHD* exhibits autosomal-dominant inheritance with maternal imprinting [101]. This means that only those who inherit a *SDHD* mutation from their fathers are at risk for paraganglioma development. Individuals who inherit a gene mutation from their mothers are at risk of passing the mutation on to their children but do not develop paragangliomas themselves.

Neurofibromatosis type 1

Neurofibromatosis type 1 is also a significant genetic contributor to pheochromocytoma development. Patients with this condition are usually easily identified because they have manifestations that are obvious on physical examination (eg, café-au-lait spots, neurofibromas, axillary and inguinal freckling) [102]. Therefore, genetic testing is almost never necessary to establish a diagnosis of neurofibromatosis type 1.

Apparently sporadic pheochromocytomas and paragangliomas

The highest mutation prevalence rates for apparently sporadic pheochromocytoma and paraganglioma have been found in patients with multifocal tumors (approximately 80% for *MEN2*, *VHL*, *SDHB*, and *SDHD* mutations combined), individuals who are age 18 years and younger at diagnosis (approximately 56% have a mutation in *VHL*, *SDHB*, or *SDHD*), and patients with malignant extra-adrenal paragangliomas (abdominal or head and neck origin) regardless of age (the mutation detection rate for *SDHB* reaches almost 50%) [90,96,103]. A moderate detection rate of 10% to 20% is seen in patients with a single benign pheochromocytoma or paraganglioma presenting between 20 and 50 years of age with no family history. The rate is slightly higher in those with extra-adrenal tumors [90,95]. Mutations are only rarely found in patients with apparently sporadic benign pheochromocytoma or paraganglioma who present after age 50 years (<2%). Table 5 provides an overview of the mutation prevalence and characteristic features of the various pheochromocytoma/paraganglioma susceptibility syndromes.

Nonmedullary thyroid cancer

The vast majority of cases of nonmedullary thyroid cancer are sporadic. However, clinicians should be aware of several rare hereditary syndromes

Table 5
Overview of familial hyperparathyroidism syndromes

Syndrome	Gene	Parathyroid features	Additional main features
MEN1	*MEN1*	Multigland primary hyperparathyroidism; young age of onset	Pituitary adenomas Pancreatic/duodenal endocrine tumors
MEN2A	*RET*	One- or two-gland primary hyperparathyroidism	Medullary thyroid cancer Pheochromocytoma
Hyperparathyroidism-jaw tumor syndrome	*HRPT2*	Cystic glands and tumors; risk for parathyroid carcinoma	Ossifying jaw tumors Kidney tumors
Familial hypocalciuric hypercalcemia	*CASR*	Normal parathyroid glands	Hypocalciuria Low to normal parathyroid hormone levels Renal calcium-to-creatinine clearance ratio <0.01 Parathyroidectomy does not cure hypercalcemia

associated with nonmedullary thyroid cancer, as affected patients may be predisposed to additional malignancies (Table 6).

Cowden syndrome

Cowden syndrome is a rare autosomal-dominant condition in which patients are predisposed to thyroid cancer and to benign and malignant tumors of the skin and oral mucosa, breast, and uterus. A wide range of other less-common tumor types have been observed, including adult-onset dysplastic gangliocytoma of the cerebellum (Lhermitte-Duclos disease, which may be pathognomonic for Cowden syndrome), hamartomatous colon polyps, lipomas, fibromas, and renal cell carcinoma [104].

Thyroid cancer in Cowden syndrome is usually follicular and less commonly papillary, though a follicular variant of papillary thyroid cancer is increasingly being recognized as a common tumor in Cowden syndrome. The risk of thyroid cancer is thought to be approximately 10% in patients with Cowden syndrome. The risk of benign thyroid disease (follicular adenomas, multinodular goiter) is much higher, at about 70%. Cowden syndrome is important to recognize so that the patient can be screened for the more common associated malignancies, including breast cancer (25%–50% risk) and endometrial cancer (5%–10% risk). Benign breast and uterine lesions are extremely common (eg, fibrocystic breast disease, uterine fibroids).

Table 6
Overview of hereditary pheochromocytoma/paraganglioma syndromes

Syndrome	Gene	Apparently sporadic tumors	Main features
VHL	*VHL*	11%	Hemangioblastoma of brain, spinal cord, and retina
			Pancreatic/kidney cysts, kidney cancer
			Secrete norepinephrine/ normetanephrine
			May be malignant; may be extra-adrenal
MEN2A	*RET*	5%	Medullary thyroid cancer
			Hyperparathyroidism
			Secrete epinephrine/metanephrine
			Usually benign; always adrenal location
Paraganglioma type 4	*SDHB*	4%	Predominantly abdominal/ extra-adrenal
			High risk of malignancy
Paraganglioma type 1	*SDHD*	4%	Predominantly head and neck
			Low risk of malignancy
			Maternal imprinting
Paraganglioma type 3	*SDHC*	Unknown	Head and neck only
			Benign
Neurofibromatosis type 1	*NF1*	Not applicable	Multiple café-au-lait macules
			Cutaneous neurofibromas
			Axillary/inguinal freckling

Cowden syndrome should be considered in thyroid cancer patients whose tumors have a follicular component and who have a personal or family history of thyroid, breast, or endometrial cancer. Clinical genetic testing for Cowden syndrome is commercially available, and approximately 80% of patients with Cowden syndrome have an identifiable *PTEN* mutation. However, the best method of evaluation for the possibility of Cowden syndrome is a formal dermatologic examination. Mucocutaneous features that are almost invariably present in patients with Cowden syndrome include facial trichilemmomas and papillomatous papules, acral keratoses, and "cobblestoning" of the gums and tongue. These skin lesions are almost always present by age 30 years but can be subtle. Patients also commonly have macrocephaly. Patients without dermatologic features are unlikely to have *PTEN* mutations.

Familial adenomatous polyposis

Familial adenomatous polyposis (FAP), also known as Gardner syndrome, is an autosomal-dominant syndrome in which the hallmark feature is the development of hundreds to thousands of adenomatous polyps in the colon starting at a young age (typically adolescence). Left untreated, FAP patients have a virtually 100% lifetime risk of colon cancer, which usually develops at a young age. Approximately 2% of FAP patients develop thyroid cancer, which is almost invariably the cribriform-morular variant of papillary thyroid cancer and usually develops by age 30 years. Thyroid cancer may be the presenting feature in FAP, so identification of papillary thyroid cancer, especially its cribriform-morular variant, in a young patient with a close relative who had early-onset colon cancer should prompt an investigation for FAP [105]. Approximately 95% of patients with FAP have an identifiable mutation of the causative gene, *APC* (Table 7).

Carney complex

Carney complex is an extremely rare autosomal-dominant condition associated mainly with characteristic spotty skin pigmentation, endocrine tumors, myxomas, and melanotic schwannomas [106]. The frequency of Carney complex in thyroid cancer patients is exceedingly low, but it should be considered in patients with suggestive skin features. The characteristic

Table 7
Overview of hereditary forms of nonmedullary thyroid carcinoma

Condition	Gene	Risk of thyroid cancer in mutation carriers	Thyroid histology	Other features
Familial adenomatous polyposis	*APC*	2%	Cribriform-morular variant of papillary	100s–1000s colon adenomas Colon, other gastrointestinal cancers Congenital hypertrophy of the retinal pigment Epithelium Desmoid tumors Osteomas, epidermoid cysts
Cowden syndrome	*PTEN*	10%	Follicular much more likely than papillary	Breast cancer, fibrocystic breasts Benign thyroid disease Uterine cancer, uterine fibroids Mucocutanous lesions
Carney complex	*PRKAR1A*	10%	Follicular or papillary	Spotty skin pigmentation Myxomas Pituitary adenomas Primary pigmented nodular adrenocortical disease Schwannomas Thyroid nodules/cysts
Familial nonmedullary thyroid cancer	Unknown	Unknown	Unknown	Unknown

skin findings include lentigines, which can range from pale brown to black, are usually slightly raised and well circumscribed, and tend to develop around the lips, eyes, and mucosal surfaces. Blue nevi and café-au-lait spots are also common, and hypopigmented areas and myxomas can occur. One or more of the skin features are almost invariably present by adolescence, are usually the first feature to develop, and are the most useful diagnostic element of Carney complex.

Although rare, Carney complex is an important entity to recognize because patients are also at risk of primary pigmented nodular adrenocortical disease, which causes clinically significant corticotropin-independent hypercortisolism–Cushing syndrome, pituitary adenomas (usually growth hormone–secreting), cardiac myxomas (which can be life-threatening), psammomatous melanotic schwannoma, and other tumor types. Carney complex is associated with *PRKAR1A* mutations, which can be identified in approximately 50% of people with a clinical diagnosis.

Familial isolated nonmedullary thyroid cancer

As many as 5% of cases of nonmedullary thyroid cancer are familial but are not associated with any of the distinguishing features of the above syndromes. The genetic basis of nonsyndromic familial nonmedullary thyroid cancer is currently unknown. However, autosomal-dominant susceptibility loci for familial isolated papillary thyroid cancer and for papillary thyroid cancer with papillary renal carcinoma have been identified [107–109]. In addition, the existence of low-penetrance susceptibility genes and multigenic inheritance has been proposed.

In the absence of a known susceptibility gene, empiric data must be used to predict unaffected family members' risk of developing thyroid cancer. If the patient is the only known affected family member, the risk for siblings is approximately 3% to 6% and that for offspring is 1% to 2%. When two family members are affected, the risk for other first degree relatives approaches 10% and, when more than two family members are affected, the risk may be as high as 50% [110]. The role of thyroid cancer screening, either by thyroid palpation or by ultrasonography, is controversial.

Summary

Clinicians need to be able to recognize the main clinical features of the MEN syndromes to ensure appropriate management. MEN patients are at risk for multiple conditions that often have a complex management and surveillance protocol involving a multidisciplinary team of endocrinologists, endocrine surgeons, and geneticists. Besides the health care management of the index patient, the risk of disease in relatives must also be adequately addressed.

References

[1] Agarwal SK, Lee Burns A, Sukhodolets KE, et al. Molecular pathology of the MEN1 gene. Ann N Y Acad Sci 2004;1014:189–98.
[2] DeLellis RA, Lloyd RV, Heitz PU, et al. Pathology and genetics: Tumours of the endocrine organs. In: Kleihues P, Sobin LH, editors. World Health Organization Classification of Tumours. Lyon (France): IARC Press; 2004;10:257.
[3] Bassett JH, Forbes SA, Pannett AA, et al. Characterization of mutations in patients with multiple endocrine neoplasia type 1. Am J Hum Genet 1998;62(2):232–44.
[4] Stratakis CA, Schussheim DH, Freedman SM, et al. Pituitary macroadenoma in a 5-year-old: an early expression of multiple endocrine neoplasia type 1. J Clin Endocrinol Metab 2000;85(12):4776–80.
[5] Trump D, Farren B, Wooding C, et al. Clinical studies of multiple endocrine neoplasia type 1 (MEN1). QJM 1996;89(9):653–69.
[6] Chandrasekharappa SC, Teh BT. Clinical and molecular aspects of multiple endocrine neoplasia type 1. Front Horm Res 2001;28:50–80.
[7] Marx S. Multiple endocrine neoplasia type 1. In: Scriber C, Sly W, Childs B, editors. The metabolic and molecular basis of inherited disease, 8. New York: McGraw-Hill Professional; 2001. p. 943–66.
[8] Hall WA, Luciano MG, Doppman JL, et al. Pituitary magnetic resonance imaging in normal human volunteers: occult adenomas in the general population. Ann Intern Med 1994; 120(10):817–20.
[9] Hai N, Aoki N, Shimatsu A, et al. Clinical features of multiple endocrine neoplasia type 1 (MEN1) phenocopy without germline MEN1 gene mutations: analysis of 20 Japanese sporadic cases with MEN1. Clin Endocrinol (Oxf) 2000;52(4):509–18.
[10] Brandi ML, Gagel RF, Angeli A, et al. Guidelines for diagnosis and therapy of MEN type 1 and type 2. J Clin Endocrinol Metab 2001;86(12):5658–71.
[11] Lairmore TC, Piersall LD, DeBenedetti MK, et al. Clinical genetic testing and early surgical intervention in patients with multiple endocrine neoplasia type 1 (MEN 1). Ann Surg 2004; 239(5):637–45 [discussion: 645–37].
[12] Clark O, Ajani J, Benson A. Neuroendocrine tumors, in NCCN oncology practice guidelines v.1.2007. Available at: www.nccn.org. Last accessed February, 2008.
[13] Hellman P, Skogseid B, Oberg K, et al. Primary and reoperative parathyroid operations in hyperparathyroidism of multiple endocrine neoplasia type 1. Surgery 1998;124(6):993–9.
[14] Elaraj DM, Skarulis MC, Libutti SK, et al. Results of initial operation for hyperparathyroidism in patients with multiple endocrine neoplasia type 1. Surgery 2003;134(6):858–64.
[15] Kivlen MH, Bartlett DL, Libutti SK, et al. Reoperation for hyperparathyroidism in multiple endocrine neoplasia type 1. Surgery 2001;130(6):991–8.
[16] Lambert LA, Shapiro SE, Lee JE, et al. Surgical treatment of hyperparathyroidism in patients with multiple endocrine neoplasia type 1. Arch Surg 2005;140(4):374–82.
[17] Carty SE, Helm AK, Amico JA, et al. The variable penetrance and spectrum of manifestations of multiple endocrine neoplasia type 1. Surgery 1998;124(6):1106–13.
[18] Verges B, Boureille F, Goudet P, et al. Pituitary disease in MEN type 1 (MEN1): data from the France-Belgium MEN1 multicenter study. J Clin Endocrinol Metab 2002;87(2): 457–65.
[19] Majewski JT, Wilson SD. The MEA-I syndrome: an all or none phenomenon? Surgery 1979;86(3):475–84.
[20] Doherty GM, Olson JA, Frisella MM, et al. Lethality of multiple endocrine neoplasia type I. World J Surg 1998;22(6):581–6.
[21] Gibril F, Schumann M, Pace A, et al. Multiple endocrine neoplasia type 1 and Zollinger-Ellison syndrome: a prospective study of 107 cases and comparison with 1009 cases from the literature. Medicine (Baltimore) 2004;83(1):43–83.

[22] Pipeleers-Marichal M, Somers G, Willems G, et al. Gastrinomas in the duodenums of patients with multiple endocrine neoplasia type 1 and the Zollinger-Ellison syndrome. N Engl J Med 1990;322(11):723–7.
[23] Norton JA, Fraker DL, Alexander HR, et al. Surgery to cure the Zollinger-Ellison syndrome. N Engl J Med 1999;341(9):635–44.
[24] Brandi ML, Marx SJ, Aurbach GD, et al. Familial multiple endocrine neoplasia type I: a new look at pathophysiology. Endocr Rev 1987;8(4):391–405.
[25] Norton JA, Cornelius MJ, Doppman JL, et al. Effect of parathyroidectomy in patients with hyperparathyroidism, Zollinger-Ellison syndrome, and multiple endocrine neoplasia type I: a prospective study. Surgery 1987;102(6):958–66.
[26] Skogseid B, Oberg K, Eriksson B, et al. Surgery for asymptomatic pancreatic lesion in multiple endocrine neoplasia type I. World J Surg 1996;20(7):872–6.
[27] Thompson NW. Current concepts in the surgical management of multiple endocrine neoplasia type 1 pancreatic-duodenal disease. Results in the treatment of 40 patients with Zollinger-Ellison syndrome, hypoglycaemia or both. J Intern Med 1998;243(6): 495–500.
[28] Bartsch DK, Langer P, Wild A, et al. Pancreaticoduodenal endocrine tumors in multiple endocrine neoplasia type 1: surgery or surveillance? Surgery 2000;128(6):958–66.
[29] Lairmore TC, Chen VY, DeBenedetti MK, et al. Duodenopancreatic resections in patients with multiple endocrine neoplasia type 1. Ann Surg 2000;231(6):909–18.
[30] Norton JA, Doppman JL, Jensen RT. Curative resection in Zollinger-Ellison syndrome. Results of a 10-year prospective study. Ann Surg 1992;215(1):8–18.
[31] Jensen RT. Management of the Zollinger-Ellison syndrome in patients with multiple endocrine neoplasia type 1. J Intern Med 1998;243(6):477–88.
[32] Norton JA, Alexander HR, Fraker DL, et al. Comparison of surgical results in patients with advanced and limited disease with multiple endocrine neoplasia type 1 and Zollinger-Ellison syndrome. Ann Surg 2001;234(4):495–505.
[33] Demeure MJ, Klonoff DC, Karam JH, et al. Insulinomas associated with multiple endocrine neoplasia type I: the need for a different surgical approach. Surgery 1991;110(6): 998–1004.
[34] Kouvaraki M, Shapiro S, Lee J, et al. Multiple endocrine neoplasia type 1. In: Von Hoff D, Evans D, Rh H, editors. Pancreatic cancer. Sudbury (MA): Jones and Bartlett Publishers; 2005. p. 631–54.
[35] Thakker RV. Multiple endocrine neoplasia type 1. Endocrinol Metab Clin North Am 2000; 29(3):541–67.
[36] Mignon M, Ruszniewski P, Podevin P, et al. Current approach to the management of gastrinoma and insulinoma in adults with multiple endocrine neoplasia type I. World J Surg 1993;17(4):489–97.
[37] Kouvaraki M, Perrier N, Rich T, et al. The surgical treatment of MEN-1. In: Pollock R, Curley S, Ross M, editors. Advanced therapy in surgical oncology. Hamilton (ON): BC Decker Inc.; 2008. p. 449–64.
[38] Teh BT, Zedenius J, Kytola S, et al. Thymic carcinoids in multiple endocrine neoplasia type 1. Ann Surg 1998;228(1):99–105.
[39] Waldmann J, Bartsch DK, Kann PH, et al. Adrenal involvement in multiple endocrine neoplasia type 1: results of 7 years prospective screening. Langenbecks Arch Surg 2007;392(4): 437–43.
[40] Nord B, Larsson C, Wong FK, et al. Sporadic follicular thyroid tumors show loss of a 200-kb region in 11q13 without evidence for mutations in the MEN1 gene. Genes Chromosomes Cancer 1999;26(1):35–9.
[41] Darling TN, Skarulis MC, Steinberg SM, et al. Multiple facial angiofibromas and collagenomas in patients with multiple endocrine neoplasia type 1. Arch Dermatol 1997;133(7): 853–7.

[42] Asgharian B, Turner ML, Gibril F, et al. Cutaneous tumors in patients with multiple endocrine neoplasm type 1 (MEN1) and gastrinomas: prospective study of frequency and development of criteria with high sensitivity and specificity for MEN1. J Clin Endocrinol Metab 2004;89(11):5328–36.
[43] McKeeby JL, Li X, Zhuang Z, et al. Multiple leiomyomas of the esophagus, lung, and uterus in multiple endocrine neoplasia type 1. Am J Pathol 2001;159(3):1121–7.
[44] Vortmeyer AO, Lubensky IA, Skarulis M, et al. Multiple endocrine neoplasia type 1: atypical presentation, clinical course, and genetic analysis of multiple tumors. Mod Pathol 1999;12(9):919–24.
[45] Asgharian B, Chen YJ, Patronas NJ, et al. Meningiomas may be a component tumor of multiple endocrine neoplasia type 1. Clin Cancer Res 2004;10(3):869–80.
[46] Calender A, Giraud S, Porchet N, et al. Clinicogenetic study of MEN1: recent physiopathological data and clinical applications. Study Group of Multiple Endocrine Neoplasia (GENEM). Ann Endocrinol (Paris) 1998;59(6):444–51.
[47] Santoro M, Carlomagno F, Melillo RM, et al. Dysfunction of the RET receptor in human cancer. Cell Mol Life Sci 2004;61(23):2954–64.
[48] Dvorakova S, Vaclavikova E, Duskova J, et al. Exon 5 of the RET proto-oncogene: a newly detected risk exon for familial medullary thyroid carcinoma, a novel germ-line mutation Gly321Arg. J Endocrinol Invest 2005;28(10):905–9.
[49] Da Silva AM, Maciel RM, Da Silva MR, et al. A novel germ-line point mutation in RET exon 8 (Gly(533)Cys) in a large kindred with familial medullary thyroid carcinoma. J Clin Endocrinol Metab 2003;88(11):5438–43.
[50] Eng C, Clayton D, Schuffenecker I, et al. The relationship between specific RET protooncogene mutations and disease phenotype in multiple endocrine neoplasia type 2. International RET mutation consortium analysis. JAMA 1996;276(19):1575–9.
[51] Lips CJ, Landsvater RM, Hoppener JW, et al. Clinical screening as compared with DNA analysis in families with multiple endocrine neoplasia type 2A. N Engl J Med 1994;331(13):828–35.
[52] Machens A, Niccoli-Sire P, Hoegel J, et al. Early malignant progression of hereditary medullary thyroid cancer. N Engl J Med 2003;349(16):1517–25.
[53] O'Riordain DS, O'Brien T, Weaver AL, et al. Medullary thyroid carcinoma in multiple endocrine neoplasia types 2A and 2B. Surgery 1994;116(6):1017–23.
[54] Ponder BA, Ponder MA, Coffey R, et al. Risk estimation and screening in families of patients with medullary thyroid carcinoma. Lancet 1988;1(8582):397–401.
[55] Schuffenecker I, Billaud M, Calender A, et al. RET proto-oncogene mutations in French MEN 2A and FMTC families. Hum Mol Genet 1994;3(11):1939–43.
[56] Mulligan LM, Eng C, Healey CS, et al. Specific mutations of the RET proto-oncogene are related to disease phenotype in MEN 2A and FMTC. Nat Genet 1994;6(1):70–4.
[57] Berndt I, Reuter M, Saller B, et al. A new hot spot for mutations in the RET protooncogene causing familial medullary thyroid carcinoma and multiple endocrine neoplasia type 2A. J Clin Endocrinol Metab 1998;83(3):770–4.
[58] Mulligan LM, Eng C, Attie T, et al. Diverse phenotypes associated with exon 10 mutations of the RET proto-oncogene. Hum Mol Genet 1994;3(12):2163–7.
[59] Schimke RN, Hartmann WH, Prout TE, et al. Syndrome of bilateral pheochromocytoma, medullary thyroid carcinoma and multiple neuromas. A possible regulatory defect in the differentiation of chromaffin tissue. N Engl J Med 1968;279(1):1–7.
[60] Wray CJ, Rich TA, Waguespack SG, et al. Failure to recognize multiple endocrine neoplasia 2B: more common than we think? Ann Surg Oncol 2008;15(1):293–301.
[61] Mulligan LM, Marsh DJ, Robinson BG, et al. Genotype-phenotype correlation in multiple endocrine neoplasia type 2: report of the International RET Mutation Consortium. J Intern Med 1995;238(4):343–6.
[62] Gimm O, Marsh DJ, Andrew SD, et al. Germline dinucleotide mutation in codon 883 of the RET proto-oncogene in multiple endocrine neoplasia type 2B without codon 918 mutation. J Clin Endocrinol Metab 1997;82(11):3902–4.

[63] Fitze G, Schierz M, Bredow J, et al. Various penetrance of familial medullary thyroid carcinoma in patients with RET protooncogene codon 790/791 germline mutations. Ann Surg 2002;236(5):570–5.
[64] Shannon KE, Gimm O, Hinze R, et al. Germline V804M mutation in the RET proto-oncogene in two apparently sporadic cases of MTC presenting in the seventh decade of life. J Endocr Genet 1999;1(1):39–45.
[65] Gimm O, Niederle BE, Weber T, et al. RET proto-oncogene mutations affecting codon 790/791: a mild form of multiple endocrine neoplasia type 2A syndrome? Surgery 2002;132(6):952–9 [discussion: 959].
[66] Gimm O, Ukkat J, Niederle BE, et al. Timing and extent of surgery in patients with familial medullary thyroid carcinoma/multiple endocrine neoplasia 2A–related RET mutations not affecting codon 634. World J Surg 2004;28(12):1312–6.
[67] Hansen HS, Torring H, Godballe C, et al. Is thyroidectomy necessary in RET mutations carriers of the familial medullary thyroid carcinoma syndrome? Cancer 2000;89(4):863–7.
[68] Brauckhoff M, Gimm O, Hinze R, et al. Papillary thyroid carcinoma in patients with RET proto-oncogene germline mutation. Thyroid 2002;12(7):557–61.
[69] Elisei R, Romei C, Cosci B, et al. RET genetic screening in patients with medullary thyroid cancer and their relatives: experience with 807 individuals at one center. J Clin Endocrinol Metab 2007;92(12):4725–9.
[70] Machens A, Ukkat J, Brauckhoff M, et al. Advances in the management of hereditary medullary thyroid cancer. J Intern Med 2005;257(1):50–9.
[71] Block MA, Jackson CE, Greenawald KA, et al. Clinical characteristics distinguishing hereditary from sporadic medullary thyroid carcinoma. Treatment implications. Arch Surg 1980;115(2):142–8.
[72] Cohen MS, Moley JF. Surgical treatment of medullary thyroid carcinoma. J Intern Med 2003;253(6):616–26.
[73] Robbins J, Merino MJ, Boice JD Jr, et al. Thyroid cancer: a lethal endocrine neoplasm. Ann Intern Med 1991;115(2):133–47.
[74] Kouvaraki M, Perrier N, Shapiro S, et al. Surgical treatment of multiple endocrine neoplasia type 2 (MEN-2). In: Pollock R, Curley S, Ross M, et al, editors. Advanced therapy in surgical oncology. Hamilton (ON): BC Decker Inc.; 2008. p. 465–73.
[75] Lenders JW, Pacak K, Walther MM, et al. Biochemical diagnosis of pheochromocytoma: Which test is best? JAMA 2002;287(11):1427–34.
[76] Sawka AM, Jaeschke R, Singh RJ, et al. A comparison of biochemical tests for pheochromocytoma: measurement of fractionated plasma metanephrines compared with the combination of 24-hour urinary metanephrines and catecholamines. J Clin Endocrinol Metab 2003;88(2):553–8.
[77] Bryant J, Farmer J, Kessler LJ, et al. Pheochromocytoma: the expanding genetic differential diagnosis. J Natl Cancer Inst 2003;95(16):1196–204.
[78] Inabnet WB, Caragliano P, Pertsemlidis D. Pheochromocytoma: inherited associations, bilaterality, and cortex preservation. Surgery 2000;128(6):1007–11.
[79] Yip L, Lee JE, Shapiro SE, et al. Surgical management of hereditary pheochromocytoma. J Am Coll Surg 2004;198(4):525–34.
[80] Heath H 3rd, Hodgson SF, Kennedy MA. Primary hyperparathyroidism. Incidence, morbidity, and potential economic impact in a community. N Engl J Med 1980;302(4):189–93.
[81] Tham E, Grandell U, Lindgren E, et al. Clinical testing for mutations in the MEN1 gene in Sweden: a report on 200 unrelated cases. J Clin Endocrinol Metab 2007;92(9):3389–95.
[82] Ellard S, Hattersley AT, Brewer CM, et al. Detection of an MEN1 gene mutation depends on clinical features and supports current referral criteria for diagnostic molecular genetic testing. Clin Endocrinol (Oxf) 2005;62(2):169–75.
[83] Cardinal JW, Bergman L, Hayward N, et al. A report of a national mutation testing service for the MEN1 gene: clinical presentations and implications for mutation testing. J Med Genet 2005;42(1):69–74.

[84] Warner J, Epstein M, Sweet A, et al. Genetic testing in familial isolated hyperparathyroidism: unexpected results and their implications. J Med Genet 2004;41(3):155–60.
[85] Cetani F, Pardi E, Ambrogini E, et al. Genetic analyses in familial isolated hyperparathyroidism: implication for clinical assessment and surgical management. Clin Endocrinol (Oxf) 2006;64(2):146–52.
[86] Warner JV, Nyholt DR, Busfield F, et al. Familial isolated hyperparathyroidism is linked to a 1.7 Mb region on chromosome 2p13.3-14. J Med Genet 2006;43(3):e12.
[87] Baysal BE, Ferrell RE, Willett-Brozick JE, et al. Mutations in SDHD, a mitochondrial complex II gene, in hereditary paraganglioma. Science 2000;287(5454):848–51.
[88] Niemann S, Muller U. Mutations in SDHC cause autosomal dominant paraganglioma, type 3. Nat Genet 2000;26(3):268–70.
[89] Astuti D, Latif F, Dallol A, et al. Gene mutations in the succinate dehydrogenase subunit SDHB cause susceptibility to familial pheochromocytoma and to familial paraganglioma. Am J Hum Genet 2001;69(1):49–54.
[90] Neumann HP, Bausch B, McWhinney SR, et al. Germ-line mutations in nonsyndromic pheochromocytoma. N Engl J Med 2002;346(19):1459–66.
[91] Eisenhofer G, Walther MM, Huynh TT, et al. Pheochromocytomas in von Hippel-Lindau syndrome and multiple endocrine neoplasia type 2 display distinct biochemical and clinical phenotypes. J Clin Endocrinol Metab 2001;86(5):1999–2008.
[92] Hull MT, Roth LM, Glover JL, et al. Metastatic carotid body paraganglioma in von Hippel-Lindau disease. An electron microscopic study. Arch Pathol Lab Med 1982;106(5):235–9.
[93] Walther MM, Linehan WM. Von Hippel-Lindau disease and pheochromocytoma. JAMA 1996;275(11):839–40.
[94] Stolle C, Glenn G, Zbar B, et al. Improved detection of germline mutations in the von Hippel-Lindau disease tumor suppressor gene. Hum Mutat 1998;12(6):417–23.
[95] Gimenez-Roqueplo AP, Lehnert H, Mannelli M, et al. Phaeochromocytoma, new genes and screening strategies. Clin Endocrinol (Oxf) 2006;65(6):699–705.
[96] Brouwers FM, Eisenhofer G, Tao JJ, et al. High frequency of SDHB germline mutations in patients with malignant catecholamine-producing paragangliomas: implications for genetic testing. J Clin Endocrinol Metab 2006;91(11):4505–9.
[97] Neumann HP, Pawlu C, Peczkowska M, et al. Distinct clinical features of paraganglioma syndromes associated with SDHB and SDHD gene mutations. JAMA 2004;292(8):943–51.
[98] Benn DE, Gimenez-Roqueplo AP, Reilly JR, et al. Clinical presentation and penetrance of pheochromocytoma/paraganglioma syndromes. J Clin Endocrinol Metab 2006;91(3):827–36.
[99] Schiavi F, Boedeker CC, Bausch B, et al. Predictors and prevalence of paraganglioma syndrome associated with mutations of the SDHC gene. JAMA 2005;294(16):2057–63.
[100] Timmers HJ, Kozupa A, Eisenhofer G, et al. Clinical presentations, biochemical phenotypes, and genotype-phenotype correlations in patients with succinate dehydrogenase subunit B–associated pheochromocytomas and paragangliomas. J Clin Endocrinol Metab 2007;92(3):779–86.
[101] Baysal BE. Genomic imprinting and environment in hereditary paraganglioma. Am J Med Genet C Semin Med Genet 2004;129(1):85–90.
[102] Gutmann DH, Aylsworth A, Carey JC, et al. The diagnostic evaluation and multidisciplinary management of neurofibromatosis 1 and neurofibromatosis 2. JAMA 1997;278(1):51–7.
[103] Boedeker CC, Neumann HP, Maier W, et al. Malignant head and neck paragangliomas in SDHB mutation carriers. Otolaryngol Head Neck Surg 2007;137(1):126–9.
[104] Eng C. Will the real Cowden syndrome please stand up: revised diagnostic criteria. J Med Genet 2000;37(11):828–30.
[105] Perrier ND, van Heerden JA, Goellner JR, et al. Thyroid cancer in patients with familial adenomatous polyposis. World J Surg 1998;22(7):738–42 [discussion: 743].

[106] Carney JA, Gordon H, Carpenter PC, et al. The complex of myxomas, spotty pigmentation, and endocrine overactivity. Medicine (Baltimore) 1985;64(4):270–83.
[107] Canzian F, Amati P, Harach HR, et al. A gene predisposing to familial thyroid tumors with cell oxyphilia maps to chromosome 19p13.2. Am J Hum Genet 1998;63(6):1743–8.
[108] McKay JD, Lesueur F, Jonard L, et al. Localization of a susceptibility gene for familial nonmedullary thyroid carcinoma to chromosome 2q21. Am J Hum Genet 2001;69(2): 440–6.
[109] Malchoff CD, Sarfarazi M, Tendler B, et al. Papillary thyroid carcinoma associated with papillary renal neoplasia: genetic linkage analysis of a distinct heritable tumor syndrome. J Clin Endocrinol Metab 2000;85(5):1758–64.
[110] Charkes ND. On the prevalence of familial nonmedullary thyroid cancer. Thyroid 1998; 8(9):857–8.

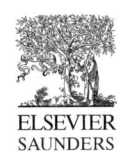

Familial Melanoma

Johan Hansson, MD, PhD

Department of Oncology-Pathology, Cancer Center Karolinska, Karolinska Institute, Karolinska University Hospital Solna, S-17176 Stockholm, Sweden

Cutaneous malignant melanoma (CMM) shows a rapidly rising incidence in white-skinned populations across the world. It has been estimated that in 2007, approximately 60,000 new cases of invasive CMM were diagnosed in the United States and over 8000 deaths from melanoma occurred [1]. There is thus a need for improved preventive strategies. One essential task is to define those at high-risk for development of melanoma who may then be enrolled in preventive programs to reduce the risk of CMM. A particular high-risk group for melanoma development includes members of families that have hereditary CMM. In this review, the clinical characteristics, genetic aspects, and guidelines for management of familial melanoma are summarized.

Risk factors for melanoma

Environmental risk factors

The major environmental risk factor for melanoma is exposure to UV radiation, both the long wavelength UVA (320–400 nm) and the intermediate wavelength UVB (290–320 nm). The increase in incidence of CMM in white-skinned populations is likely caused to a large degree by changing sun exposure patterns, however, the relationship between sun exposure and CMM is complex. In a recent meta-analysis of the published data, the most consistent relationship to increased risk of CMM was seen between intermittent sun exposure, particularly in early life, and a history of sunburns [2]. In contrast, increased levels of chronic sun exposure showed no significant association with increased risk of CMM.

This work was supported by the Swedish Cancer Society, the Swedish Medical Research Council, the Radiumhemmet Research Funds, the National Institutes of Health (RO1-CA-083115-06), and the European Commission (Sixth Framework Program, GenoMEL).

E-mail address: johan.hansson@ki.se

Host risk factors

The presence of large numbers of melanocytic nevi is an important risk factor for CMM [3]. In addition to large numbers of common nevi, the presence of atypical moles/dysplastic nevi (DN) is a melanoma risk factor. For the clinical diagnosis of DN, the established ABCD(E) criteria may be used. Nevi are judged DN if they have an asymmetrical form (Asymmetry), irregular borders (Border), composite multicolor pigmentation (Color), and a diameter of more than 6 mm (Diameter) [4]. Elevation of the nevus (Elevation), that is, the simultaneous presence of macular and papular components, is a further criterion [5]. It should be noted that these criteria are also used to identify CMM, indicating the difficulty in the differential diagnosis of DN and CMM. In trained hands, dermatoscopy (epiluminescence microscopy) is a useful technique to increase the diagnostic accuracy [6].

Although DN were originally described in the context of familial melanoma [7], DN are not infrequent in the adult population. In a German study, at least 5% of individuals had at least one DN [8], whereas in a Swedish study, this figure was as high as 19% [9].

Other phenotypic risk factors include skin type with an inability to tan, presence of many freckles, red or blond hair, blue/gray eyes, indicators of actinic skin damage, and a history of a previous premalignant or skin cancer lesions (melanoma or nonmelanoma) [10].

Familial melanoma

There is evidence for familial clustering of cases of CMM. It is estimated that 5% to 10% of all cases of CMM occur in kindreds that have a hereditary predisposition for CMM [11,12]. In population-based studies, 1% to 13% of melanoma cases report melanoma in at least one first-degree relative [13,14]. The risk of melanoma is increased in relatives of CMM patients. Thus, according to a recent report from the Genetic Epidemiology of Melanoma Group, individuals who have a first-degree relative who has CMM have a markedly increased risk of developing melanoma, with a cumulative risk of 6% to 7% at age 80 years [15]. Increased CMM risk in biologic relatives of CMM patients may be caused by genetic factors and by shared environmental exposure. Ultimately, the individual risk is a result of gene–gene and gene–environment interactions, which are just beginning to be elucidated.

The occurrence of families that have increased melanoma risk has been recognized for nearly 2 centuries. In the first description of CMM in the English language in 1820, Norris [16] reported a family in which two members had CMM and several relatives had large moles. In 1978, Clark and colleagues [7] reported six melanoma-prone families in which CMM patients and their relatives had large "funny-looking" nevi, which were designated as potential precursors of CMM. The syndrome was subsequently entitled dysplastic nevus syndrome (DNS) (Figs. 1 and 2) [14]. In parallel, Lynch and colleagues [17] reported the same syndrome, which was entitled familial atypical multiple-mole melanoma syndrome. The syndrome is also called atypical mole syndrome [18].

Familial melanoma patients tend to have an earlier age at first melanoma diagnosis, thinner tumors, and a higher frequency of multiple primary melanomas (MPMs) than patients who have sporadic melanoma [19]. In some melanoma families, there is also an increased risk of pancreatic carcinoma (see later discussion).

In the original descriptions of melanoma families, there was an association between melanoma risk and the DNS phenotype, and DN were considered precursor lesions of CMM [7]. For instance, in an early study, 14 families that had familial melanoma and DNS were reported [20]. Approximately 95% of the melanoma patients and 50% of the family members had DN. During follow-up, new cases of CMM were diagnosed only in individuals who had DN. It has now become clear that a variation between families exists as to whether they exhibit the DNS phenotype. Moreover, although risk of melanoma is higher in family members who have DNS (and it is clear that DN may be precursor lesions of CMM; see Fig. 2) [21], CMM also develops in individuals who do not have DNS. Therefore, all members of melanoma families should be considered at increased risk for CMM.

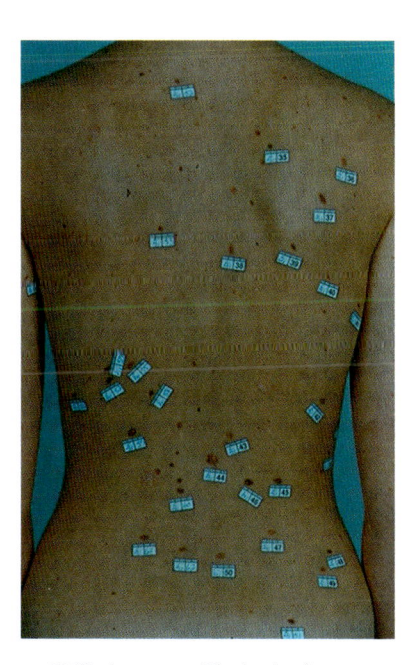

Fig. 1. Familial melanoma—DNS phenotype. The back of a young woman belonging to a kindred with familial melanoma who exhibits numerous DN.

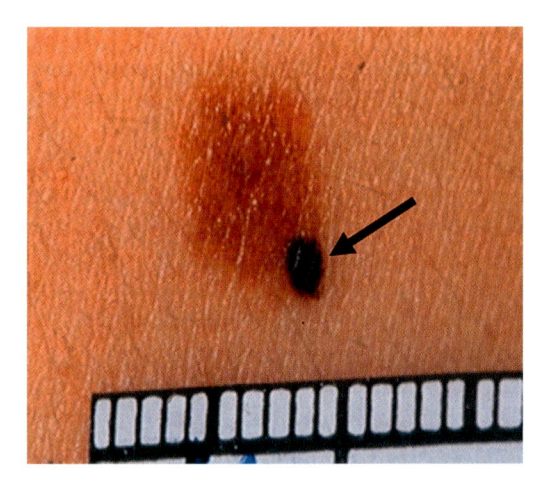

Fig. 2. Development of an early melanoma in a DN. During follow-up of this member of a kindred that had familial melanoma, a dark pigmentation arose in the lower part of this DN (*arrow*). Histopathologic examination of the excised nevus showed that the darkly pigmented area corresponded to an early CMM: a superficial spreading melanoma with a tumor thickness of 0.5 mm (T1a, according to the American Joint Committee on Cancer classification).

Molecular genetics of familial cutaneous melanoma

In recent years, considerable efforts have been made to unravel the genetic alterations responsible for familial CMM. For instance, the Melanoma Genetics Consortium (GenoMEL) has been active as a nonprofit consortium since 1997 in this area. GenoMEL comprises most research groups worldwide working on the genetics of familial CMM. The mission of GenoMEL is to develop and support collaborations between member groups to identify melanoma susceptibility genes, to evaluate gene–environment interactions, and to assess the risk of CMM and other cancers related to variations in these genes. More detailed information on GenoMEL and its activities can be obtained at http://www.genomel.org.

High-risk melanoma genes

CDKN2A

In 1994, it was demonstrated that affected members in some kindreds that have familial CMM harbor germline mutations in the *CDKN2A* gene on chromosome 9p21 [22,23]. Remarkably, the *CDKN2A* gene encodes two unrelated proteins, which are tumor suppressors and which play key roles in cell cycle regulation (Fig. 3) (reviewed in Ref. [24]). Thus, the p16INK4 protein is encoded by exons 1a, 2, and 3 and negatively regulates cell cycle progression by inhibiting the cyclin-dependent kinases CDK4 and CDK6. Inhibition of the kinases prevents phosphorylation of the retinoblastoma protein pRb, thereby preventing entry into the S-phase of the cell cycle.

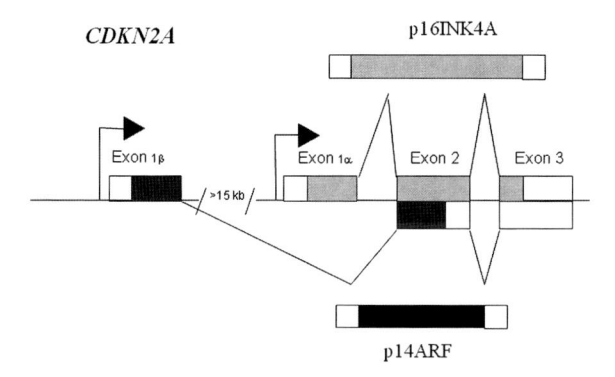

Fig. 3. The *CDKN2A* locus on chromosome 9p21. This gene encodes two different proteins: p16INK4A and p14ARF. p16INK4A is encoded by exons 1a, 2, and 3, whereas the p14ARF protein is encoded by alternative splicing of an alternative exon 1b to exon 2. The two proteins have different amino acid sequences because they are translated in different reading frames.

Recently, it was suggested that p16INK4 normally causes senescence in melanocytes and in nevi containing activating BRAF proto-oncogene mutations [25,26]. Germline loss of one *CDKN2A* allele would thus weaken this protective mechanism against melanoma development and may contribute to the development of increased numbers of nevi later in life in affected individuals compared with healthy persons [27]. The second *CDKN2A* protein product, p14ARF, is encoded by splicing of an alternative exon 1b to exon 2. This protein is translated in an alternative reading frame (hence the acronym ARF) and therefore shows no amino acid homology to p16INK4. p14ARF blocks HDM2-mediated degradation of p53. Mutations in *CDKN2A* thus have the capacity to target negative regulators in two key signaling pathways, the pRb and p53 pathways, which have central roles in cell cycle regulation. In addition, p14ARF has been implicated in sumoylation of several of its binding proteins and in inhibiting the transcriptional activator E2F-1 and promoting its degradation [28,29].

A large number of different germline CDKN2A mutations have been identified in members of kindreds that have familial melanoma and in patients who have multiple primary CMM [30–33]. Most mutations are missense mutations and are scattered throughout the gene without any clear hotspots. Mutations in exon 1a alter the p16INK4 protein only; those in exon 1b target the p14 ARF protein. Exon 2 mutations, however, may affect both proteins. Most mutations have been reported in exons 1a and 2, which is consistent with inactivation of the p16INK4 protein as the main predisposing factor for CMM. More recently, however, alterations affecting exon 1b only have been described in melanoma families in which neural system tumors (NSTs) also occur, including deletions, insertions, and splice site mutations [34–38]. Therefore, it seems that mutations affecting either protein may be involved in development of familial CMM.

Worldwide, it has been estimated that approximately 20% to 40% of kindreds that have familial melanoma are related to germline CDKN2A mutations [39]. GenoMEL recently reported a large study that included 466 families (2137 patients) with at least three melanoma patients from 17 centers [40]. Overall, 41% (n = 190) of families had mutations; most involved p16INK4A (n = 178), whereas mutations in CDK4 (n = 5) (see later discussion) and p14ARF (n = 7) occurred at similar frequencies (2%–3%). There were striking differences in mutations across geographic areas. Specific founder CDKN2A mutations have been described in several countries, and the proportion of families that had such mutations differed significantly among geographic regions ($P = .0009$). Single founder CDKN2A mutations are predominant in Sweden (p.R112_L113insR, 92% of familial mutations) [41], the Netherlands (c.225_243del19, 90% of familial mutations) [42], and Iceland (p.G89D) [43]. France, Spain, and Italy have the same most frequent mutation (p.G101W) [44]. Similarly, Australia and United Kingdom share the same most common mutations (p.M53I, c.IVS2-105A>G, p.R24P, and p.L32P).

In another recent international GenoMEL study of 385 families that had three or more melanoma cases, frequencies of germline CDKN2A mutations in different continents were analyzed [43]. Overall, 39% of families had CDKN2A mutations, ranging from 20% (32/162) in Australia to 45% (29/65) in North America and to 57% (89/157) in Europe. The lower frequencies of CDKN2A mutations in areas with high CMM incidence, such as Australia, may be explained by a higher frequency of clustering of sporadic cases or by cases associated with low-penetrance genes in geographic areas with high environmental UV exposure.

An analysis of factors predictive of germline CDKN2A mutations was performed using the major factors individually reported to be associated with an increased frequency of CDKN2A mutations: increased number of patients who had melanoma in a family, early age at melanoma diagnosis, and family members who had MPMs or pancreatic cancer. All four features in each group, except pancreatic cancer in Australia ($P = .38$), individually showed significant associations with CDKN2A mutations, but the effects varied widely across continents. Multivariate examination also showed different predictors of mutation risk across continents. In Australian families, the predictors of more than two patients who had MPM, median age at melanoma diagnosis of 40 years or younger, and six or more patients who had melanoma in a family jointly predicted the mutation risk. In European families, all four factors concurrently predicted the risk, but with less stringent criteria than in Australia. In North American families, only 1 or more patient who had MPM and age at diagnosis of 40 years or younger simultaneously predicted the mutation risk. The variation in CDKN2A mutations for the four features across continents is consistent with the lower melanoma incidence rates in Europe and the higher rates of sporadic melanoma in Australia.

CDK4

Worldwide, only a small number of kindreds that have familial CMM and germline mutations in the *CDK4* gene encoding a cyclin-dependent kinase, which normally interacts with p16INK4A, have been described (reviewed in Ref. [24]). In all cases, the mutations occur in exon 2 and affect codon 24 (p.R24C, p.R24H), which is essential for binding to p16INK4A. The phenotype of these families seems to be similar to those that have *CDKN2A* mutations.

Candidate loci for novel genes predisposing to familial cutaneous malignant melanoma

GenoMEL has performed a genome-wide screen of microsatellite markers in 82 melanoma families, most of who were from Australia. This screen yielded a significant linkage to a marker on chromosome 1p22 [45]. Although loss of heterozygosity studies indicate that a tumor suppressor gene may be present at this locus, so far, no susceptibility gene has been identified, despite considerable efforts [46].

More recently, a linkage analysis of three Danish kindreds that had ocular and cutaneous melanoma yielded a suggested linkage to markers on chromosome 9q21.32, but the putative gene responsible for the syndrome has not been identified [47].

Risk of melanoma and of other cancers in melanoma families that have germline *CDKN2A* mutations

For genetic counseling, it is important to obtain an estimate of the penetrance of a certain germline gene mutation, that is, the risk of developing the disease among carriers of the gene mutation. The penetrance of germline *CDKN2A* mutations for melanoma development in kindreds that have familial melanoma has been the subject of a large collaborative study by GenoMEL. In this study, members of 80 kindreds that had familial melanoma from different parts of the world were investigated. Overall, *CDKN2A* mutation penetrance was estimated to be 0.30 (95% confidence interval [CI], 0.12–0.62) by age 50 years and 0.67 (95% CI, 0.31–0.96) by age 80 years. Penetrance with respect to melanoma development was not statistically significantly modified by sex or by whether the *CDKN2A* mutation altered the p14ARF protein; however, there was a statistically significant effect of residing in a location with a high population incidence rate of melanoma ($P = .003$). By age 50 years, *CDKN2A* mutation penetrance reached 0.13 in Europe, 0.50 in the United States, and 0.32 in Australia; by age 80 years, it was 0.58 in Europe, 0.76 in the United States, and 0.91 in Australia. Thus, the same factors that affect population incidence of melanoma may also modulate *CDKN2A* penetrance. These data strongly support an interaction between the presence of a germline CDKN2A mutation and environmental UV exposure.

The risk of melanoma in carriers of germline *CDKN2A* mutations in the general population is lower, however, as reported in a recent publication from the Genes, Environment and Melanoma study [48]. This investigation was based on analyses of 3550 population-based melanoma patients and 23,485 of their first-degree relatives. The risk of melanoma in carriers of germline *CDKN2A* mutations was 14% (95% CI, 8%–22%) by age 50 years, 24% (95% CI, 15%–34%) by age 70 years, and 28% (95% CI, 18%–40%) by age 80 years. Thus, carriers of *CDKN2A* germline mutations in the general population seem to have a considerably lower melanoma risk than those who belong to kindreds that have familial melanoma. This is most likely due to the influence of other, unknown melanoma predisposing factors in melanoma kindreds that interact with and increase the penetrance of *CDKN2A* mutations.

Apart from CMM, an increased risk for pancreatic carcinoma has been documented in several families, including families that have the Dutch p16 Leiden mutation and the Mediterranean p.G101W and the Swedish p.R112_L113insR founder mutations [42,49–51]. In the recent study from GenoMEL addressing risk of other cancers, there was a strong association between the presence of pancreatic cancer and CDKN2A germline mutations in melanoma families ($P<.0001$); however, this relationship differed between mutations and also between geographic areas because there was no significant association between pancreatic carcinoma and CDKN2A mutations in Australian families, which may reflect a different spectrum of mutations in Australian compared with European or North American families. Although the data indicate a possible relationship between the type of CDKN2A mutation and risk of pancreatic cancer, with more mutations affecting p16 and p14ARF in kindreds that have pancreatic cancer compared with those that do not, further studies are needed to further explore this association. The cumulative risk for development of pancreatic cancer in individuals who have the p16-Leiden deletion was 17%, with a mean age at diagnosis of 58 years [52]. Although the risk of pancreatic cancer is lower than that of melanoma, a study of Dutch melanoma families showed nearly equal mortality rates owing to melanoma and pancreatic cancer in these families [53].

In a small number of families, the incidence of CMM and NSTs has been associated with large deletions of CDKN2A/ARF, mutations that affect p14ARF, or both [34–38]. In the recent GenoMEL study, there was no significant association between CDKN2A mutations and NSTs ($P = .52$) and a marginally significant association of NSTs with mutations affecting the p14ARF transcript ($P = .05$), thus giving some support for the impact of germline ARF alterations, NSTs, and melanoma [40]. This analysis, however, has low power and requires further confirmation. Furthermore, there was no significant association between CDKN2A germline mutations in families and the occurrence of uveal melanoma ($P = .25$). Thus, rare families that have clustering of uveal and cutaneous melanoma may have a different underlying genetic alteration such as the putative chromosome 9q21 gene mentioned earlier [47].

Gene testing in familial melanoma

Gene testing for familial melanoma remains controversial. Although it is practised in certain health care systems, it has, until recently, been the view of GenoMEL that testing is premature [54], but this remains under review and family members should be counseled regarding the advantages and disadvantages of genetic testing [55].[1] There are several arguments against genetic testing. First, many melanoma families that have several affected members still lack identifiable germline mutations in known high-risk genes. Therefore, a negative test result is uninformative. Second, the risk of melanoma and other cancers in individuals who have germline mutations is still insufficiently characterized, making the implications of a positive test result imprecise. Third, because non–gene carriers in CDKN2A-positive families may have DNS and develop CMM, there is an increased risk of CMM in family members who do not have mutations. A negative test result could thus lead to false reassurance and possibly have a negative impact on preventive activities, although there is no evidence for this from genetic testing for other familial cancers [56,57]. Ultimately, in the absence of a validated screening method for pancreatic cancer, a positive CDKN2A test will have little impact on the management of melanoma kindreds.

Arguments in favor of gene testing have been given. First, provided that the limitations of the test are explained to family members, the information obtained may be valuable to them. Second, a positive test result may improve the compliance of some family members in preventive programs. Finally, a negative test result in a member of a high-risk family who has relatives who have died from melanoma or pancreatic cancer is reassuring.

Gene testing for melanoma should be offered only in conjunction with qualified genetic counseling and education and be performed at departments of clinical genetics or equivalent centers. Gene testing for germline CDKN2A mutations should be considered only when there is a reasonable likelihood of finding a positive result. At this time, it is not possible to define the exact criteria for such testing in melanoma. CDKN2A testing is not meaningful in patients who have single sporadic CMM without a family history of melanoma, even if the melanoma has occurred at an early age, due to the low frequency of mutations [58]. For the same reason, testing is not meaningful in patients who have MPMs in the absence of a family history

---

[1] For a directory of cancer genetics professionals—the National Cancer Institute PDQ Cancer Genetics Services Directory—visit www.cancer.gov/search/results_geneticsservices.aspx.

[30–33]. CDKN2A mutations are more prevalent in the setting of familial CMM. As discussed previously, although there are geographic variations, the likelihood of the presence of a CDKN2A mutation increases with (1) the number of affected CMM cases in a family, (2) a lower median age of diagnosis of CMM, (3) the occurrence of MPMs, and (4) an incidence of pancreatic carcinoma. Thus, although testing for germline CDKN2A mutations may be considered in families that have two first- or second-degree relatives who have CMM, the likelihood of a positive test in such kindreds is very low, below 10% in most areas [11]. Thus, the main-candidate families for genetic testing are those that have three or more affected members, particularly when there is a low age of diagnosis of CMM, individuals who have MPMs, and occurrence of pancreatic carcinoma.

Management of familial melanoma

There is a long-standing consensus that members of kindreds that have familial melanoma should be invited to participate in preventive programs [59]. A consensus statement on the management and counseling of such individuals has been published by GenoMEL [60]. In the absence of data from randomized controlled clinical trials, the evidence for these measures is level 4 (Oxford Center for Evidence-Based Medicine Levels of Evidence, www.cebm.net).

To identify kindreds that have familial melanoma, it is important to question all newly diagnosed patients who have CMM regarding family history of melanoma and other malignancies. Verified diagnoses of CMM and other cancers, preferably through histopathology reports, and age at diagnosis should be documented. Such verification of diagnoses is essential because family members often confuse nonmelanoma skin cancers and DN with melanoma. When a family history of melanoma has been established, the health care provider should establish a careful extended pedigree of the family in collaboration with the proband of the family (Fig. 4). The pedigree should be revised annually in collaboration with the proband.

At present, due to the limitations of testing for germline CDKN2A mutations, it is recommended that members of melanoma families be managed in a similar manner regardless of CDKN2A mutation status. It is recommended that in melanoma families, at least all first-degree relatives of patients affected with CMM are offered to participate in a preventive program. This recommendation also applies to members of CDKN2A mutation–negative families with multiple melanoma cases in whom it can be assumed that an unidentified high-penetrance gene is present. First-degree relatives of CMM patients in such families have a 50% likelihood of carrying the unknown melanoma risk gene.

Primary prevention of cutaneous malignant melanoma

An essential part of primary prevention is education of family members regarding sun protection. Support for a role of sun exposure on melanoma

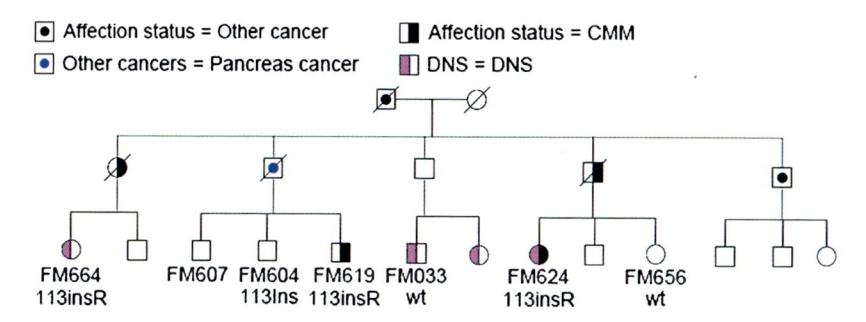

Fig. 4. Pedigree of a familial melanoma kindred that has CMM and pancreatic carcinoma in which affected members carry the Swedish CDKN2A founder mutation. Four members were diagnosed with CMM and one individual died from pancreatic carcinoma. The two living individuals who have CMM tested positive for CDKN2A mutations, whereas the two deceased melanoma patients and the patient who had pancreatic carcinoma were obligate carriers of the CDKN2A mutation. In contrast, the DNS phenotype is seen in mutation-positive and in mutation-negative family members.

risk in CDKN2A germline mutation carriers comes from the observation that CDKN2A penetrance is higher in Australia than in the United States or Europe [61]. Case-control studies in sporadic melanoma strongly support the role of intermittent sun exposure, particularly in early life and when associated with sunburns [2]. The efforts should aim to reduce sun exposure in all members of melanoma families, particularly in early life. Thus, parents should be educated about sun-protective measures for infants and children [59,62], including the use of sun-protective clothing, hats, and sunglasses; avoidance of sun exposure during peak UV conditions; and absolute avoidance of sunburns. The use of sunscreens remains controversial but may be considered as a complement to other sun-protective measures. If used, it must be ensured that sunscreens have a sufficient level of broad-spectrum protection for UVA and UVB [63].

Secondary prevention of cutaneous malignant melanoma

Because many melanomas develop from precursor lesions such as DN, and because melanomas that are detected and treated early have an excellent prognosis, there is a clear role for monitoring of pigmented skin lesions in members of melanoma families. Family members should be instructed in skin self-examination and be given the opportunity to participate in regular screening by trained health care professionals. Commencing at age 10 years, members of kindreds that have familial CMM should have a baseline whole-skin examination with characterization of moles. The skin examination must include examination of the scalp and the external genitals. The examination should focus on detection and characterization of nevi and any suspicious melanoma lesions. Documentation, with overview photographs of the entire skin and close-up pictures of DN, is very useful for follow-up (see Figs. 1 and 2). Melanoma family members should be followed by an appropriately trained health care provider, with skin examinations approximately every 6 months, at least until the nevi are stable and the person is judged competent in self-surveillance. Subsequently, the individual should be examined annually or have prompt access to the health provider as necessary. Individuals who have large numbers of DN and unstable and rapidly changing nevi may require more frequent skin examinations. Such examinations may also be necessary, for instance, during pregnancy, when nevi may be particularly unstable. Skin-surface microscopy (epiluminescence microscopy) using conventional dermatoscopes or digital equipment is helpful during skin examinations [6,64,65].

Any changing nevus should be considered for excision for histopathologic diagnosis. There is, however, no justification for prophylactic removal of nevi because the probability of progression to melanoma is low for every individual lesion and, over time, many nevi mature and disappear. Furthermore, because melanomas may occur on previously normal skin, removal of nevi would not change the guidelines for skin surveillance by the patient or the health care provider [66].

Family members should be taught about routine self-examination of the skin and may be provided with their own set of photographs and be instructed on how to use them in self-examination. A monthly self-examination or examination by a parent, a partner, or another family member is recommended. Information regarding the significance of change in shape and size of pigmented lesions should be given, and instruction on the ABCD(E) rules may be useful [4,5,67]. It should be noted, however, that these criteria do not apply to all melanomas because a considerable fraction of early melanomas have a diameter less than 6 mm [68]. Moreover, because some CMM tumors apparently arise de novo and not by progression of a precursor lesion, the individuals must also be informed to be watchful regarding novel skin lesions [66].

Because no prospective studies of the outcome of preventive programs in high-risk groups for CMM have been reported, the benefits remain unproven. There are reports, however, that indicate that preventive activities may result in early diagnosis of CMM, as indicated by a low tumor thickness of tumors detected during follow-up [69–71]. In a more recent report on long-term follow-up of 844 members of 33 kindreds that had familial melanoma, of which 19 had germline mutations in *CDKN2A* or *CDK4*, 86 new CMMs were identified [72]. Of these, 72 were classified as T1a lesions (tumor thickness ≤1.0 mm; Clark level ≤3; no ulceration) with an average thickness of 0.3 mm. Similarly, in an analysis of 2080 family members of 280 Swedish familial CMM kindreds who were followed between 1987 and 2001, 41 CMM tumors were detected during follow-up. Of these, 15 (37%) were in situ tumors, and among the 26 invasive CMMs, 22 were

T1a tumors. Overall, 27 of the 41 CMM tumors (66%) lacked vertical growth phase and thus, by definition, lacked metastatic capacity [73]. The existing data support the hypothesis that preventive programs as previously described can lead to the diagnosis of early melanomas with an excellent prognosis and can efficiently reduce the risk of potentially metastatic CMMs in melanoma families.

Pancreatic carcinoma surveillance

At present there are no efficient screening methods to detect pancreatic carcinoma at a curable stage. Surveillance of pancreatic cancer in familial melanoma kindreds affected with this second malignancy is therefore a difficult task [74–76]. Serum markers, such as CA 19-9 are of limited value in asymptomatic individuals. Likewise, noninvasive imaging techniques such as abdominal CT or MRI are inadequate for the detection of pancreatic carcinoma at an early stage. Endoscopic retrograde cholangiopancreatography (ERCP) is considered the gold standard for visualization of pancreatic carcinoma. Due to the risk of serious complications such as bleeding, intestinal perforation, and pancreatitis, however, ERCP cannot be used in routine surveillance. Endoscopic ultrasound is a novel technique that may be able to detect early pancreatic cancer and precursor lesions. More recently, MRI combined with magnetic resonance cholangiopancreatography has been proposed as a screening tool. Parker and colleagues [74] described a pancreatic carcinoma screening algorithm for familial melanoma kindreds affected with pancreatic cancer in which CDKN2A mutation carriers are offered surveillance with endoscopic ultrasound and CA 19-9 beginning at age 50 years, or 10 years before the first diagnosis of pancreatic carcinoma in the family. Individuals who have abnormal findings are further investigated with ERCP. The benefits of such screening programs need to be investigated in prospective studies, and there are a number of research programs in the United States and Europe addressing this. For improved future surveillance, development of improved noninvasive methods such as serum markers would be very useful.

Other cutaneous malignant melanoma–predisposing genes

Low-penetrance risk–modifying genes: MC1R *and* OCA2

The melanocortin 1 receptor gene, *MC1R*, encodes the membrane receptor for a-melanocyte-stimulating hormone (a-MSH). On binding of a-MSH to the receptor, the levels of cyclic AMP increase, which in turn results in a shift in melanin synthesis from reddish pheomelanin to brown-black eumelanin [77]. Several variants—single nucleotide polymorphisms (SNPs)—have been described in the *MC1R* gene, and some of these may alter the function of the receptor, thereby shifting melanin synthesis from eumelanin toward pheomelanin [78–80]. Such variants, which are common in Caucasian populations, are associated with red hair, fair skin, and freckling. Certain SNPs, so-called "RHC alleles," are associated with a significant, although modest (approximately twofold) increased risk of CMM (these RHC alleles include D84E, R151C, R160W, and D294H) [81]. Other frequent, non–RHC alleles are not associated with significantly increased CMM risk. An independent association between some *MC1R* SNPs and melanoma risk after adjustment for phenotype has also been reported [81,82]. This association suggests that that the a-MSH receptor may have functions apart from its role in pigment metabolism. There are reports that a-MSH, through the receptor, may affect the growth of melanocytic cells and may have immunomodulatory and anti-inflammatory effects, although the role, if any, of such effects for CMM risk remains to be established [83–86]. Although each RHC allele is associated with an approximately twofold risk for CMM, each individual may carry two or more RHC SNPs, which further increases the CMM risk [79]. In the context of familial melanoma with germline CDKN2A mutations, *MC1R* RHC variants increase the gene penetrance. In conclusion, the *MC1R* gene is the most commonly altered low-penetrance gene for CMM.

The *OCA2* gene, which is a gene of importance for eye color, is mutated in oculo-cutaneous albinism [87,88]. More recently, variants of the *OCA2* gene have been implicated as low-risk melanoma genes [89,90]. In a recent report of Icelandic and Dutch individuals, other SNPs in genes of importance for skin pigmentation were reported [91]. Whether these SNPs have an implication for melanoma risk remains to be established.

Other inherited syndromes associated with increased risk for cutaneous malignant melanoma

Familial retinoblastoma is caused by a germline mutation in the *RB1* gene and is characterized by early-onset retinoblastoma, which is frequently bilateral. In reported series of retinoblastoma patients, there is an elevated risk for melanoma [79,92–95]. It is likely that the risk of melanoma in *RB1* mutation carriers is considerably elevated.

The Li-Fraumeni syndrome is characterized by an increased risk of several tumor types including sarcomas, brain tumors, adenocarcinomas, and childhood tumors [96] and is associated with germline mutations in the *TP53* tumor suppressor gene [96]. An association with CMM has been reported in some [97–99], but not other [100,101], Li-Fraumeni kindreds. Thus, the association with CMM remains controversial.

Neurofibromatosis 1 is caused by germline mutations in the *NF1* gene and is characterized by alterations of cells of neural crest origin, resulting in neurofibromas, café-au-lait spots, freckling in non–sun-exposed areas, and bone lesions. In some affected kindreds, CMM has been reported, and there have been reports of extracutaneous melanomas such as ocular and mucosal melanomas [102]. The occurrence of melanomas is not unexpected because they represent tumors of neural crest–derived cells.

Xeroderma pigmentosum (XP) is a rare autosomal recessive syndrome associated with hypersensitivity to UV light due to defects in DNA repair. XP is subclassified into seven genetic complementation groups, XPA through XPG, each associated with defects in separate genes involved in nucleotide excision repair [103]. XP patients have more than a 1000-fold increased risk of developing skin cancers, predominantly nonmelanoma skin cancers, and CMM is diagnosed in approximately 5% to 20% of XP patients [103]. Of interest, a large proportion of melanomas in XP patients are lentigo maligna melanomas on chronically sun-exposed sites, indicating that chronic, rather than intermittent, UV radiation damage is the major cause of melanoma in XP.

Werner syndrome is caused by a defect in the *WRN* gene encoding a DNA helicase with a putative role in DNA repair. The syndrome is characterized by premature aging and by increased cancer incidence, including CMM. In a Japanese study, a large number of acral lentiginous and mucosal melanomas were found [104].

BRCA2-associated familial breast/ovarian carcinoma is characterized by greatly increased risk of breast and ovarian carcinoma. Some of these families are reported to have a modestly increased risk of CMM [105], whereas other groups of families do not [105–107].

Summary

Because CMM is rapidly increasing in white-skinned populations, there is a need for improved preventive strategies. Identification of risk groups for CMM is a central task. Familial melanoma represents 5% to 10% of cases of CMM. Such kindreds are characterized by multiple cases of CMM in biologic relatives, an earlier age at diagnosis, and a larger proportion of MPMs in affected individuals compared with sporadic CMM cases. In many families, members exhibit DN, some of which may be precursor lesions for CMM. In approximately 20% to 40% of familial melanoma kindreds, germline mutations in the CDKN2A gene are identified. Intense efforts are ongoing to identify novel melanoma-predisposing genes. The likelihood of CDKN2A mutations is increased in families that have three or more CMM cases, members who have an early onset of melanoma, and members who have MPMs or pancreatic carcinoma. In such families, genetic testing for germline CDKN2A mutations may be considered if combined with adequate information and counseling. Members of melanoma families should be invited to participate in preventive programs, including education regarding sun protection, skin self-examination, and regular skin examinations by trained professionals. There is a need for improved methods for surveillance of pancreatic cancer in families that have germline CDKN2A mutations and occurrence of pancreatic carcinoma. Members of such families should have the opportunity to be enrolled in research programs aiming to improve such surveillance.

References

[1] Jemal A, Siegel R, Ward E, et al. Cancer statistics, 2007. CA Cancer J Clin 2007;57(1): 43–66.
[2] Gandini S, Sera F, Cattaruzza MS, et al. Meta-analysis of risk factors for cutaneous melanoma: II. Sun exposure. Eur J Cancer 2005;41(1):45–60.
[3] Gandini S, Sera F, Cattaruzza MS, et al. Meta-analysis of risk factors for cutaneous melanoma: I. Common and atypical naevi. Eur J Cancer 2005;41(1):28–44.
[4] Friedman RJ, Rigel DS, Kopf AW. Early detection of malignant melanoma: the role of physician examination and self-examination of the skin. CA Cancer J Clin 1985;35(3): 130–51.
[5] Hofmann-Wellenhof R, Blum A, Wolf IH, et al. Dermoscopic classification of Clark's nevi (atypical melanocytic nevi). Clin Dermatol 2002;20(3):255–8.
[6] Roesch A, Burgdorf W, Stolz W, et al. Dermatoscopy of "dysplastic nevi": a beacon in diagnostic darkness. Eur J Dermatol 2006;16(5):479–93.
[7] Clark WH Jr, Reimer RR, Greene M, et al. Origin of familial malignant melanomas from heritable melanocytic lesions. 'The B-K mole syndrome'. Arch Dermatol 1978;114(5): 732–8.
[8] Garbe C, Kruger S, Stadler R, et al. Markers and relative risk in a German population for developing malignant melanoma. Int J Dermatol 1989;28(8):517–23.
[9] Augustsson A, Stierner U, Suurkula M, et al. Prevalence of common and dysplastic naevi in a Swedish population. Br J Dermatol 1991;124(2):152–6.
[10] Gandini S, Sera F, Cattaruzza MS, et al. Meta-analysis of risk factors for cutaneous melanoma: III. Family history, actinic damage and phenotypic factors. Eur J Cancer 2005;41(14):2040–59.
[11] Platz A, Ringborg U, Hansson J. Hereditary cutaneous melanoma. Semin Cancer Biol 2000;10(4):319–26.
[12] Florell SR, Boucher KM, Garibotti G, et al. Population-based analysis of prognostic factors and survival in familial melanoma. J Clin Oncol 2005;23(28):7168–77.
[13] Ford D, Bliss JM, Swerdlow AJ, et al. Risk of cutaneous melanoma associated with a family history of the disease. The International Melanoma Analysis Group (IMAGE). Int J Cancer 1995;62(4):377–81.
[14] Greene MH, Clark WH Jr, Tucker MA, et al. Precursor naevi in cutaneous malignant melanoma: a proposed nomenclature. Lancet 1980;2(8202):1024.
[15] Begg CB, Hummer A, Mujumdar U, et al. Familial aggregation of melanoma risks in a large population-based sample of melanoma cases. Cancer Causes Control 2004;15(9):957–65.
[16] Norris W. Case of fungoid disease. Edinburgh Med Surg J 1820;16:562–5.
[17] Lynch HT, Frichot BC 3rd, Lynch JF. Familial atypical multiple mole-melanoma syndrome. J Med Genet 1978;15(5):352–6.
[18] Newton Bishop JA, Bataille V, Pinney E, et al. Family studies in melanoma: identification of the atypical mole syndrome (AMS) phenotype. Melanoma Res 1994;4(4):199–206.
[19] Goldstein AM, Fraser MC, Clark WH Jr, et al. Age at diagnosis and transmission of invasive melanoma in 23 families with cutaneous malignant melanoma/dysplastic nevi. J Natl Cancer Inst 1994;86(18):1385–90.
[20] Greene MH, Clark WH Jr, Tucker MA, et al. High risk of malignant melanoma in melanoma-prone families with dysplastic nevi. Ann Intern Med 1985;102(4):458–65.
[21] Marks R, Dorevitch AP, Mason G. Do all melanomas come from "moles"? A study of the histological association between melanocytic naevi and melanoma. Australas J Dermatol 1990;31(2):77–80.

[22] Hussussian CJ, Struewing JP, Goldstein AM, et al. Germline p16 mutations in familial melanoma. Nat Genet 1994;8(1):15–21.
[23] Kamb A, Gruis NA, Weaver-Feldhaus J, et al. A cell cycle regulator potentially involved in genesis of many tumor types. Science 1994;264(5157):436–40.
[24] de Snoo FA, Hayward NK. Cutaneous melanoma susceptibility and progression genes. Cancer Lett 2005;230(2):153–86.
[25] Michaloglou C, Vredeveld LC, Soengas MS, et al. BRAFE600-associated senescence-like cell cycle arrest of human naevi. Nature 2005;436(7051):720–4.
[26] Gray-Schopfer VC, Cheong SC, Chong H, et al. Cellular senescence in naevi and immortalisation in melanoma: a role for p16? Br J Cancer 2006;95(4):496–505.
[27] Florell SR, Meyer LJ, Boucher KM, et al. Longitudinal assessment of the nevus phenotype in a melanoma kindred. J Invest Dermatol 2004;123(3):576–82.
[28] Rizos H, Woodruff S, Kefford RF. p14ARF interacts with the SUMO-conjugating enzyme Ubc9 and promotes the sumoylation of its binding partners. Cell Cycle 2005;4(4):597–603.
[29] Rizos H, Scurr LL, Irvine M, et al. p14ARF regulates E2F-1 ubiquitination and degradation via a p53-dependent mechanism. Cell Cycle 2007;6(14):1741–7.
[30] Monzon J, Liu L, Brill H, et al. CDKN2A mutations in multiple primary melanomas. N Engl J Med 1998;338(13):879–87.
[31] MacKie RM, Andrew N, Lanyon WG, et al. CDKN2A germline mutations in U.K. patients with familial melanoma and multiple primary melanomas. J Invest Dermatol 1998;111(2):269–72.
[32] Hashemi J, Platz A, Ueno T, et al. CDKN2A germ-line mutations in individuals with multiple cutaneous melanomas. Cancer Res 2000;60(24):6864–7.
[33] Auroy S, Avril MF, Chompret A, et al. Sporadic multiple primary melanoma cases: CDKN2A germline mutations with a founder effect. Genes Chromosomes Cancer 2001; 32(3):195–202.
[34] Bahuau M, Vidaud D, Jenkins RB, et al. Germ-line deletion involving the INK4 locus in familial proneness to melanoma and nervous system tumors. Cancer Res 1998;58(11): 2298–303.
[35] Hewitt C, Lee Wu C, Evans G, et al. Germline mutation of ARF in a melanoma kindred. Hum Mol Genet 2002;11(11):1273–9.
[36] Petronzelli F, Sollima D, Coppola G, et al. CDKN2A germline splicing mutation affecting both p16(ink4) and p14(arf) RNA processing in a melanoma/neurofibroma kindred. Genes Chromosomes Cancer 2001;31(4):398–401.
[37] Randerson-Moor JA, Harland M, Williams S, et al. A germline deletion of p14(ARF) but not CDKN2A in a melanoma-neural system tumour syndrome family. Hum Mol Genet 2001;10(1):55–62.
[38] Rizos H, Puig S, Badenas C, et al. A melanoma-associated germline mutation in exon 1beta inactivates p14ARF. Oncogene 2001;20(39):5543–7.
[39] Hayward NK. Genetics of melanoma predisposition. Oncogene 2003;22(20):3053–62.
[40] Goldstein AM, Chan M, Harland M, et al. High-risk melanoma susceptibility genes and pancreatic cancer, neural system tumors, and uveal melanoma across GenoMEL. Cancer Res 2006;66(20):9818–28.
[41] Platz A, Hansson J, Mansson-Brahme E, et al. Screening of germline mutations in the CDKN2A and CDKN2B genes in Swedish families with hereditary cutaneous melanoma. J Natl Cancer Inst 1997;89(10):697–702.
[42] Gruis NA, Sandkuijl LA, van der Velden PA, et al. CDKN2 explains part of the clinical phenotype in Dutch familial atypical multiple-mole melanoma (FAMMM) syndrome families. Melanoma Res 1995;5(3):169–77.
[43] Goldstein AM, Stacey SN, Olafsson JH, et al. CDKN2A mutations and melanoma risk in the icelandic population. J Med Genet 2008;45:284–9.
[44] Ciotti P, Struewing JP, Mantelli M, et al. A single genetic origin for the G101W CDKN2A mutation in 20 melanoma-prone families. Am J Hum Genet 2000;67(2):311–9.

[45] Gillanders E, Juo SH, Holland EA, et al. Localization of a novel melanoma susceptibility locus to 1p22. Am J Hum Genet 2003;73(2):301–13.
[46] Walker GJ, Indsto JO, Sood R, et al. Deletion mapping suggests that the 1p22 melanoma susceptibility gene is a tumor suppressor localized to a 9-Mb interval. Genes Chromosomes Cancer 2004;41(1):56–64.
[47] Jonsson G, Bendahl PO, Sandberg T, et al. Mapping of a novel ocular and cutaneous malignant melanoma susceptibility locus to chromosome 9q21.32. J Natl Cancer Inst 2005;97(18):1377–82.
[48] Begg CB, Orlow I, Hummer AJ, et al. Lifetime risk of melanoma in CDKN2A mutation carriers in a population-based sample. J Natl Cancer Inst 2005;97(20):1507–15.
[49] Goldstein AM, Fraser MC, Struewing JP, et al. Increased risk of pancreatic cancer in melanoma-prone kindreds with p16INK4 mutations. N Engl J Med 1995;333(15): 970–4.
[50] Borg A, Sandberg T, Nilsson K, et al. High frequency of multiple melanomas and breast and pancreas carcinomas in CDKN2A mutation-positive melanoma families. J Natl Cancer Inst 2000;92(15):1260–6.
[51] Goldstein AM. Familial melanoma, pancreatic cancer and germline CDKN2A mutations. Hum Mutat 2004;23(6):630.
[52] Vasen HF, Gruis NA, Frants RR, et al. Risk of developing pancreatic cancer in families with familial atypical multiple mole melanoma associated with a specific 19 deletion of p16 (p16-Leiden). Int J Cancer 2000;87(6):809–11.
[53] Hille ET, van Duijn E, Gruis NA, et al. Excess cancer mortality in six Dutch pedigrees with the familial atypical multiple mole-melanoma syndrome from 1830 to 1994. J Invest Dermatol 1998;110(5):788–92.
[54] Kefford R, Bishop JN, Tucker M, et al. Genetic testing for melanoma. Lancet Oncol 2002; 3(11):653–4.
[55] Newton Bishop JA, Gruis NA. Genetics: what advice for patients who present with a family history of melanoma? Semin Oncol 2007;34(6):452–9.
[56] Botkin JR, Smith KR, Croyle RT, et al. Genetic testing for a BRCA1 mutation: prophylactic surgery and screening behavior in women 2 years post testing. Am J Med Genet A 2003; 118(3):201–9.
[57] Hadley DW, Jenkins JF, Dimond E, et al. Colon cancer screening practices after genetic counseling and testing for hereditary nonpolyposis colorectal cancer. J Clin Oncol 2004; 22(1):39–44.
[58] Berg P, Wennberg AM, Tuominen R, et al. Germline CDKN2A mutations are rare in child and adolescent cutaneous melanoma. Melanoma Res 2004;14(4):251–5.
[59] National Institutes of Health Consensus Development Conference Statement on Diagnosis and Treatment of Early Melanoma, January 27–29, 1992. Am J Dermatopathol 1993;15(1): 34–43 [discussion: 46–51].
[60] Kefford RF, Newton Bishop JA, Bergman W, et al. Counseling and DNA testing for individuals perceived to be genetically predisposed to melanoma: a consensus statement of the Melanoma Genetics Consortium. J Clin Oncol 1999;17(10):3245–51.
[61] Bishop DT, Demenais F, Goldstein AM, et al. Geographical variation in the penetrance of CDKN2A mutations for melanoma. J Natl Cancer Inst 2002;94(12):894–903.
[62] Ferrini RL, Perlman M, Hill L. American College of Preventive Medicine practice policy statement: skin protection from ultraviolet light exposure. The American College of Preventive Medicine. Am J Prev Med 1998;14(1):83–6.
[63] Krien PM, Moyal D. Sunscreens with broad-spectrum absorption decrease the trans to cis photoisomerization of urocanic acid in the human stratum corneum after multiple UV light exposures. Photochem Photobiol 1994;60(3):280–7.
[64] Kenet RO, Kang S, Kenet BJ, et al. Clinical diagnosis of pigmented lesions using digital epiluminescence microscopy. Grading protocol and atlas. Arch Dermatol 1993;129(2): 157–74.

[65] Menzies SW, Ingvar C, McCarthy WH. A sensitivity and specificity analysis of the surface microscopy features of invasive melanoma. Melanoma Res 1996;6(1):55–62.

[66] Kelly JW, Yeatman JM, Regalia C, et al. A high incidence of melanoma found in patients with multiple dysplastic naevi by photographic surveillance. Med J Aust 1997;167(4):191–4.

[67] McGovern TW, Litaker MS. Clinical predictors of malignant pigmented lesions. A comparison of the Glasgow seven-point checklist and the American Cancer Society's ABCDs of pigmented lesions. J Dermatol Surg Oncol 1992;18(1):22–6.

[68] Shaw HM, McCarthy WH. Small-diameter malignant melanoma: a common diagnosis in New South Wales, Australia. J Am Acad Dermatol 1992;27(5 Pt 1):679–82.

[69] Rhodes AR. Intervention strategy to prevent lethal cutaneous melanoma: use of dermatologic photography to aid surveillance of high-risk persons. J Am Acad Dermatol 1998;39(2 Pt 1):262–7.

[70] Masri GD, Clark WH Jr, Guerry Dt, et al. Screening and surveillance of patients at high risk for malignant melanoma result in detection of earlier disease. J Am Acad Dermatol 1990;22(6 Pt 1):1042–8.

[71] MacKie RM, McHenry P, Hole D. Accelerated detection with prospective surveillance for cutaneous malignant melanoma in high-risk groups. Lancet 1993;341(8861):1618–20.

[72] Tucker MA, Fraser MC, Goldstein AM, et al. A natural history of melanomas and dysplastic nevi: an atlas of lesions in melanoma-prone families. Cancer 2002;94(12):3192–209.

[73] Hansson J, Bergenmar M, Hofer PA, et al. Monitoring of kindreds with hereditary predisposition for cutaneous melanoma and dysplastic nevus syndrome: results of a Swedish preventive program. J Clin Oncol 2007;25(19):2819–24.

[74] Parker JF, Florell SR, Alexander A, et al. Pancreatic carcinoma surveillance in patients with familial melanoma. Arch Dermatol 2003;139(8):1019–25.

[75] Brand RE, Lerch MM, Rubinstein WS, et al. Advances in counselling and surveillance of patients at risk for pancreatic cancer. Gut 2007;56(10):1460–9.

[76] Lynch HT, Fusaro RM, Lynch JF, et al. Pancreatic cancer and the FAMMM syndrome. Fam Cancer 2008;7(1):103–12.

[77] Salazar-Onfray F, Lopez M, Lundqvist A, et al. Tissue distribution and differential expression of melanocortin 1 receptor, a malignant melanoma marker. Br J Cancer 2002;87(4):414–22.

[78] Kennedy C, ter Huurne J, Berkhout M, et al. Melanocortin 1 receptor (MC1R) gene variants are associated with an increased risk for cutaneous melanoma which is largely independent of skin type and hair color. J Invest Dermatol 2001;117(2):294–300.

[79] Palmer JS, Duffy DL, Box NF, et al. Melanocortin-1 receptor polymorphisms and risk of melanoma: is the association explained solely by pigmentation phenotype? Am J Hum Genet 2000;66(1):176–86.

[80] Valverde P, Healy E, Sikkink S, et al. The Asp84Glu variant of the melanocortin 1 receptor (MC1R) is associated with melanoma. Hum Mol Genet 1996;5(10):1663–6.

[81] Sturm RA, Duffy DL, Box NF, et al. The role of melanocortin-1 receptor polymorphism in skin cancer risk phenotypes. Pigment Cell Res 2003;16(3):266–72.

[82] Matichard E, Verpillat P, Meziani R, et al. Melanocortin 1 receptor (MC1R) gene variants may increase the risk of melanoma in France independently of clinical risk factors and UV exposure. J Med Genet 2004;41(2):e13.

[83] Abdel-Malek Z, Swope VB, Suzuki I, et al. Mitogenic and melanogenic stimulation of normal human melanocytes by melanotropic peptides. Proc Natl Acad Sci U S A 1995;92(5):1789–93.

[84] Suzuki I, Cone RD, Im S, et al. Binding of melanotropic hormones to the melanocortin receptor MC1R on human melanocytes stimulates proliferation and melanogenesis. Endocrinology 1996;137(5):1627–33.

[85] Haycock JW, Rowe SJ, Cartledge S, et al. Alpha-melanocyte-stimulating hormone reduces impact of proinflammatory cytokine and peroxide-generated oxidative stress on keratinocyte and melanoma cell lines. J Biol Chem 2000;275(21):15629–36.

[86] Luger TA, Scholzen T, Brzoska T, et al. Cutaneous immunomodulation and coordination of skin stress responses by alpha-melanocyte-stimulating hormone. Ann N Y Acad Sci 1998;840:381–94.

[87] Rebbeck TR, Kanetsky PA, Walker AH, et al. P gene as an inherited biomarker of human eye color. Cancer Epidemiol Biomarkers Prev 2002;11(8):782–4.

[88] Duffy DL, Montgomery GW, Chen W, et al. A three-single-nucleotide polymorphism haplotype in intron 1 of OCA2 explains most human eye-color variation. Am J Hum Genet 2007;80(2):241–52.

[89] Duffy DL, Box NF, Chen W, et al. Interactive effects of MC1R and OCA2 on melanoma risk phenotypes. Hum Mol Genet 2004;13(4):447–61.

[90] Jannot AS, Meziani R, Bertrand G, et al. Allele variations in the OCA2 gene (pink-eyed-dilution locus) are associated with genetic susceptibility to melanoma. Eur J Hum Genet 2005;13(8):913–20.

[91] Sulem P, Gudbjartsson DF, Stacey SN, et al. Genetic determinants of hair, eye and skin pigmentation in Europeans. Nat Genet 2007;39(12):1443–52.

[92] Eng C, Li FP, Abramson DH, et al. Mortality from second tumors among long-term survivors of retinoblastoma. J Natl Cancer Inst 1993;85(14):1121–8.

[93] Moll AC, Imhof SM, Bouter LM, et al. Second primary tumors in patients with hereditary retinoblastoma: a register-based follow-up study, 1945–1994. Int J Cancer 1996;67(4):515–9.

[94] Sanders BM, Jay M, Draper GJ, et al. Non-ocular cancer in relatives of retinoblastoma patients. Br J Cancer 1989;60(3):358–65.

[95] Albert LS, Sober AJ, Rhodes AR. Cutaneous melanoma and bilateral retinoblastoma. J Am Acad Dermatol 1990;23(5 Pt 2):1001–4.

[96] Malkin D, Li FP, Strong LC, et al. Germ line p53 mutations in a familial syndrome of breast cancer, sarcomas, and other neoplasms. Science 1990;250(4985):1233–8.

[97] Hisada M, Garber JE, Fung CY, et al. Multiple primary cancers in families with Li-Fraumeni syndrome. J Natl Cancer Inst 1998;90(8):606–11.

[98] Nichols KE, Malkin D, Garber JE, et al. Germ-line p53 mutations predispose to a wide spectrum of early-onset cancers. Cancer Epidemiol Biomarkers Prev 2001;10(2):83–7.

[99] Birch JM, Alston RD, McNally RJ, et al. Relative frequency and morphology of cancers in carriers of germline TP53 mutations. Oncogene 2001;20(34):4621–8.

[100] Frebourg T, Barbier N, Yan YX, et al. Germ-line p53 mutations in 15 families with Li-Fraumeni syndrome. Am J Hum Genet 1995;56(3):608–15.

[101] Birch JM, Blair V, Kelsey AM, et al. Cancer phenotype correlates with constitutional TP53 genotype in families with the Li-Fraumeni syndrome. Oncogene 1998;17(9):1061–8.

[102] Guillot B, Dalac S, Delaunay M, et al. Cutaneous malignant melanoma and neurofibromatosis type 1. Melanoma Res 2004;14(2):159–63.

[103] Cleaver JE. Cancer in xeroderma pigmentosum and related disorders of DNA repair. Nat Rev Cancer 2005;5(7):564–73.

[104] Goto M, Miller RW, Ishikawa Y, et al. Excess of rare cancers in Werner syndrome (adult progeria). Cancer Epidemiol Biomarkers Prev 1996;5(4):239–46.

[105] Cancer risks in BRCA2 mutation carriers. The Breast Cancer Linkage Consortium. J Natl Cancer Inst 1999;91(15):1310–6.

[106] Thorlacius S, Olafsdottir G, Tryggvadottir L, et al. A single BRCA2 mutation in male and female breast cancer families from Iceland with varied cancer phenotypes. Nat Genet 1996;13(1):117–9.

[107] Phelan CM, Lancaster JM, Tonin P, et al. Mutation analysis of the BRCA2 gene in 49 site-specific breast cancer families. Nat Genet 1996;13(1):120–2.

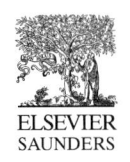

Index

Note: Page numbers of article titles are in **boldface** type.

A

AAPC. See *Attenuated adenomatous polyposis coli (AAPC)*.

Acetylsalicylic acid (ASA;aspirin), for FAP, 829

Age, as factor in cancer, 683, 685

American Gastroenterological Association, in screening/surveillance for FAP, 825–826

American Management Association, 725

American Society of Clinical Oncologists (ASCO), on genetic testing for cancer susceptibility, 710

Americans with Disabilities Act, 728

Amsterdam I criteria, for Lynch syndrome, 834

Amsterdam II criteria, for Lynch syndrome, 834

Anemia, Fanconi, genes in, 684

Angiofibroma(s), benign facial, in MEN1 patients, 872–873

Anti-inflammatory drugs, nonsteroidal, for FAP, 829

APC gene, in FAP, 823–824

Apoptosis, mutations in genes regulating, 700

Apparently sporadic pheochromocytomas and paragangliomas, genetic risk assessment of patients with, 885

ASA. See *Acetylsalicylic acid (ASA; aspirin)*.

ASCO. See *American Society of Clinical Oncologists (ASCO)*.

Ataxia telangiectasia, genes in, 684

Attenuated adenomatous polyposis coli (AAPC), 820

B

Bannayan-Riley-Ruvalbaba syndrome, **800–807**
  anomalies associated with, 803–804
  cancer predisposition for, 804–805
  clinical features of, 801–804
  colorectal cancer and, 804
  genetic counseling in, 807
  genetic(s) of, 806–807
  histopathology of, 804
  history of, 800–801
  management of, 805–806
  reproductive organ–related cancers and, 804–805
  thyroid cancer and, 804–805

Basal cell nevus syndrome, genes in, 684

Benign facial angiofibromas, in MEN1 patients, 872–873

Bethesda guidelines, for Lynch syndrome, 834–835

Bloom syndrome, genes in, 684

BRCA–associated breast and ovarian cancer syndrome, hereditary predisposition for, 744

Breast cancer
  genetic predisposition for
    BRCA–associated breast and ovarian cancer syndrome, 744
    described, 744
    genetic testing for, 848–849
  hereditary breast and ovarian cancer syndrome, 846–847
  management of women with, **845–861**
    chemoprevention in, 855–856
    options for mutation carriers, 849
    prophylactic surgery in, 744–747, 753, 853–855
  prevalence of, 845
  screening for, 849–853

Breast cancer (*continued*)
  HDGC and, lobular carcinoma, 774–775
  prevalence of, 845
  treatment of, 856–857
Burlington Northern Santa Fe Railroad, 726
Bush administration, on GINA, 732–733

C

Cancer(s). See also specific types, e.g., *Colon cancer*.
  age as factor in, 683, 685
  cell cycle checkpoints and, 694
  genetics of, **681–704**, 744
    alterations in, 689–690
    cancer cell origins, 686–688
    chromosomal translocations, 693
    epigenetics, 700–701
    gene amplifications, 693–694
    genetic instability, 690–693
    instability in, 690–693. See also *Genetic instability*.
    mutations in
      genes regulating apoptosis and cell death pathways, 700
      types of, 689–690
    oncogenes, 694–697
    tumor suppressor genes, 697–700
  hereditary predisposition for
    described, 739–740
    genetic testing for, 741–742
    management of, prophylactic surgery in, **739–758**
      approach to patient, 742–743, 753
      breast cancer, 744–747, 753
      colon cancer, 748–750, 753
      FAP, 748–749, 753
      HDGC, 751–753
      HNPCC, 749–750, 753
      MEN2, 750–751, 753
      penetrance as factor in, 741
      timing of, 744
  inherited forms of, 683
  JPS and, 783–784
  mortality due to, 739
  PJS and, 789–793
  sporadic forms of, 683
  susceptibility to, genetic testing for, **705–721**. See also *Genetic testing, for cancer susceptibility*.

Cancer cells, origin of, 686–688
  cancer stem cell hypothesis, 688
  monoclonal theory of, 687–688
  stem cells, 686–687

Cancer genes, 682

Cancer stem cell hypothesis, 688
Carcinogenesis, 683–686
  defined, 683
  described, 681
Caretaker genes, 691
Carney complex, genetic risk assessment of patients with, 865, 888–889
CDH1 mutations carriers, unaffected, in HDGC, identification of, 760–762
CDK4 gene, in familial melanoma, 903
CDKN2A gene, in familial melanoma, 900–902
CDKN2A mutations, germline, melanoma families with, familial melanoma risk factor in, 903–905
Cell(s), cancer, origin of, 686–688. See also *Cancer cells, origin of*.
Cell cycle checkpoints, cancer and, 694
Cell death pathways, mutations in genes regulating, 700
Children, genetic testing for cancer susceptibility in, criteria for, 713–714
Chromosomal instability, 691–692
Chromosomal translocations, 689–690, 693
Chromosome(s), normal diploid number of, changes in, 689
Civil Rights Act of 1963, Title VII of, 728
CMM. See *Cutaneous malignant melanoma (CMM)*.
Colon cancer, hereditary predisposition for
  described, 748
  management of, prophylactic surgery in, 748–750, 753
Colorectal cancer
  Bannayan-Riley-Ruvalbaba syndrome and, 804
  Cowden syndrome and, 804
  Cronkhite-Canada syndrome and, 809–810
  JPS and, 783
  PJS and, 789–791
  PTEN hemartoma tumor syndrome and, 804
Concerted Action for Polyp Preventions (CAPP1) trial, 829
Consent, informed
  basic elements of, 714
  in genetic testing for cancer susceptibility, 713

Counseling, genetic. See *Genetic counseling.*

Cowden syndrome, 800–807
 anomalies associated with, 803–804
 cancer predisposition for, 804–805
 clinical features of, 801–804
 colorectal cancer and, 804
 genes in, 684
 genetic counseling in, 807
 genetic(s) of, 806–807
 genetic risk assessment of patients with, 865, 886–887
 histopathology of, 804
 history of, 800–801
 management of, 805–806
 reproductive organ–related cancers and, 804–805
 thyroid cancer and, 804–805

Cronkhite-Canada syndrome, 808–810
 cancer predisposition for, 809–810
 clinical features of, 808–809
 colorectal cancer and, 809–810
 gastric cancer and, 810
 histopathology of, 809
 history of, 808
 management of, 810

Cutaneous malignant melanoma (CMM). See also *Familial melanoma.*
 CDK4 gene in, 903
 CDKN2A gene in, 900–902
 described, 898–899
 familial clustering of cases of, 898–899
 incidence of, 897
 low-penetrance risk–modifying genes in, 909–910
 MC1R gene in, 909–910
 molecular genetics of, 900
 mortality due to, 897
 novel genes predisposing to, candidate loci for, 903
 OCA2 gene in, 909–910
 predisposing genes for, 909–910
 prevention of
  primary, 906–907
  secondary, 907–909
 risk factors for, inherited syndromes, 910–911

Cytoplasmic protein tyrosine kinases, as oncogenes, 696

Cytoplastic tumor suppressor genes, 699

D

Department of Energy, 724

Department of Health and Human Services, 724, 728

DGC. See *Diffuse gastric cancer (DGC).*

Diffuse gastric cancer (DGC), screening for, inadequacies of, 762–764

Discrimination, genetic, **723–738**. See also *Genetic discrimination.*

"Dor Yeshorim," 725

Duodenal tumors, in MEN1 patients, 869–872

E

Employee Retirement and Security Act (ERISA), 728

Environment, as factor in melanoma, 897

Epigenetic(s), 700–701

Epigenetic changes, 690

ERISA. See *Employee Retirement and Security Act (ERISA).*

F

Familial adenomatous polyposis (FAP), **819–829**
 AAPC, 820
 APC gene in, 823–824
 clinical features of, 820–822
 described, 819
 diagnosis of, 822–824
 extraintestinal manifestations of, 820–821
 gastric polyps in, 820–821
 genes in, 684
 genetic(s) in, 822–824
 genetic risk assessment of patients with, 865, 887–888
 history of, 819
 malignancies associated with, 821
 management of
  nonsurgical, 828–829
  NSAIDs in, 829
  prophylactic surgery in, 748–749, 753
  surgery in, 826–828
   of colon, 826–827
   of desmoid, 828
   of duodenum, 827–828
   of rectum, 826–827
 MYH gene in, 823–824
 prevalence of, 819
 screening/surveillance in, 825–826
 Turcot syndrome and, 821

Familial breast ovarian cancer, genes in, 684

Familial cancer syndromes, genes in, 684

Familial isolated nonmedullary thyroid cancer, genetic risk assessment of patients with, 889

Familial medullary thyroid carcinoma (FMTC), in MEN2 patients, 864, 875–876

Familial melanoma, **897–916**. See also *Cutaneous malignant melanoma (CMM)*.
  CDK4 gene in, 903
  CDKN2A gene in, 900–902
  described, 898–899
  genetic testing in, 905–906
  high-risk melanoma genes in, 900–903
  management of, 906–909
    CMM prevention in, 906–909
  molecular genetics of, 900
  novel genes predisposing to, candidate loci for, 903
  risk factors for, in melanoma families with germline *CDKN2A* mutations, 903–905

Familial paraganglioma syndromes, genetic risk assessment of patients with, 884–885

Familial retinoblastoma, genes in, 684

Fanconi anemia, genes in, 684

FAP. See *Familial adenomatous polyposis (FAP)*.

Federal legislation, genetic discrimination–related, need for, 727–729

FMTC. See *Familial medullary thyroid carcinoma (FMTC)*.

G

Gallbladder cancer, PJS and, 792–793

Gastrectomy, prophylactic total, for HDGC, 768–772
  benefits of, 768–770
  complications of, 768–770

Gastric cancer
  Cronkhite-Canada syndrome and, 810
  diffuse, screening for, inadequacies of, 762–764
  hereditary diffuse. See *Hereditary diffuse gastric cancer (HDGC)*.
  incidence of, 759
  JPS and, 783–784
  mortality due to, 759
  PJS and, 791–792
  types of, 759

Gastric polyps, in FAP, 820–821

Gastrinoma(s), in MEN1 patients, 869–870

Gatekeeper genes, 691

Gene(s)
  APC, in FAP, 823–824
  cancer, 682
  caretaker, 691
  CDK4, in familial melanoma, 903
  CDKN2A, in familial melanoma, 900–902
  cytoplasmic tumor suppressor, 699
  gatekeeper, 691
  in familial cancer syndromes, 684
  low-penetrance risk–modifying, in CMM, 909–910
  MC1R, in CMM, 909–910
  melanoma, high-risk, 900–903
  MYH, in FAP, 823–824
  OCA2, in CMM, 909–910
  receptor tumor suppressor, 699–700
  tumor suppressor, 697–700. See also *Tumor suppressor genes*.

Gene amplifications, 690, 693–694

Genetic(s)
  discrimination related to, **723–738**. See also *Genetic discrimination*.
  in Bannayan-Riley-Ruvalbaba syndrome, 806–807
  in breast cancer, 744, **845–861**. See also *Breast cancer, genetic predisposition for*.
  in colon cancer, 748
  in Cowden syndrome, 806–807
  in FAP, 822–824
  in HDGC, 751–752
  in HMPS, 798–799
  in JPS, 786–787
  in Lynch syndrome, 831–835
  in MEN 2, 750
  in PJS, 795–796
  in PTEN hamartoma tumor syndrome, 806–807
  molecular, of familial cutaneous melanoma, 900

Genetic counseling
  as criterion for genetic testing for cancer susceptibility, 711–713
  for HDGC, 766–768
  in Bannayan-Riley-Ruvalbaba syndrome, 807
  in Cowden syndrome, 807
  in HMPS, 799–800
  in JPS, 787
  in PJS, 795–796
  in PTEN hamartoma tumor syndrome, 807

Genetic discrimination, **723–738**

federal legislation related to, need for, 727–729
implications for America's public health and scientific research, 726–727
pervasiveness of, 725–726

Genetic Discrimination Task Force, 728

Genetic education, as criterion for genetic testing for cancer susceptibility, 711–713

Genetic Information Nondiscrimination Act (GINA), **723–738**. See also *Genetic discrimination*.
Bush administration on, 732–733
described, 729
future directions for, 736–737
implications of, 731–734
legislative process related to, overview of, 731
National Institutes of Health on, 733
opponents of, 733–734
opposition to, refuting of, 734–736
political influence of, 731–734
supporters of, 733
Title I–health insurers, 729–730
Title II–employers, 730–731
to US House of Representatives, 731–732
to US Senate, 732
to White House, 732–733

Genetic instability, 690–693
chromosomal instability, 691–692
nucleotide instability, 692–693

Genetic testing
advantages of, 724–725
challenges facing, 724–725
defined, 724
for cancer susceptibility, **705–721**, 741–742
breast cancer, 848–849
criteria for, 710–715
ASCO on, 710–715
genetic education and counseling, 711–713
in children, 713–714
informed consent, 713, 714
patient selection, 711
selection of testing laboratory, 714–715
establishing differential diagnosis, 705–710
future challenges for, 718
test results interpretation, 715–718
in familial melanoma, 905–906

Germline CDKN2A mutations, melanoma families with, familial melanoma risk factor in, 903–905

GINA. See *Genetic Information Nondiscrimination Act (GINA)*.

Gorlin syndrome, genes in, 684

Growth factor production, tumor growth related to, 681–682

H

Hamartomatous polyposis syndromes, **779–817**. See also specific syndromes, e.g., *Juvenile polyposis syndrome (JPS)*.
Bannayan-Riley-Ruvalbaba syndrome, 800–807
Cowden syndrome, 800–807
Cronkhite-Canada syndrome, 808–810
described, 779
HMPS, 796–800
JPS, 779–787
PJS, 787–796
PTEN hemartoma tumor syndrome, 800–807
types of, 779

HDGC. See *Hereditary diffuse gastric cancer (HDGC)*.

Health Insurance Portability and Accountability Act (HIPAA), Executive Order 13145, 728

Hemartomatous colorectal cancer syndromes, **819–844**. See also specific disorders, e.g., *Familial adenomatous polyposis (FAP)*.
FAP, **819–829**
Lynch syndrome, 829–838
management of, ASA in, 829

Hereditary breast and ovarian cancer syndrome, 846–847

Hereditary diffuse gastric cancer (HDGC), **759–778**
breast cancer and, lobular carcinoma, 774–775
described, 760
genetic counseling for, 766–768
prophylactic surgery for, 751–753
prophylactic surgery in
future directions in, 775
implications of discussion of, 765–775
Newfoundland experience with, 764–765
prophylactic total gastrectomy

Hereditary diffuse (*continued*)
  benefits of, 768–770
  complications of, 768–772
  sentinel node mapping, 772–774
  screening for, inadequacies of, 762–764
  unaffected *CDH1* mutation carriers in, identification of, 760–762

Hereditary mixed polyposis syndrome (HMPS), 796–800
  cancer predisposition for, 797–798
  clinical features of, 796–797
  genetic counseling in, 799–800
  genetic(s) in, 798–799
  histopathology of, 797
  history of, 796
  management of, 798

Hereditary nonpolyposis colon cancer (HNPCC), 829–838. See also *Lynch syndrome.*

Hereditary papillary renal cancer, genes in, 684

HIPAA 13145, 728

HMPS. See *Hereditary mixed polyposis syndrome (HMPS).*

HNPCC. See *Hereditary nonpolyposis colon cancer (HNPCC).*

Human Genome Project

I

Informed consent
  basic elements of, 714
  in genetic testing for cancer susceptibility, 713

Insulinoma(s), in MEN1 patients, 870–871

International Breast Intervention Study-1 trial, 855

Italian trial, 855

J

John Hopkins University Genetics and Public Policy Center, 724

JPS. See *Juvenile polyposis syndrome (JPS).*

Juvenile polyposis, genes in, 684

Juvenile polyposis syndrome (JPS), 779–787
  anomalies associated with, 781–782
  cancer predisposition for, 783–784
  clinical features of, 780–782
  colorectal cancer and, 783
  gastric cancer and, 783–784
  genetic counseling for, 787

  genetic(s) of, 786–787
  histopathology of, 782
  history of, 779–780
  management of, 784–786
  pancreatic cancer and, 784

K

Kidney cancer, hereditary papillary, genes in, 684

L

Lawrence Livermore Laboratories, 726

Li Fraumeni syndrome, genes in, 684

Lobular carcinoma of breast, HDGC and, 774–775

Low-penetrance risk–modifying genes, in CMM, 909–910

Lynch syndrome, 829–838
  Amsterdam I criteria for, 834
  Amsterdam II criteria for, 834
  Bethesda guidelines for, 710, 834–835
  cancer risks associated with, 831
  cancer surveillance for, 835–836
  cardinal features of, 830
  described, 829–830
  diagnosis of, 710, 831–835
  genes in, 684
  genetics of, 831–835
  history of, 829–830
  management of
    nonsurgical, 837–838
    prophylactic surgery in, 749–750, 753
    surgical, 836–837
  testing for, Bethesda guidelines for, revised, 710, 834–835
  Turcot syndrome and, 821

M

MC1R gene, in CMM, 909–910

Medullary thyroid carcinoma (MTC), in MEN2 patients, 864, 876–879

Melanoma(s)
  cutaneous malignant. See *Cutaneous malignant melanoma (CMM).*
  familial, **897–916.** See also *Familial melanoma.*
  risk factors for, 897–898
    environmental, 897
    host-related, 898

Melanoma genes, high-risk, 900–903

MEN1. See *Multiple endocrine neoplasia type 1 (MEN1).*

MEN2. See *Multiple endocrine neoplasia type 2 (MEN2)*.

Molecular genetics, of familial cutaneous melanoma, 900

MTC. See *Medullary thyroid carcinoma (MTC)*.

Multiple endocrine neoplasia (MEN) syndromes, **863–895**
  described, 863–864
  FMTC and, 864, 875–876
  genetic risk assessment of patients with, 880–889
    apparently sporadic pheochromocytomas and paragangliomas, 885
    Carney complex, 865, 888–889
    Cowden syndrome, 865, 886–887
    familial isolated nonmedullary thyroid cancer, 889
    familial paraganglioma syndromes, 884–885
    FAP, 865, 887–888
    neurofibromatosis type 1, 864, 885
    nonmedullary thyroid cancer, 885–886
    overview of, 880–881
    paragangliomas, 882–883
    parathyroid disease, 881–882
    pheochromocytomas, 882–883
    von Hippel–Lindau syndrome, 883–884
  MEN1, 864–873. See also *Multiple endocrine neoplasia type 1 (MEN1)*.
  MEN2, 864, 873–889. See *Multiple endocrine neoplasia type 2 (MEN2)*.
  MTC and, 864, 876–879
  overview of, 864–865
  parathyroid tumors and, 864, 880
  pheochromocytomas and, 864, 879–880

Multiple endocrine neoplasia type 1 (MEN1), 865–873
  benign facial angiofibromas and, 872–873
  component tumors in, diagnosis and management of, 867–873
  duodenal tumors and, 869–872
  gastrinomas and, 869–870
  genes in, 684
  insulinomas and, 870–871
  manifestations of, 872–873
  overview of, 865–866
  pancreatic tumors and, 869–872
  parathyroid tumors and, 867–868

  pituitary tumors and, 868–869
  risk assessment for, 866–867
  somatostatinomas and, 871–872
  surveillance of, 866–867
  thyroid tumors and, 872
  VIPomas and, 871
  Zollinger-Ellison syndrome and, 869–870

Multiple endocrine neoplasia type 2 (MEN2), 864–865, 873–889
  component tumors in, diagnosis and management of, 864, 876–889
  described, 750
  FMTC, 864, 875–876
  genes in, 684
  genetics of, 750
  hallmark of, 873
  management of, prophylactic surgery in, 750–751, 753
  MEN2A, 864, 873–874
    genetic risk assessment of patients with, 883
  MEN2B, 864, 874–875
  MTC, 864, 876–879
  overview of, 873
  pheochromocytomas and, 864, 879–880
  risk assessment for, 876
  surveillance of, 876

Mutation(s)
  CDKN2A, germline, melanoma families with, familial melanoma risk factor in, 903–905
  genetic alterations and, 689–690
  in genes regulating apoptosis, 700
  in genes regulating cell death pathways, 700

Mutation carriers, *CDH1*, unaffected, in HDGC, identification of, 760–762

MYH gene, in FAP, 823–824

N

National Comprehensive Cancer network guidelines, in primary hyperparathyroidism in MEN1 patients management, 867–868

National Institutes of Health, 726
  on GINA, 733

National Surgical Adjuvant Breast and Bowel Project (NSABP) P-1 trial, 855

Neurofibromatosis
  genes in, 684
  type 1, genetic risk assessment of patients with, 864, 885

Nonmedullary thyroid cancer, genetic risk assessment of patients with, 885–886

NSAIDs. See *Anti-inflammatory drugs, nonsteroidal.*

Nuclear proteins, as oncogenes, 696–697

Nucleotide instability, 692–693

Nucleotide sequence, changes in, 689

O

OCA2 gene, in CMM, 909–910

Oncogene(s), 694–697
cytoplasmic protein tyrosine kinases as, 696
described, 694–695
nuclear proteins as, 696–697
receptor protein tyrosine kinases as, 695–696

P

Pancreatic cancer
JPS and, 784
PJS and, 792–793

Pancreatic tumors, in MEN1 patients, 869–872

Paraganglioma(s), genetic risk assessment of patients with, 882–883

Parathyroid disease, genetic risk assessment of patients with, 881–882

Parathyroid tumors
in MEN1 patients, 867–868
in MEN2 patients, 864, 880

Peutz-Jeghers syndrome (PJS), 787–796
anomalies associated with, 789
cancer predisposition for, 789–793
clinical features of, 788–789
colorectal cancer and, 789–791
gallbladder cancer and, 792–793
gastric cancer and, 791–792
genes in, 684
genetic(s) and, 795–796
genetic counseling in, 795–796
histopathology of, 789
history of, 787
management of, 793–794
pancreatic cancer and, 792–793
reproductive organ–related cancers and, 792
small bowel cancer and, 791–792

Pheochromocytoma(s)
genetic risk assessment of patients with, 882–883
in MEN2 patients, 864, 879–880

Pituitary tumors, in MEN1 patients, 868–869

PJS. See *Peutz-Jeghers syndrome (PJS).*

Polyp(s), gastric, in FAP, 820–821

Polyposis
familial adenomatous. See *Familial adenomatous polyposis (FAP).*
juvenile, genes in, 684

Prophylactic total gastrectomy, for HDGC, 768–772
benefits of, 768–770
complications of, 768–770

Protein(s), nuclear, as oncogenes, 696–697

PTEN hemartoma tumor syndrome, 800–807
anomalies associated with, 803–804
cancer predisposition for, 804–805
clinical features of, 801–804
colorectal cancer and, 804
genetic counseling in, 807
genetic(s) of, 806–807
histopathology of, 804
history of, 800–801
management of, 805–806
reproductive organ–related cancers and, 804–805
thyroid cancer and, 804–805

Public health, genetic discrimination effects on, 726–727

R

Receptor protein tyrosine kinases, as oncogenes, 695–696

Receptor tumor suppressor genes, 699–700

Renal cancer, hereditary papillary, genes in, 684

Reproductive organs, cancer of
Bannayan-Riley-Ruvalbaba syndrome and, 804–805
Cowden syndrome and, 804–805
PJS and, 792
PTEN hemartoma tumor syndrome and, 804–805

Retinoblastoma, familial, genes in, 684

Royal Marsden trial, 855

S

Scientific research, genetic discrimination effects on, 726–727

Sclerosis, tuberous, genes in, 684

Secretary's Advisory Committee on Genetics, Health, and Society, 725–726, 728

Sentinel node mapping, in HDGC, 772–774

Small bowel cancer, PJS and, 791–792

Somatostatinoma(s), in MEN1 patients, 871–872

Stem cells, origin of, 686–687

T

Tamoxifen, in breast cancer prevention, 855–856

Telangiectasia(s), ataxis, genes in, 684

Testing laboratory, in genetic testing for cancer susceptibility, 714–715

Thyroid cancer
  Bannayan-Riley-Ruvalbaba syndrome and, 804–805
  Cowden syndrome and, 804–805
  nonmedullary
    familial isolated, genetic risk assessment of patients with, 889
    genetic risk assessment of patients with, 885–886
  PTEN hemartoma tumor syndrome and, 804–805

Thyroid tumors, in MEN1 patients, 872

Title VII of Civil Rights Act of 1963, 728

Transcriptional factors, as tumor suppressor genes, 698–699

Tuberous sclerosis, genes in, 684

Tumor(s)
  duodenal, in MEN1 patients, 869–872
  growth of, growth factor production and, 681–682
  pancreatic, in MEN1 patients, 869–872
  parathyroid
    in MEN1 patients, 867–868
    in MEN2 patients, 864, 880
  pituitary, in MEN2 patients, 868–869
  thyroid, in MEN1 patients, 872
  Wilms, genes in, 684

Tumor suppressor genes, 697–700
  cytoplastic, 699
  described, 697–698
  receptor, 699–700
  transcriptional factors as, 698–699

Turcot syndrome
  FAM and, 821
  Lynch syndrome and, 821

2006 Cogent Research poll, 726–727

V

Vasoactive intestinal peptide tumors (VIPomas), in MEN1 patients, 871

VIPomas. See *Vasoactive intestinal peptide tumors (VIPomas)*.

von Hippel–Lindau syndrome
  genes in, 684
  genetic risk assessment of patients with, 883–884

W

Wilms tumor, genes in, 684

X

Xeroderma pigmentosum, genes in, 684

Z

Zollinger-Ellison syndrome, in MEN1 patients, 869–870

Moving?

Make sure your subscription moves with you!

To notify us of your new address, find your **Clinics Account Number** (located on your mailing label above your name), and contact customer service at:

E-mail: elspcs@elsevier.com

800-654-2452 (subscribers in the U.S. & Canada)
1-407-563-6020 (subscribers outside of the U.S. & Canada)

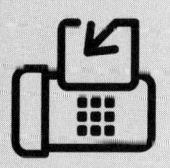

Fax number: 407-363-9661

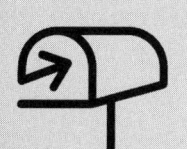

Elsevier Periodicals Customer Service
6277 Sea Harbor Drive
Orlando, FL 32887-4800

*To ensure uninterrupted delivery of your subscription, please notify us at least 4 weeks in advance of move.

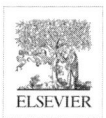